W9-DGX-815

Saunders PRINCIPLES OF MEDICINE Series

Lookingbill & Marks
PRINCIPLES OF DERMATOLOGY

Brenner, Rector, & Coe
PRINCIPLES OF RENAL MEDICINE

Lockey and Bukantz
PRINCIPLES OF ALLERGY AND IMMUNOLOGY

Principles of
PULMONARY
MEDICINE

STEVEN E. WEINBERGER, M.D.

Assistant Professor of Medicine, Harvard Medical School and
Beth Israel Hospital, Boston, Massachusetts

W.B. SAUNDERS COMPANY
Philadelphia □ London □ Toronto □ Mexico City
Rio de Janeiro □ Sydney □ Tokyo □ Hong Kong

W. B. SAUNDERS COMPANY
Harcourt Brace Jovanovich, Inc.

The Curtis Center
Independence Square West
Philadelphia, PA 19106

Library of Congress Cataloging in Publication Data

Weinberger, Steven E.

Principles of pulmonary medicine.

Includes index.

1. Lungs—Diseases.   I. Title. [DNLM: 1. Lung diseases.
   WF 600 W423p]

RC756.W45 1986   616.2′4   85–10822

ISBN 0–7216–1559–7

Listed here is the latest translated edition of this book together
with the language of the translation and the publisher.

Spanish *(1st edition)*—Editorial Medica Panamericana, Buenos Aires, Argentina.

Editor: Dana Dreibelbis
Designer: Bill Donnelly
Production Manager: Bill Preston
Manuscript Editor: Steven Albert
Illustrator: Karen McGarry
Illustration Coordinator: Peg Shaw
Page Layout Artist: Patti Maddaloni
Indexer: Dennis Dolan

Principles of Pulmonary Medicine   ISBN 0-7216-1559-7

Last digit is the print number: 9   8   7   6   5   4   3   2

Introduction

Gaining an understanding of the patient with pulmonary disease requires not only in-depth knowledge of the disease itself but also an appreciation of how lung function is affected. This close relationship of disease to disordered function often makes the study of lung disease particularly complicated for the beginning student, but also especially rewarding for the student who has mastered the basic physiology of breathing. Once a framework of fundamental principles is established, it becomes much easier to expand one's knowledge of the pathophysiology and clinical features of specific diseases.

This book has been written with the goal of synthesizing disease processes with the relevant aspects of normal physiology that they affect. It is directed primarily at students who wish to learn about respiratory disease—not only medical students, but also students from such other disciplines as respiratory therapy and chest physical therapy, who will be caring for patients with lung disease. Ideally, the student exposed to pulmonary medicine for the first time will have an opportunity to build his or her knowledge of clinical pulmonary medicine around a pathophysiologic framework. The student, physician, or therapist who already has some background should have the opportunity to increase and consolidate his or her understanding of the respiratory system by integrating basic principles with a clinical approach.

Before attempting to learn about disease processes affecting the lungs, it is essential that the student acquire an overview of pulmonary physiology above and beyond those aspects relevant to specific diseases. Consequently, the first chapter in this book is designed to present those basic concepts of pulmonary physiology that should initially be mastered by the reader, since they will become an important part of the language used for discussions about disease. Similarly, the clinical presentation and fundamentals of approaching the patient with pulmonary disease are discussed in Chapters 2 and 3, respectively. The approach to the patient will be considered on three levels—assessing the patient's disease from macroscopic, microscopic, and functional points of view. Again, the points covered in Chapters 2 and 3 will be useful for approaching any patient with respiratory complaints, and they will be referred to repeatedly in subsequent chapters.

The bulk of the book deals with disease processes and is organized primarily by anatomic areas—airways, pulmonary parenchyma, pulmonary vasculature, pleura and mediastinum, and neural, muscular, and chest wall interactions with the lungs. Within each of these major sections, the basic physiology of the particular anatomic area is discussed in some depth, followed by a presentation of the major disorders affecting that area. For each disease, emphasis is placed on (1) etiology and pathogenesis; (2) pathology; (3) pathophysiology; (4) clinical features; (5) diagnostic approach; and (6) general principles of the therapeutic approach.

Several topics that pertain to more than one anatomic area are considered in separate sections, namely, infection and lung cancer. Finally, a section is devoted to a discussion of respiratory failure, including its pathophysiology and management. Patients with respiratory failure provide some of the most difficult management problems for the physician handling critically ill patients, and it is here that the application of pulmonary physiologic principles to patient management is most evident and most crucial.

Although a broad spectrum of pulmonary diseases is covered in this book, it is not aimed at presenting a comprehensive description of all aspects of pulmonary medicine. Consequently, it is not a reference textbook, nor is it solely a textbook of basic pulmonary physiology. Rather, its intent is to bridge the gap between basic physiology and clinical pulmonary medicine and to provide a readable format for introducing the student to the principles involved in pulmonary medicine.

During the writing of this book, I have been assisted by many of my colleagues, to whom I am deeply indebted. Valuable comments and suggestions were provided by Drs. Vladimir Fencl, Roland Ingram, Scott Johnson, Earl Kasdon, Mark Kelley, Bohdan Pichurko, Arthur Saari, Richard Schwartzstein, Ira Tager, Scott Weiss, and Woodrow Weiss. In addition, Dr. Earl Kasdon was extremely kind in providing most of the illustrations of pathology presented in the book. The editors at W. B. Saunders, specifically Dana Dreibelbis, Steven Albert, and Albert Meier, were most helpful throughout preparation of the book and contributed immensely to making the experience an enjoyable one. Finally, I am most grateful to my wife Janet and son Eric for their invaluable inspiration, support, and patience.

Contents

Pulmonary Anatomy and Physiology—The Basics

Anatomy
Mechanical Aspects of the Lungs and Chest Wall
Ventilation
Circulation
Diffusion
Oxygen Transport
Carbon Dioxide Transport
Ventilation-Perfusion Relationships
Abnormalities in Gas Exchange
   Hypoxemia
   Hypercapnia

In order to be effective at gas exchange, the lungs cannot act in isolation but must participate in a well-coordinated fashion with the central nervous system (which provides the rhythmic drive to breathe), the diaphragm and muscular apparatus of the chest wall (which respond to signals from the central nervous system and act as a "bellows" for movement of air), and the circulatory system (which provides blood flow and hence gas transport between the tissues and the lungs). The processes of oxygen uptake and carbon dioxide elimination by the lungs depend upon adequate functioning of all of these interrelated systems, and a disturbance in any one can result in clinically important abnormalities in gas transport and thus arterial blood gases. In this chapter, we will initially present an overview of pulmonary anatomy, followed by a discussion of mechanical properties of the lungs and chest wall, and a consideration of some aspects of the contribution of the lungs and the circulatory system to gas exchange. Additional discussion about pulmonary and circulatory physiology will be presented in Chapters 4, 8, and 12, and neurologic, muscular, and chest wall interactions with the lungs will be discussed further in Chapter 17.

ANATOMY

It is most appropriate when discussing the anatomy of the respiratory system to include the entire pathway for airflow from the mouth or nose down to the alveolar sacs. En route to the alveoli, gas must flow through the oro- or nasopharynx, the larynx, the trachea, and finally a progressively arborizing system of bronchi and bronchioles (Fig. 1–1). The trachea divides at the carina into right and left mainstem bronchi, which subsequently branch into lobar bronchi (three on the right, two on the left), segmental bronchi, and an extensive system of subsegmental and smaller bronchi. These conducting airways divide approximately 15 to 20 times down to the level of terminal bronchioles, which are the smallest units that do not actually participate in gas exchange.

Conducting airways include all airways down to the level of the terminal bronchioles.

Beyond the terminal bronchioles, further divisions include respiratory bronchioles, alveolar ducts, and finally alveoli themselves. These smallest units, from the respiratory bronchioles on, form the portion of the lung involved in gas exchange and collectively constitute the terminal respiratory unit or *acinus*. At this level, inhaled gas comes into contact with alveolar walls (septae), and pulmonary capillary blood loads oxygen and unloads carbon dioxide as it courses through the septae.

The acinus includes structures distal to a terminal bronchiole: respiratory bronchioles, alveolar ducts, and alveoli (alveolar sacs).

The surface area for gas exchange provided by the alveoli is enormous. It is estimated that the adult human lung has on the order of 300 million alveoli, with a total surface area approximately the size

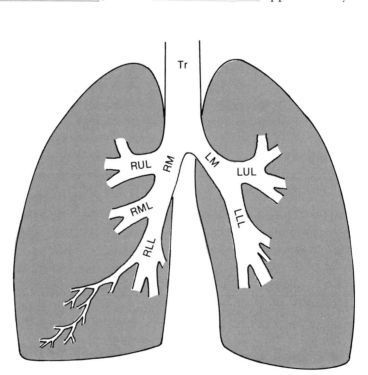

Figure 1–1. Schematic diagram of airway branching. Abbreviations: Tr = trachea; RM = right mainstem bronchus; LM = left mainstem bronchus; RUL = right upper lobe bronchus; RML = right middle lobe bronchus; RLL = right lower lobe bronchus; LUL = left upper lobe bronchus; LLL = left lower lobe bronchus.

of a tennis court. This vast surface area of gas in contact with alveolar walls is a most efficient mechanism for oxygen and carbon dioxide transfer between alveolar spaces and pulmonary capillary blood.

The pulmonary capillary network and the blood within provide the other crucial requirement for gas exchange, namely a transportation system for oxygen and carbon dioxide to and from other body tissues and organs. After blood arrives at the lungs via the pulmonary artery, it courses through a widely branching system of smaller pulmonary arteries and arterioles to the major locale for gas exchange, the pulmonary capillary network. The capillaries generally allow red blood cells to flow through only in single file, so that gas exchange between each cell and alveolar gas is facilitated. Upon completion of gas exchange and travel through the pulmonary capillary bed, oxygenated blood then flows through pulmonary venules and veins and finally arrives at the left side of the heart, whereupon pumping to the systemic circulation and distribution to the tissues are initiated.

Further details about the anatomy of airways, alveoli, and the pulmonary vasculature, particularly with regard to structure-function relationships and cellular anatomy, are found in Chapters 4, 8, and 12.

MECHANICAL ASPECTS OF THE LUNGS AND CHEST WALL

We will start our discussion of pulmonary physiology by introducing a few concepts about the mechanical properties of the respiratory system; these will have important implications for assessment of pulmonary function and its derangement in disease states. When considering certain aspects of respiratory function in health and disease, one should realize that both the lungs and the chest wall have elastic properties. That is, these structures have a particular resting size (or volume) that they would assume if no internal or external pressure were exerted upon them, and any deviation from this volume requires some additional influencing force.

In the case of the lungs, we must think of the size the lungs would take if they were removed from the chest and no longer had the external influences of the chest wall and the pleural space acting on them. Under these conditions, the lungs would be almost airless, and would have a much lower volume than they have within the thoracic cage. In order to expand these isolated lungs, positive pressure would have to be exerted on the airspaces, as could be done by putting positive pressure through the airway. We can actually draw an analogy between this behavior and that of a balloon. A balloon is essentially airless unless positive pressure has been exerted upon the opening to distend the elastic wall and fill it with air.

Alternatively, instead of positive pressure exerted on alveoli through the airways, negative pressure could be applied outside of the lungs and would also cause their expansion. Thus, what increases the volume of the isolated lungs from the resting, essentially airless state is the application of a positive *transpulmonary pressure*, i.e., the pressure inside the lungs relative to the pressure outside. Either internal pressure can be made positive, or external pressure can be made negative; the net effect is the same. If we go back to the "real-life" situation with the lungs inside the chest wall, the internal pressure is alveolar pressure, whereas external pressure is the pressure within the pleural space (Fig. 1–2). Therefore, transpulmonary pressure is now defined as alveolar pressure (P_{alv}) minus pleural pressure (P_{pl}), and the presence of air in the lungs requires that pleural pressure be relatively negative compared with alveolar pressure.

We can go one step further and describe the relationship between transpulmonary pressure and lung volume for a range of transpulmonary pressures. A plot of this relationship, shown in Figure 1–3A, is called the *compliance curve* of the lung. As transpulmonary pressure increases, lung volume naturally increases. However, the relationship is not linear, but rather curvilinear; at relatively high lung volumes, the lungs reach their limit of distensibility, and even rather large increases in transpulmonary pressure do not result in significant increases in lung volume.

Switching from the lungs to the chest wall, we find that if the lungs were removed from the chest, the chest wall would expand to a larger size when no external or internal pressures were exerted upon it. Thus, there is a "spring-like" character to the chest wall; the resting volume is relatively high, and distortion to either a smaller or larger volume requires an alteration of either the external or internal pressures acting on the chest wall. The pressure across the chest wall is akin to the transpulmonary pressure. If we again go back to the real-life situation in which the lungs occupy the region inside of the chest wall, then the pressure across the chest wall is the pleural pressure (internal

Transpulmonary pressure = $P_{alv} - P_{pl}$

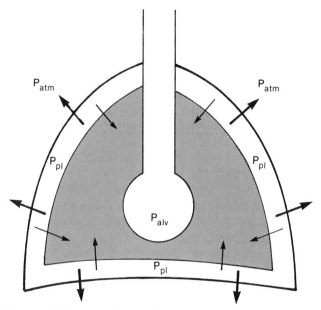

Figure 1–2. Simplified diagram showing the pressures on either side of the chest wall (heavy line) and the lung (shaded area). P_{pl} = pleural pressure; P_{alv} = alveolar pressure; P_{atm} = atmospheric pressure. Thin arrows show the direction of elastic recoil of the lung (at the resting end-expiratory position); thick arrows show the direction of elastic recoil of the chest wall.

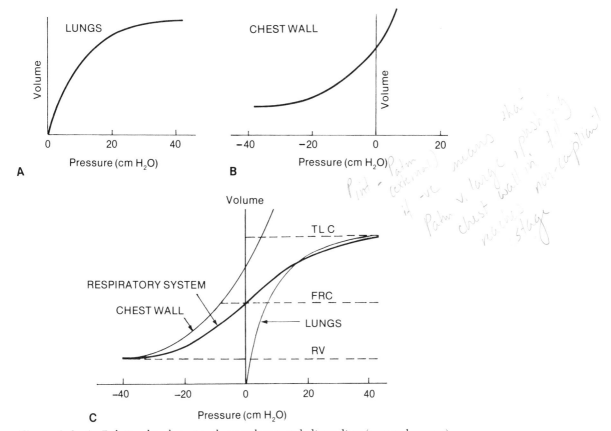

Figure 1–3. *A*, Relationship between lung volume and distending (transpulmonary) pressure, i.e., compliance curve of the lung. *B*, Relationship between volume enclosed by the chest wall and distending (trans–chest wall) pressure, i.e., compliance curve of the chest wall. *C*, Combined compliance curves of the lung and chest wall, showing relationship between respiratory system volume and distending (trans–respiratory system) pressure. RV = residual volume; FRC = functional residual capacity; TLC = total lung capacity.

pressure) minus the external pressure surrounding the chest wall (i.e., atmospheric pressure).

We can now also construct a compliance curve of the chest wall, relating the volume enclosed by the chest wall to the pressure across it. As we can see from Figure 1–3B, the curve becomes relatively flat at low lung volumes, at which the chest wall becomes quite stiff; further changes in the pressure across the chest wall cause little further decrement in volume.

In order to examine how the lungs and chest wall behave in situ, we must remember that the elastic properties of each are acting in opposite directions. At the normal resting end-expiratory position of the respiratory system (which is called *functional residual capacity* or FRC), the lung is expanded to a volume greater than the resting volume it would have in isolation. On the other hand, the chest wall is contracted to a volume smaller than it would have in isolation. However, at FRC the tendency of the lung to become smaller (the inward or elastic recoil of the lung) is exactly balanced by the tendency

At FRC, the inward elastic recoil of the lung is balanced by the outward elastic recoil of the chest wall.

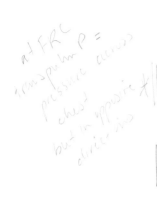

at FRC P = transpulm pressure across chest but in opposite dir'n

of the chest wall to expand (the outward recoil of the chest wall). In other words, by looking at Figure 1–3C we see that the transpulmonary pressure at FRC is equal in magnitude to the pressure across the chest wall but acts in an opposite direction. Pleural pressure is therefore negative, a consequence of the inward recoil of the lungs and the outward recoil of the chest wall.

We can also consider the chest wall and the lungs together as a unit, for this purpose called the "respiratory system." The respiratory system has its own compliance curve, which is essentially a combination of the individual compliance curves of the lungs and chest wall (Fig. 1–3C). The transrespiratory system pressure, again defined as internal minus external pressure, is therefore airway pressure minus atmospheric pressure. At a transrespiratory system pressure of 0, the respiratory system is at its normal resting end-expiratory position, and the volume within the lungs is FRC.

We can now define two additional lung volumes and discuss the factors that determine each of them. The first, *total lung capacity* or TLC, is the volume of gas within the lungs at the end of a maximal inhalation. At this point, the lungs are stretched well above their resting position, and even the chest wall is stretched beyond its resting position. We are able to distort both the lungs and the chest wall so far from FRC by using our inspiratory muscles, which exert an outward force to counterbalance the inward elastic recoil of the lung and, at TLC, the chest wall. However, at TLC it is primarily the extreme stiffness of the lungs that prevents even further expansion by inspiratory muscle action. We can therefore define the primary determinants of TLC—the expanding action of the inspiratory musculature balanced by the inward elastic recoil of the lung.

At the other extreme, when we exhale as much as possible, we reach *residual volume* or RV. At this point, there is still a significant amount of gas remaining within the lungs; that is, we can never exhale far enough to empty our lungs entirely of gas. Again, the reason can be seen by looking at the compliance curves in Figure 1–3C. The chest wall becomes so stiff at low volumes that additional effort by the expiratory muscles is unable to decrease the volume any further. Therefore, RV is determined primarily by the balance of the outward recoil of the chest wall and the contracting action of the expiratory musculature. As we will see, this simple model for RV applies only to the young individual with normal lungs and airways. With age or with disease of the airways, further expulsion of gas during expiration is limited not by the outward recoil of the chest wall, but rather by the tendency for airways to close during expiration and for gas to be trapped behind the closed airways.

At TLC, the expanding action of the inspiratory musculature is limited primarily by the inward elastic recoil of the lung.

rather than inward action of chest wall

At RV, either outward recoil of the chest wall or closure of airways prevents further expiration.

VENTILATION

In order to maintain normal gas exchange to the tissues, an adequate volume of air must pass through the lungs for provision of oxygen to and removal of carbon dioxide from the blood. A normal subject under resting conditions typically breathes approximately 500 ml of air per breath at a frequency of 12 to 16 times per minute, resulting in a ventilation of 6 to 8 liters per minute (termed the minute ventilation and commonly abbreviated $\dot{V}_E$).* The volume of each breath, or the tidal volume (V_T), is not used entirely for gas exchange, as a portion stays in the conducting airways and does not reach the distal part of the lung capable of gas exchange. This portion of the tidal volume that is wasted (in the sense of gas exchange) is termed *dead space* (V_D), while the volume that reaches the gas-exchanging portion of the lung is called the *alveolar volume* (V_A). The dead space, which includes the larynx, trachea, and bronchi down to the level of the terminal bronchioles, is approximately 150 ml in a normal person, so that 30 percent of a tidal volume of 500 ml is "wasted."

The volume of each breath (tidal volume or V_T) is divided into dead space volume (V_D) and alveolar volume (V_A).

In terms of CO_2 elimination by the lung, it is the alveolar ventilation ($\dot{V}_A$), which is equal to the breathing frequency (f) multiplied by V_A, that bears a direct relationship to the amount of CO_2 removed from the body. In fact, the partial pressure of CO_2 in arterial blood ($PaCO_2$) is inversely proportional to $\dot{V}_A$, so that as $\dot{V}_A$ increases, $PaCO_2$ decreases. Additionally, $PaCO_2$ is affected by the body's rate of carbon dioxide production ($\dot{V}CO_2$); if $\dot{V}CO_2$ increases without any change in $\dot{V}_A$, $PaCO_2$ shows a proportional increase as well. Hence, it is easy to understand the relationship in Equation 1–1:

$$PaCO_2 \propto \frac{\dot{V}CO_2}{\dot{V}_A} \qquad (1-1)$$

which defines the major factors determining $PaCO_2$. When a normal individual exercises, $\dot{V}CO_2$ increases, but $\dot{V}_A$ increases proportionately, so that $PaCO_2$ remains relatively constant.

Arterial PCO_2 ($PaCO_2$) is inversely proportional to alveolar ventilation ($\dot{V}_A$) and directly proportional to CO_2 production ($\dot{V}CO_2$).

As mentioned above, the dead space comprises that amount of each breath going to parts of the tracheobronchial tree not involved in gas exchange. The "anatomic dead space" consists of the conducting airways and is generally about 150 ml in a normal person. However, in disease states, areas of lung that normally participate in gas exchange (i.e., parts of the terminal respiratory unit) may not receive normal blood flow, even though they continue to be ventilated. In these areas, some of the ventilation is thus wasted; such regions contribute additional volume to the dead space.

Hence, a more useful clinical concept than "anatomic dead space" is "physiologic dead space," which takes into account the volume of each breath not involved in gas exchange, whether at the level of the conducting airways or the terminal respiratory units. Primarily in certain disease states, where areas of normal ventilation arise but with decreased or no perfusion, the physiologic dead space is larger than the anatomic dead space.

Quantitation of the physiologic dead space, or more precisely, the fraction of the tidal volume that is represented by the dead space (V_D/V_T), can be made by measurement of PCO_2 in arterial blood ($PaCO_2$) and expired gas ($PECO_2$) and by use of Equation 1–2, known as the *Bohr equation* for physiologic dead space:

$$\frac{V_D}{V_T} = \frac{PaCO_2 - PECO_2}{PaCO_2} \qquad (1-2)$$

---

*By convention, a dot over a letter adds a time dimension. Hence, $\dot{V}_E$ stands for volume of expired gas per minute, i.e., minute ventilation. Other similar abbreviations that will be used in this chapter include $\dot{V}CO_2$ (volume of CO_2 produced per minute) and $\dot{Q}$ (blood flow per minute).

For gas coming directly from alveoli that have participated in gas exchange, the P_{CO_2} approximates that of arterial blood. For gas coming from the dead space, the P_{CO_2} is 0, since the gas never came into contact with pulmonary capillary blood.

Let's look at the two extremes. If the expired gas came entirely from perfused alveoli, P_{ECO_2} would equal Pa_{CO_2}, and, according to the equation, V_D/V_T would equal 0. On the other hand, if expired gas came totally from the dead space, it would contain no CO_2, P_{ECO_2} would equal 0, and V_D/V_T would equal 1. In practice, this equation is used in situations between these two extremes, and quantitates the proportion of expired gas coming from alveolar gas ($P_{CO_2} = Pa_{CO_2}$) versus dead space gas ($P_{CO_2} = 0$).

The Bohr equation can be used to quantitate the fraction of each breath that is wasted, the dead space to tidal volume ratio (V_D / V_T).

In summary, each normal or tidal volume breath can be divided into alveolar volume and dead space, just as the total minute ventilation can be divided into alveolar ventilation and wasted (or dead space) ventilation. Elimination of CO_2 by the lungs is proportional to the alveolar ventilation, and therefore Pa_{CO_2} is inversely proportional to the alveolar ventilation, not to the minute ventilation. The wasted ventilation can be quantitated by the Bohr equation, using the principle that increasing amounts of dead space ventilation augment the difference between P_{CO_2} in arterial blood and expired gas.

CIRCULATION

Since the entire cardiac output flows from the right ventricle to the lungs and back to the left side of the heart, the pulmonary circulation handles a blood flow of approximately 5 liters per minute. If the pulmonary vasculature were similar in structure to the systemic vasculature, large pressures would need to be generated because of the thick walls and high resistance offered by systemic-type arteries. However, pulmonary arteries are quite different in structure from systemic arteries, with thin walls that provide much less resistance to flow. Hence, despite equal right and left ventricular outputs, the normal mean pulmonary artery pressure of 15 mm Hg is strikingly different from the normal mean aortic pressure of approximately 95 mm Hg.

One important feature of blood flow in the pulmonary capillary bed is the distribution of flow observed in different areas of the lung. The pattern of flow is easily explained by the effects of gravity and the need for blood to be pumped "uphill" to reach the apices of the lungs. In the upright person, the apex of each lung is approximately 25 cm higher than the base, so that the pressure in pulmonary vessels at the apex is 25 cm water (19 mm Hg) lower than in pulmonary vessels at the bases. Since flow through these vessels is dependent on the perfusion pressure, the capillary network at the bases receives much more flow than capillaries at the apices. In fact, flow at the lung apices falls to zero during the part of the cardiac cycle at which pulmonary artery pressure is insufficient to pump blood up to the apex.

As a result of gravity, there is more blood flow to dependent regions of the lung.

West has developed a model of pulmonary blood flow that divides the lung into zones, based on the relationship among pulmonary arterial, venous, and alveolar pressures (Fig. 1–4). As stated above, the

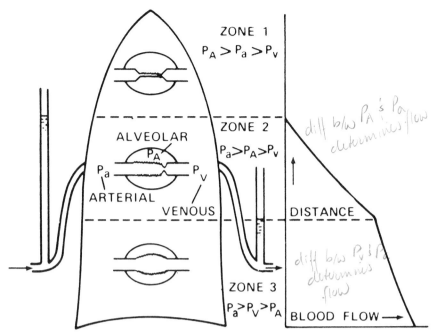

ZONE 1
$P_A > P_a > P_v$

ALVEOLAR
P_A
P_a P_v
ARTERIAL
VENOUS

ZONE 2
$P_a > P_A > P_v$

DISTANCE

diff b/w P_A & P_a determines flow

ZONE 3
$P_a > P_v > P_A$

BLOOD FLOW →

diff b/w P_v & P_a determines flow

Figure 1–4. Three-zone model of pulmonary blood flow, showing the relationships between alveolar pressure (PA), arterial pressure (Pa), and venous pressure (Pv) in each zone. On the right side of the figure, blood flow (per unit volume of lung) is shown as a function of vertical distance. (From West, J. B., Dollery, C. T., and Naimark, A.: J. Appl. Physiol. 19:713–724, 1964. Reproduced with permission).

vascular pressures, i.e., pulmonary arterial and venous, depend in part on the vertical location of the vessels in the lung because of the hydrostatic effect. Apical vessels have much lower pressure than basilar vessels, the difference being the vertical distance between them (divided by a correction factor of 1.3 to convert from cm water to mm Hg).

At the apex of the lung (zone 1), alveolar pressure exceeds both arterial and venous pressures, and no flow results. Normally, such a condition does not arise, unless pulmonary arterial pressure is decreased or alveolar pressure is increased (by exogenous pressure applied to the airways and alveoli). In zone 2, arterial but not venous pressure exceeds alveolar pressure, and the driving force for flow is determined by the difference between arterial and alveolar pressures. In zone 3, both arterial and venous pressures exceed alveolar pressure, and the driving force is the difference between arterial and venous pressures, as is seen in the systemic vasculature.

When cardiac output is increased, as with exercise, the normal pulmonary vasculature is able to handle the increase in flow primarily by recruiting previously unperfused vessels. The ability to expand the pulmonary vascular bed and thus decrease vascular resistance allows major increases in cardiac output with exercise to be accompanied by only small increments in mean pulmonary artery pressure. However, in disease states affecting the pulmonary vascular bed, the ability to recruit additional vessels with increased flow may not be available, and significant increases in pulmonary artery pressure may result.

DIFFUSION

In order for oxygen and carbon dioxide to be transferred between the alveolar space and blood in the pulmonary capillary, diffusion through several compartments must take place—alveolar gas, alveolar and capillary walls, plasma, and membrane and cytoplasm of the red blood cell. Under normal circumstances, the process of diffusion of both gases is relatively rapid, and full equilibration occurs during the transit time of blood flowing through the pulmonary capillary bed. In fact, the P_{O_2} in capillary blood rises from the mixed venous level of 40 torr* to the end-capillary level of 100 torr in approximately 0.25 seconds, or one-third of the total transit time (0.75 seconds) that an erythrocyte spends within the pulmonary capillaries. Similarly, CO_2 transfer is complete within an approximately equal period of time.

Normally, equilibration of O_2 and CO_2 between alveolar gas and pulmonary capillary blood is complete in one-third the time spent by blood in the pulmonary capillary bed.

total transit time
= 0.75 sec

exercise ↓
transit
time

Though diffusion of oxygen is normally a rapid process, it is not instantaneous. The "resistance" to diffusion is provided primarily by the alveolar-capillary membrane and by the reaction by which oxygenated hemoglobin forms within the erythrocyte. Each of these two factors provides approximately equal resistance to the transfer of oxygen, and each can be disturbed in various disease states. However, as will be discussed later in this chapter, even when diffusion is measurably impaired, it is rarely a cause of impaired gas exchange. There is still generally sufficient time for full equilibration of O_2 or CO_2 to occur, unless transit time is significantly shortened, as with exercise.

Even though diffusion limitation rarely contributes to hypoxemia, an abnormality in diffusion may be a useful marker for diseases of the pulmonary parenchyma affecting the alveolar-capillary membrane and/or the volume of blood in the pulmonary capillaries. Rather than using O_2 to measure diffusion within the lung, clinicians generally resort to use of carbon monoxide, which also combines with hemoglobin and provides a technically easier test to perform and interpret. The usefulness and meaning of the measurement of diffusing capacity will be discussed further in Chapter 3.

OXYGEN TRANSPORT

Since the eventual goal of tissue oxygenation requires transport of oxygen from the lungs to the peripheral tissues and organs, any discussion of oxygenation is incomplete without consideration of these transport mechanisms.

In preparation for this discussion, an understanding of the concepts of partial pressure, gas content, and percent saturation is essential, and these principles will therefore be covered first. The *partial pressure* of any gas is the product of the ambient total gas pressure and the proportion of total gas composition made up by the specific gas of interest. For example, air is composed of approximately 21 percent oxygen; assuming a total pressure of 760 mm Hg (760 torr) at sea level and no water vapor pressure, the partial pressure of oxygen (P_{O_2}) is 0.21 × 760, or 160 torr. If the gas is saturated with water vapor at body temperature (37° C), the water vapor has a partial pressure of 47

---

*The terms *torr* and *mm Hg* are used interchangeably throughout the text, i.e., 1 torr = 1 mm Hg.

torr; the partial pressure of oxygen is then calculated on the basis of the remaining pressure, or $760 - 47 = 713$ torr. Therefore, when room air is saturated at body temperature, the P_{O_2} is $0.21 \times 713 = 150$ torr. Since inspired gas is normally humidified by the upper airway, it becomes fully saturated by the time it reaches the trachea and bronchi, where inspired P_{O_2} is approximately 150 torr.

In clinical situations, we are faced not only with the concept of partial pressure of a gas mixed with other gases, e.g., oxygen as a component of room air, but also with the partial pressure of a gas within a body fluid, primarily blood. When a liquid is in contact with a gas mixture, the partial pressure of a particular gas in the liquid is the same as its partial pressure in the gas mixture, assuming full equilibration has taken place. Therefore, the partial pressure of the gas acts as the "driving force" for the gas to be carried by the liquid phase.

However, the quantity of a gas that can be carried by the liquid medium depends on the "capacity" of the liquid for that particular gas. If a specific gas is quite soluble within a liquid, more of that gas is carried for a given partial pressure than a less soluble gas. In addition, if a component of the liquid is able to bind the gas of interest, then again more of the gas is transported at a particular partial pressure. The latter circumstance holds with the interaction of hemoglobin and oxygen, as will be discussed in more detail.

The *content* of a gas in a liquid, such as blood, is the actual amount of the gas contained within the liquid. For oxygen in blood, one generally refers to milliliters O_2 per 100 ml blood. The percent *saturation* of a gas is the ratio between the actual content of the gas and the maximum possible content if there is a limit or plateau in the amount that can be carried.

Oxygen is transported in blood in two distinct ways, either dissolved in blood or bound to the heme portion of hemoglobin. Oxygen is not very soluble in plasma, and only a small amount of oxygen is carried this way under normal conditions. The amount dissolved is proportional to the partial pressure of oxygen, with 0.0031 ml dissolved per mm Hg partial pressure. The amount bound to hemoglobin is a function of the *oxyhemoglobin dissociation curve*, which relates the driving pressure or P_{O_2} to the quantity of oxygen bound. As can be seen in Figure 1–5, this curve reaches a plateau, indicating that hemoglobin can hold only so much oxygen before it becomes fully saturated. At a P_{O_2} of 60 torr, hemoglobin is approximately 90 percent saturated, so that only relatively small amounts of additional oxygen are transported at a P_{O_2} above this level.

Almost all oxygen transported in the blood is bound to hemoglobin; a small fraction is dissolved in plasma.

Hemoglobin is 90 percent saturated with oxygen at an arterial P_{O_2} of 60 torr.

However, it is important to note that this curve can shift to the right or left, depending on a variety of conditions. Thus, the relationships between arterial P_{O_2} and saturation are not fixed. For instance, a decrease in pH or an increase in P_{CO_2} (largely via a pH effect), temperature, or 2,3-diphosphoglycerate (2,3-DPG) levels each shifts the oxyhemoglobin dissociation curve to the right, making it easier to unload (or harder to bind) oxygen for any given P_{O_2} (Fig. 1–5). Conversely, the opposite changes in pH, P_{CO_2}, temperature, or 2,3-DPG shift the curve to the left and make it harder to unload (or easier to bind) oxygen for any given P_{O_2}.

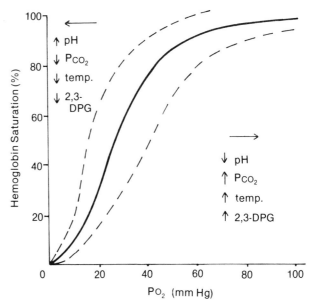

Figure 1–5. Oxyhemoglobin dissociation curve, relating percent hemoglobin saturation and P_{O_2}. The oxygen content can then be determined on the basis of the hemoglobin concentration and the percent hemoglobin saturation (see text). The normal curve is depicted with a solid line; the curves shifted to the right or left (along with conditions leading to them), with dotted lines.

At this point, perhaps the easiest way to understand oxygen transport is to follow the fate of oxygen and hemoglobin as they course through the circulation in a normal person. When blood leaves the pulmonary capillaries, it has already been oxygenated by equilibration with alveolar gas, and the P_{O_2} should be identical to that in the alveoli. Because of oxygen uptake at the level of the alveolar-capillary interface, alveolar P_{O_2} is less than the 150 torr that we calculated for inspired gas within the airways. As we will find shortly when we discuss the alveolar gas equation, alveolar P_{O_2} in a normal individual (breathing air at sea level) is approximately 100 torr. However, the P_{O_2} measured in arterial blood is actually slightly lower than this value for alveolar P_{O_2}, partly because of the presence of small amounts of "shunted" blood that do not participate in gas exchange at the alveolar level—e.g., desaturated blood from the bronchial circulation draining into pulmonary veins, and venous blood from the coronary circulation draining into the left ventricle via Thebesian veins.

Assuming a P_{O_2} of 95 torr in arterial blood, the total oxygen content is the sum of the quantity of oxygen bound to hemoglobin plus the amount dissolved. To calculate the quantity bound to hemoglobin, one needs to know the patient's hemoglobin level and the percent saturation of the hemoglobin with oxygen. Since each gram of hemoglobin can carry 1.34 ml O_2 when fully saturated, the oxygen content is calculated by the following equation:

$$O_2 \text{ content bound to hemoglobin}$$
$$= 1.34 \times \text{hemoglobin} \times \text{saturation} \qquad (1\text{--}3)$$

Let us assume that hemoglobin is 97 percent saturated at a $P_{O_2} = 95$, and that the subject has a hemoglobin level of 15 gm per 100 ml blood. Hence,

$$O_2 \text{ content bound to hemoglobin} = 1.34 \times 15 \times 0.97$$
$$= 19.5 \text{ ml } O_2/100 \text{ ml blood} \qquad (1\text{–}4)$$

In contrast, the amount of dissolved O_2 is much smaller and is proportional to the P_{O_2}, with 0.0031 ml O_2 dissolved per 100 ml blood per torr P_{O_2}. Therefore, at an arterial P_{O_2} of 95 torr:

$$\text{Dissolved } O_2 \text{ content} = 0.0031 \times 95$$
$$= 0.3 \text{ ml } O_2/100 \text{ ml blood} \qquad (1\text{–}5)$$

The total O_2 content is the sum of the hemoglobin-bound O_2 plus the dissolved O_2, or $19.5 + 0.3 = 19.8$ ml O_2 per 100 ml blood.

It is important to realize that the arterial P_{O_2} is not the sole determinant of O_2 content, as the hemoglobin level is also crucial. With anemia, i.e., a reduced hemoglobin level, there are fewer binding sites available for O_2, and the O_2 content falls even though the P_{O_2} remains unchanged. Additionally, the O_2 content of blood is a "static" measurement of the quantity of O_2 per 100 ml blood. The actual O_2 delivery to tissues is "dynamic" and dependent upon blood flow, i.e., cardiac output, as well as O_2 content. Hence, there are three factors that determine tissue O_2 delivery—arterial P_{O_2}, hemoglobin level, and cardiac output—and disturbances in any one of these can result in decreased or insufficient O_2 delivery.

Oxygen content in arterial blood depends upon arterial P_{O_2} and the hemoglobin level; tissue oxygen delivery depends upon these two factors and cardiac output.

When blood reaches the systemic capillaries, oxygen is unloaded to the tissues, and P_{O_2} falls. The extent to which P_{O_2} falls is dependent upon the balance of O_2 supply and demand—the local venous P_{O_2} of blood leaving a tissue falls to a greater degree if more oxygen is extracted per volume of blood because of increased tissue requirements or decreased supply (e.g., as a result of decreased cardiac output).

On the average, in a resting subject the P_{O_2} falls to approximately 40 torr after oxygen extraction occurs at the tissue capillary level. Since a P_{O_2} of 40 torr is associated with a 75 percent saturation of hemoglobin, the total oxygen content in venous blood is calculated by the following:

$$\text{Venous } O_2 \text{ content} = (1.34 \times 15 \times 0.75) + (0.0031 \times 40)$$
$$= 15.2 \text{ ml } O_2/100 \text{ ml blood} \qquad (1\text{–}6)$$

The quantity of oxygen consumed at the tissue level is the difference between the arterial and venous O_2 contents, or $19.8 - 15.2 = 4.6$ ml O_2 per 100 ml blood. The total oxygen consumption (abbreviated $\dot{V}_{O_2}$) is the product of cardiac output and the above arterial-venous oxygen content difference. Since normal resting cardiac output for a young male is about 5 to 6 liters per minute, and since 46 ml O_2 are extracted per liter of blood flow (note difference in units), the resting O_2 consumption is approximately 250 ml per min.

When venous blood returns to the lungs, oxygenation of this desaturated blood occurs at the level of the pulmonary capillaries, and the entire cycle can then be repeated.

CARBON DIOXIDE TRANSPORT

Carbon dioxide is transported through the circulation in three different forms: (1) as bicarbonate (HCO_3^-), the quantitatively largest component; (2) as CO_2 dissolved in plasma; and (3) as carbaminohemoglobin, bound to terminal amino groups on hemoglobin. The first of these, bicarbonate, results from the combination of CO_2 with H_2O to form H_2CO_3, catalyzed by the enzyme carbonic anhydrase, and the subsequent dissociation to H^+ and HCO_3^-. This reaction takes place primarily within the red blood cell, but HCO_3^- then diffuses out into the plasma in exchange for Cl^-.

CO$_2$ is carried in blood as:
(1) bicarbonate
(2) dissolved CO$_2$
(3) carbaminohemoglobin

Though dissolved CO_2, the second form in which CO_2 is transported, comprises only a small portion of the total CO_2 transported, it is quantitatively more important for CO_2 transport than dissolved O_2 is for O_2 transport, since CO_2 is approximately 20 times more soluble in plasma than is O_2. Carbaminohemoglobin, formed by the combination of CO_2 with hemoglobin, is the third of the transport mechanisms available for CO_2. The oxygenation status of hemoglobin is important in determining the quantity of CO_2 that can be bound, deoxygenated hemoglobin having a greater affinity for CO_2 than oxygenated hemoglobin (known as the Haldane effect). Therefore, oxygenation of hemoglobin in the pulmonary capillaries decreases its ability to bind CO_2 and facilitates the elimination of CO_2 by the lungs.

In the same way that the oxyhemoglobin dissociation curve depicts the relationship between Po_2 and O_2 content of blood, a curve can be constructed relating the total CO_2 content to the Pco_2 of blood. However, within the range of gas tensions encountered under physiologic circumstances, the Pco_2 – CO_2 content relationship is almost linear, compared with the curvilinear relationship between Po_2 and O_2 content (Fig. 1–6).

The Pco_2 in mixed venous blood is approximately 46 torr, whereas normal arterial Pco_2 is approximately 40 torr. This decrease of 6 torr in going from mixed venous to arterial blood, combined with the effect of oxygenation of hemoglobin on release of CO_2, corresponds to a change in CO_2 content of approximately 3.6 ml per 100 ml blood.

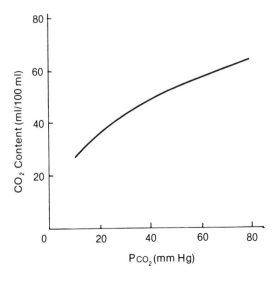

Figure 1–6. Relationship between Pco_2 and CO_2 content. The curve shifts slightly to the left as the O_2 saturation of blood decreases; the curve shown is for blood completely saturated with oxygen.

Assuming a cardiac output of 5 to 6 liters per minute, the CO_2 production can be calculated as the product of the cardiac output and the arterial-venous CO_2 content difference, or approximately 200 ml per min.

VENTILATION-PERFUSION RELATIONSHIPS

The earlier topics of ventilation, blood flow, and diffusion and their relationship to gas exchange (O_2 uptake and CO_2 elimination) are actually more complicated than initially presented, since we did not consider how the total ventilation and blood flow are distributed within the lung. Effective gas exchange depends critically on the relationship between ventilation and perfusion in individual gas-exchanging units; a disturbance in this relationship, even if the total amounts of ventilation and blood flow are normal, is frequently responsible for markedly abnormal gas exchange in disease states.

The optimal efficiency for gas exchange would be provided by an even distribution of ventilation and perfusion throughout the lung, so that a matching of ventilation and perfusion is always present. In reality, such a circumstance does not exist, even in normal lungs. Since blood flow is determined to a large extent by hydrostatic forces, the dependent regions of the lung receive a disproportionately large share of the perfusion, while the uppermost regions are relatively underperfused. Similarly, there is a gradient of ventilation throughout the lung, with greater amounts again going to the dependent areas. However, even though ventilation and perfusion are both greater in the gravity-dependent regions of lung, this gradient is more marked for perfusion than for ventilation. Consequently, the ratio of ventilation (V) to perfusion (Q̇) is higher in apical regions of lung than in basal regions. As a result, gas exchange throughout the lung is not uniform, but varies depending on the V̇/Q̇ ratio of each region.

From top to bottom of the lung the ventilation and perfusion gradient is more marked for perfusion (Q̇) than for ventilation (V̇), thus the V̇/Q̇ ratio is lower in the dependent regions of lung.

In order to understand the effects of altering the V̇/Q̇ ratio on gas exchange, it is first worthwhile to consider the individual alveolus, and then to proceed to the more complex model with multiple alveoli and variable V̇/Q̇ ratios. In a single alveolus, a continuous spectrum exists for the possible relationships between V̇ and Q̇ (Fig. 1–7). At one

Figure 1–7. Spectrum of ventilation-perfusion ratios within a single alveolar-capillary unit. In *A*, ventilation is obstructed but perfusion preserved, and the alveolar-capillary unit is behaving as a shunt. In *B*, ventilation and perfusion are well matched. In *C*, no blood flow is reaching the alveolus, so that ventilation is wasted, i.e., serving as dead-space ventilation. (Adapted from West, J. B.: Ventilation/Blood Flow and Gas Exchange. 3rd ed. Oxford, Blackwell Scientific Publications, 1977, p. 36. Reproduced with permission.)

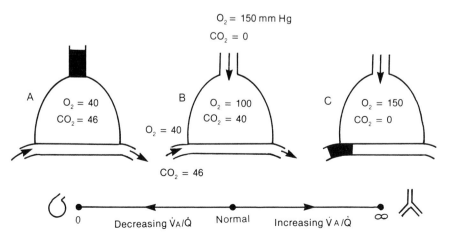

$O_2 = 150$ mm Hg
$CO_2 = 0$

A $O_2 = 40$ $CO_2 = 46$

B $O_2 = 100$ $CO_2 = 40$ $O_2 = 40$

C $O_2 = 150$ $CO_2 = 0$

$CO_2 = 46$

0   Decreasing V̇A/Q̇   Normal   Increasing V̇A/Q̇   ∞

extreme, where $\dot{V}$ is maintained and $\dot{Q}$ approaches 0, the $\dot{V}/\dot{Q}$ ratio approaches infinity. When there is actually no perfusion ($\dot{Q} = 0$), the ventilation is "wasted" insofar as gas exchange is concerned, and the alveolus is part of the "dead space." At the other extreme, $\dot{V}$ approaches 0 while $\dot{Q}$ is preserved, and the $\dot{V}/\dot{Q}$ ratio approaches 0. When there is no ventilation ($\dot{V} = 0$), a "shunt" exists, oxygenation does not take place during transit through the pulmonary circulation, and the hemoglobin is still desaturated when it leaves the pulmonary capillary.

Again dealing with the extremes, for an alveolar-capillary unit acting as dead space ($\dot{V}/\dot{Q} = \infty$), P_{O_2} in the alveolus is equal to that in air, i.e., 150 torr (taking into account the fact that air in the alveolus is saturated with water vapor), while P_{CO_2} is 0, since no blood and therefore no CO_2 are in contact with alveolar gas. With a region of true dead space, there is no blood flow, so one does not speak of gas tensions in blood leaving the alveolus. If there were a minutely small amount of blood flow, i.e., the $\dot{V}/\dot{Q}$ ratio approached but did not reach ∞, then the blood would also have a P_{O_2} approaching (but slightly less than) 150 torr and a P_{CO_2} approaching (but slightly more than) 0 torr. At the other extreme, for an alveolar-capillary unit acting as a shunt ($\dot{V}/\dot{Q} = 0$), blood leaving the capillary has gas tensions identical to those in mixed venous blood, i.e., $P_{O_2} = 40$ torr, $P_{CO_2} = 46$ torr, assuming the rest of the lung functioned well enough to maintain normal arterial and mixed venous gas tensions.

In reality, alveolar-capillary units may fall anywhere along this continuum of $\dot{V}/\dot{Q}$ ratios. With normal breathing, the higher the $\dot{V}/\dot{Q}$ ratio in an alveolar-capillary unit, the closer the unit comes to behaving like an area of dead space, and the more the P_{O_2} approaches 150 torr and the P_{CO_2} approaches 0 torr. The lower the $\dot{V}/\dot{Q}$ ratio, the closer the unit comes to behaving like a shunt, and the more the P_{O_2} and P_{CO_2} of blood leaving the capillary approach the gas tensions in mixed venous blood (40 and 46 torr, respectively). This continuum is depicted in Figure 1–8, where moving to the left signifies lowering the $\dot{V}/\dot{Q}$ ratio, and moving to the right means an increase in the $\dot{V}/\dot{Q}$ ratio. The ideal circumstance lies between these extremes, where $P_{O_2} = 100$ torr and $P_{CO_2} = 40$ torr.

Ventilation-perfusion ratios within each alveolar-capillary unit range from $V/\dot{Q} = \infty$ (dead space) to $V/\dot{Q} = 0$ (shunt).

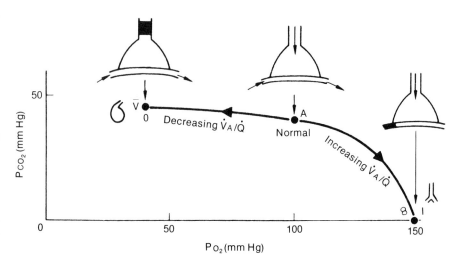

Figure 1–8. Continuum of alveolar gas composition at different ventilation-perfusion ratios within a single alveolar–capillary unit. The line is called the "ventilation-perfusion ratio line"; at the extreme left side of the line, $\dot{V}/\dot{Q} = 0$ (shunt), while at the extreme right side of the line, $\dot{V}/\dot{Q} = \infty$ (dead space). (Adapted from West, J. B.: Ventilation/Blood Flow and Gas Exchange. 3rd ed. Oxford, Blackwell Scientific Publications, 1977, p. 37. Reproduced with permission.)

In multiple alveolar-capillary units, the net P_{O_2} and P_{CO_2} of the resulting pulmonary venous blood depend on the total O_2 or CO_2 content and the total volume of blood collected from each of the contributing units. Considering P_{CO_2} first, areas with relatively high $\dot{V}/\dot{Q}$ ratios contribute blood with a lower P_{CO_2} than areas with low $\dot{V}/\dot{Q}$ ratios. However, since the relationship between CO_2 content and P_{CO_2} is nearly linear over the range of concern, if blood having a higher P_{CO_2} and CO_2 content mixes with an equal volume of blood having a lower P_{CO_2} and CO_2 content, an intermediate P_{CO_2} and CO_2 content (approximately halfway in between) result.

In contrast, a high P_{O_2} in blood coming from a region with a high $\dot{V}/\dot{Q}$ ratio cannot compensate for blood with a low P_{O_2} from a region with a low $\dot{V}/\dot{Q}$ ratio. The difference stems from the shape of the oxyhemoglobin dissociation curve; once hemoglobin is nearly saturated with O_2, increasing the P_{O_2} does not boost the O_2 content. Therefore, blood with a higher than normal P_{O_2} does not have a correspondingly higher content, and cannot compensate for blood with a low P_{O_2} and low O_2 content.

Regions of the lung with a high $\dot{V}/\dot{Q}$ ratio and a high P_{O_2} cannot compensate for regions with a low $\dot{V}/\dot{Q}$ ratio and low P_{O_2}.

In the normal lung, regional differences in $\dot{V}/\dot{Q}$ ratio affect gas tensions in blood coming from specific regions as well as gas tensions in the resulting arterial blood. At the apices, where the $\dot{V}/\dot{Q}$ ratio is approximately 3.3, P_{O_2} = 132 torr and P_{CO_2} = 28 torr; at the bases, where the $\dot{V}/\dot{Q}$ ratio is approximately 0.63, P_{O_2} = 89 torr and P_{CO_2} = 42 torr. As discussed, the net P_{O_2} and P_{CO_2} of the combined blood coming from the apices, the bases, and the areas in between is a function of the relative amounts of blood from each of these areas and the gas contents of each.

In disease states, ventilation-perfusion mismatch is frequently much more extreme, resulting in clinically significant gas exchange abnormalities. When an area of lung behaves as a shunt or even as a region of very low $\dot{V}/\dot{Q}$ ratio, blood coming from this area has a low O_2 content and saturation, which cannot be compensated for by blood from relatively preserved regions of lung. If $\dot{V}/\dot{Q}$ mismatch is severe, particularly with areas of high $\dot{V}/\dot{Q}$, this can effectively produce dead space and therefore decrease the alveolar ventilation to other areas of the lung carrying a disproportionate share of the perfusion. Since CO_2 excretion depends on alveolar ventilation, P_{CO_2} may rise unless there is an overall increase in the minute ventilation to restore the effective alveolar ventilation.

ABNORMALITIES IN GAS EXCHANGE

The net effect of disturbances in the normal pattern of gas exchange can be assessed by measurement of the gas tensions (P_{O_2} and P_{CO_2}) in arterial blood. Though the information that can be obtained from arterial blood gas measurement will be discussed further in Chapter 3, the mechanisms of hypoxemia (decreased arterial P_{O_2}) and hypercapnia (increased P_{CO_2}) will be considered here, as they relate to the physiologic principles just discussed.

Hypoxemia

As mentioned previously, blood that has traversed pulmonary capillaries leaves with a P_{O_2} that should be in equilibrium with and almost identical to the P_{O_2} in companion alveoli. Though it is difficult to measure the oxygen tension in alveolar gas, it can be conveniently calculated by a formula known as the *alveolar gas equation.* A simplified version of this formula is relatively easy to use and can prove extremely useful in the clinical setting, particularly when one is trying to deduce why a patient is hypoxemic. According to this formula, the alveolar oxygen tension (P_{AO_2})* can be calculated by the following:

$$P_{AO_2} = F_{IO_2} (P_B - P_{H_2O}) - \frac{P_{ACO_2}}{R} \qquad (1-7)$$

where F_{IO_2} is the fractional content of inspired oxygen (F_{IO_2} of air = 0.21), P_B is barometric pressure (approximately 760 torr at sea level), P_{H_2O} is the vapor pressure of water in the alveoli (at full saturation at 37° C, $P_{H_2O} = 47$ torr), P_{ACO_2} is alveolar CO_2 tension (which can be assumed to be identical to arterial CO_2 tension, P_{aCO_2}), and R is the respiratory quotient (CO_2 production divided by O_2 consumption, usually about 0.8). In practice, the equation is often simplified to a less cumbersome form; when numbers are substituted for P_B and P_{H_2O}, and P_{aCO_2} is used instead of P_{ACO_2}, the resulting equation (at sea level) is:

$$P_{AO_2} = 713 \times F_{IO_2} - \frac{P_{aCO_2}}{0.8} \qquad (1-8)$$

The simplified alveolar gas equation (Equation 1–8) can be used for calculation of alveolar P_{O_2} (P_{AO_2}).

By calculating the P_{AO_2}, one can then determine what the expected P_{aO_2} should be. Even in a normal person, P_{AO_2} is greater than P_{aO_2} by an amount that is called the *alveolar-arterial oxygen difference* or *gradient* (commonly abbreviated AaD_{O_2}). There are two main reasons why a gradient exists even in normal individuals: (1) A small amount of the cardiac output behaves as a shunt, without ever going through the pulmonary capillary bed. This includes venous blood from the bronchial circulation, which drains into the pulmonary veins, and coronary venous blood draining via Thebesian veins directly into the left ventricle. Desaturated blood from these sources lowers the oxygen tension in the resulting arterial blood. (2) Ventilation-perfusion gradients from the top to the bottom of the lung result in somewhat less oxygenated blood from the bases combining with better oxygenated blood from the apices.

The AaD_{O_2} is normally less than approximately 15 torr, though it increases with age. There are several reasons why it may be elevated in disease. First, a shunt may be present, so that some desaturated blood combines with fully saturated blood and lowers the P_{O_2} in the resulting arterial blood. The following are common causes of a shunt:

1. Intracardiac lesions, with a right-to-left shunt at the atrial or ventricular level, e.g., atrial or ventricular septal defect. Note that a left-to-right shunt does not affect either the AaD_{O_2} or the arterial P_{O_2}, since its net effect is to "recycle" already oxygenated blood through the pulmonary vasculature, not to dilute oxygenated blood with desaturated blood.

---

* By convention, "A" refers to alveolar, "a" to arterial.

2. Structural abnormalities of the pulmonary vasculature resulting in direct communication between pulmonary arterial and venous systems, e.g., pulmonary arteriovenous malformations.

3. Pulmonary diseases that result in filling of the alveolar spaces with fluid, e.g., pulmonary edema, or complete alveolar collapse. Either process can result in complete loss of ventilation to the affected alveoli, while some perfusion through the associated capillaries may continue.

Another cause of an elevated $AaDo_2$ is ventilation-perfusion mismatch. Even when total ventilation and perfusion to both lungs is normal, if some areas receive less ventilation and more perfusion (low $\dot{V}/\dot{Q}$) while others receive more ventilation and less perfusion (high $\dot{V}/\dot{Q}$), then the $AaDo_2$ increases and hypoxemia results. As we just mentioned, the reason for this phenomenon is that areas of low $\dot{V}/\dot{Q}$ provide relatively desaturated blood with a low oxygen content. Blood coming from regions with a high $\dot{V}/\dot{Q}$ ratio cannot compensate for this problem, since the hemoglobin is already fully saturated and cannot increase its O_2 content further by the increased ventilation (see Fig. 1–9).

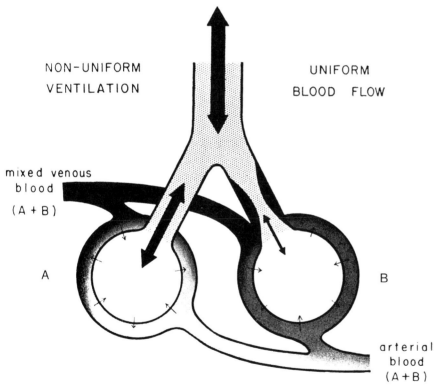

NON-UNIFORM VENTILATION

UNIFORM BLOOD FLOW

mixed venous blood (A + B)

A

B

arterial blood (A + B)

	A	B	A + B
Alveolar ventilation (l/min)	3.2	0.8	4.0
Pulmonary blood flow (l/min)	2.5	2.5	5.0
Ventilation / blood flow ratio	1.3	0.3	0.8
Mixed venous O_2 saturation (%)	75.0	75.0	75.0
Arterial O_2 saturation (%)	98.2	91.7	95.0
Mixed venous O_2 tension (mm Hg)	40.0	40.0	40.0
Alveolar O_2 tension (mm Hg)	116.0	66.0	106.0
Arterial O_2 tension (mm Hg)	116.0	66.0	84.0
Alveolar-arterial Po_2 difference (mm Hg)	0.0	0.0	22.0

Figure 1–9. Example of nonuniform ventilation producing $\dot{V}/\dot{Q}$ mismatch in a two-alveolus model. In this particular instance, perfusion is equally distributed between the two alveoli. The calculations demonstrate how $\dot{V}/\dot{Q}$ mismatch lowers arterial Po_2 and causes an elevated alveolar-arterial oxygen difference. (Adapted from Comroe, J. H., et al.: The Lung. 2nd ed. Chicago, Year Book Medical Publishers, Inc., 1962, p. 94. Reproduced with permission.)

Ventilation-perfusion mismatch and shunting are the two important mechanisms for elevation of the alveolar–arterial O_2 difference (AaDO_2).

In practice, one can distinguish a true shunt ($\dot{V}/\dot{Q} = 0$) and $\dot{V}/\dot{Q}$ mismatch (with areas of $\dot{V}/\dot{Q}$ that are low but not 0) by having the patient inhale 100 percent O_2. In the former case, increasing the inspired PO_2 does not add further O_2 to the shunted blood, and O_2 content does not increase significantly. In the latter case, the alveolar and capillary PO_2 rises considerably with additional O_2, fully saturating blood coming even from regions with a low $\dot{V}/\dot{Q}$ ratio, and arterial PO_2 rises substantially.

A third cause for an elevated AaDO_2 can be postulated on a theoretical basis, though in reality it very rarely occurs. This final cause is a "diffusion block," in which the PO_2 in pulmonary capillary blood does not reach equilibrium with alveolar gas. If the interface (i.e., the tissue within the alveolar wall) between the capillary and the alveolar lumen were thickened, it could be hypothesized that O_2 would not diffuse as readily, and that PO_2 in pulmonary capillary blood would never reach the PO_2 of alveolar gas. However, even with a thickened alveolar wall, there is still sufficient time for this equilibrium; unless the transit time of erythrocytes is also significantly shortened, failure to equilibrate does not appear to be a problem. One of the rare times this occurs may be during exercise in a patient with interstitial lung disease, as will be discussed later. For most practical purposes, a "diffusion block" should be considered only a hypothetical rather than a realistic mechanism for increasing the AaDO_2 and causing hypoxemia.

Increasing the difference between alveolar and arterial PO_2 is not the only mechanism resulting in hypoxemia. One can also decrease the alveolar PO_2, which must necessarily lower arterial PO_2 if the AaDO_2 remains constant. Referring back to the alveolar gas equation, it is relatively easy to see that alveolar PO_2 drops if barometric pressure falls (e.g., with altitude) or if the alveolar PCO_2 rises (e.g., with hypoventilation). In the latter circumstance, when the total alveolar ventilation falls, PCO_2 in alveolar gas rises, while alveolar PO_2 falls. This last mechanism, i.e., hypoventilation, is relatively common in lung disease, and can easily be identified by the presence of a high PCO_2 accompanying the hypoxemia. If the AaDO_2 is normal, then hypoventilation is the exclusive cause of the low PO_2. If AaDO_2 is elevated, then either $\dot{V}/\dot{Q}$ mismatch or shunting also contributes to the hypoxemia.

When hypoventilation is the sole cause of hypoxemia, AaDO_2 is normal.

In summary, lung disease can eventuate in hypoxemia for multiple reasons. Shunting and ventilation-perfusion mismatch are both associated with an elevated AaDO_2 and can often be distinguished if necessary by inhalation of 100 percent O_2, which markedly increases PaO_2 with $\dot{V}/\dot{Q}$ mismatch but not with true shunting. In contrast, both hypoventilation (identified by a high PaCO_2) and a low inspired PO_2 lower alveolar PO_2 and cause hypoxemia, though AaDO_2 remains normal. Since many of the disease processes we will be examining have several pathophysiologic abnormalities, it is not at all uncommon to see more than one of the above mechanisms producing hypoxemia in a particular patient.

Mechanisms of hypoxemia:
(1) Shunt
(2) V/Q mismatch
(3) Hypoventilation
(4) Low inspired PO_2

Hypercapnia

As mentioned earlier under Ventilation, alveolar ventilation is the prime determinant of arterial PCO_2, assuming that CO_2 production remains constant. It is clear that alveolar ventilation is compromised either by decreasing the total minute ventilation (without changing the relative proportions of dead space and alveolar ventilation) or by keeping the total minute ventilation constant and increasing the relative proportion of dead space to alveolar ventilation. A simple way to produce the latter circumstance is to change the pattern of breathing, i.e., by decreasing the tidal volume and increasing the frequency of breathing. With a lower tidal volume, a larger proportion of each breath ventilates the anatomic dead space, and the proportion of alveolar ventilation to total ventilation must decrease.

In addition, if significant ventilation-perfusion mismatching is present, well-perfused areas may be underventilated, while underperfused areas receive a disproportionate amount of ventilation. The net effect of having a large proportion of ventilation go to poorly perfused areas is similar to that of increasing the dead space. By wasting this ventilation, the remainder of the lung with the large share of the perfusion is underventilated, and the net effect is to decrease the effective alveolar ventilation. Under many disease conditions, when such significant $\dot{V}/\dot{Q}$ mismatch exists, any increase in the P_{CO_2} stimulates breathing, increases the total minute ventilation, and compensates for the effectively wasted ventilation.

Therefore, one can define several causes of hypercapnia, all of which have in common a decrease in the effective alveolar ventilation. A decrease in the minute ventilation, an increase in the proportion of wasted ventilation, and significant ventilation-perfusion mismatch may all result in CO_2 retention. However, by increasing the total minute ventilation, a patient is often capable of compensating for the latter two situations, so that CO_2 retention does not result.

A decrease in alveolar ventilation is the primary mechanism causing hypercapnia.

One must also remember that increasing CO_2 production necessitates an increase in alveolar ventilation to avoid CO_2 retention. Hence, if alveolar ventilation cannot rise to compensate for additional CO_2 production, hypercapnia will also result.

As is the case with hypoxemia, pathophysiologic explanations for hypercapnia do not necessarily follow such simple rules, in which each case can be fully explained by one of the mechanisms. In practice, several of these mechanisms may be operative, even in a particular patient.

REFERENCES

Comroe, J. H.: Physiology of Respiration. 2nd ed. Chicago, Year Book Medical Publishers, 1974.

Murray, J. F.: The Normal Lung: The Basis for Diagnosis and Treatment of Pulmonary Disease. Philadelphia, W. B. Saunders Co., 1976.

West, J. B.: Respiratory Physiology—The Essentials. 2nd ed. Baltimore, Williams & Wilkins, 1979.

West, J. B.: Ventilation/Blood Flow and Gas Exchange. 3rd ed. Oxford, Blackwell Scientific Publications, 1977.

2

Presentation of the Patient with Pulmonary Disease

Dyspnea
Cough
Hemoptysis
Chest Pain

The patient with a pulmonary problem generally comes to the attention of the clinician in either of two ways—by complaining of a symptom that can be traced back to a respiratory etiology, or by incidentally having an abnormal chest radiograph. Though the former presentation is more common, the latter is certainly not uncommon when a roentgenogram is done either as part of a routine examination or for evaluation of a seemingly unrelated problem. In this chapter, we will focus on the first case, the patient who comes to the physician with a respiratory-related complaint. In the next and in subsequent chapters, we will often refer to the abnormal roentgenogram as the clue to the presence of pulmonary pathology.

There are four particularly common (as well as a number of less common) symptoms that bring the patient with lung disease to the physician—dyspnea (and its variants), cough (with or without sputum production), hemoptysis, and chest pain. However, all of these symptoms, to a greater or lesser extent, may result from nonpulmonary pathology, especially primary cardiac disease. For each symptom, we will discuss some of the important clinical features, followed by the pathophysiology and the differential diagnosis.

DYSPNEA

Dyspnea, or shortness of breath, is frequently a difficult symptom for the physician to evaluate, since it is such a subjective feeling experienced by the patient. Patients may describe this complaint in a variety of ways, including shortness of breath, difficulty in getting air, or difficulty catching their breath. To a large degree, the symptom of dyspnea reflects an uncomfortable awareness of one's own breathing, which is normally a phenomenon to which we pay little attention.

Not only is the symptom very subjective, but the patient's appreciation of it and its importance to the physician depend heavily on the stimulus or amount of activity required to precipitate it. The physician must also take into account how the stimulus, when quantified, compares with the patient's usual level of activity. For example, a patient who is limited in exertion by a nonpulmonary problem may not experience any shortness of breath even if he additionally has significant lung disease; if he were more active, however, dyspnea would become readily apparent. Or, to give another example, a marathon runner who experiences a new symptom of shortness of breath after 10 miles of running may warrant much more concern than an elderly man who has for many years had a stable symptom of shortness of breath after 3 blocks of walking.

It is also important to distinguish dyspnea from several other signs or symptoms that may have an entirely different significance. First of all, the term *tachypnea* refers to a rapid respiratory rate (i.e., greater than the usual value of 12 to 20 per minute); tachypnea may be present with or without dyspnea, just as dyspnea does not necessarily entail the finding of tachypnea on physical examination. Secondly, the term *hyperventilation* refers to ventilation that is greater than the amount required to maintain normal CO_2 elimination. Hence the P_{CO_2} in arterial blood is lowered, and this decrease in P_{CO_2} is the hallmark of hyperventilation. Finally, the symptom of exertional fatigue must be distinguished from dyspnea. Fatigue may be due to cardiovascular, neuromuscular, or other nonpulmonary diseases, and the implication of this symptom is quite different from that of true shortness of breath.

Dyspnea is distinct from tachypnea, hyperventilation, and external fatigue.

There are also some variations on the basic theme of dyspnea. *Orthopnea*, or shortness of breath on assuming the recumbent position, is often quantitated by the number of pillows or angle of elevation necessary to relieve or prevent the sensation. One of the main causes of orthopnea is an increase in venous return and central intravascular volume upon assuming the recumbent position. In patients with cardiac decompensation and either overt or subclinical congestive heart failure, the increment in left atrial and left ventricular filling may result in pulmonary vascular congestion and pulmonary interstitial or alveolar edema. Hence orthopnea frequently suggests cardiac disease and some element of congestive heart failure. However, some patients with primary pulmonary disease experience orthopnea, such as those with a significant amount of secretions, who have more difficulty handling their secretions when they are in the supine position.

Orthopnea, often associated with left ventricular failure, may accompany primary pulmonary disease.

The term *paroxysmal nocturnal dyspnea* refers to awakening from sleep with dyspnea. As with orthopnea the recumbent position is important, but this symptom differs from orthopnea in that it does not occur soon after lying down. Though the implication with regard to underlying cardiac decompensation still applies, the increase in central intravascular volume is due more to a slow mobilization of tissue fluid, such as peripheral edema, than to a rapid redistribution of intravascular volume from peripheral to central vessels.

Other variants that are much more uncommon and will just be mentioned but not discussed in detail are platypnea and trepopnea. *Platypnea* is the symptom of shortness of breath in the upright position, i.e., the opposite of orthopnea. *Trepopnea*, on the other hand, is shortness of breath when lying on one's side; patients experiencing this symptom complain of dyspnea on either the right or the left side, which can be relieved by moving to the opposite lateral position.

Returning to the more general symptom of dyspnea, it is difficult to identify a unifying mechanism that can explain the sensation of shortness of breath. Finding a common denominator among the diverse conditions that produce dyspnea has been extremely difficult, and it appears that different mechanisms may be involved in different disorders. In some subjects, an increase in airways resistance seems to be important, while in others an abnormally stiff lung may be the problem. In still other cases, such as pulmonary embolic disease, neither of these explanations is satisfactory. A reasonable but still not totally satisfactory hypothesis suggests that an imbalance of work to ventilatory output may be important. For example, dyspnea may be the sensation produced by an amount of respiratory work (or muscular effort) that is disproportionate either to ventilatory demands or to the level of ventilation actually produced. An attractive feature of this hypothesis is that it explains why the sensation of breathing hard with exercise in a normal subject is distinct from the uncomfortable sensation of dyspnea, since the amount of respiratory work performed when a normal subject exercises is appropriate for the ventilatory demands.

No totally satisfactory explanation for dyspnea is yet available.

There is a broad differential diagnosis of disorders resulting in dyspnea (Table 2–1), and it is perhaps best to separate them into the major categories of respiratory, cardiovascular, and anxiety-related or

Table 2–1. DIFFERENTIAL DIAGNOSIS OF DYSPNEA

Respiratory
    Airways disease
        Asthma
        Chronic obstructive lung disease
        Upper airway obstruction
    Parenchymal lung disease
        Adult respiratory distress syndrome
        Pneumonia
        Interstitial lung disease
    Pulmonary vascular disease
        Pulmonary emboli
    Pleural disease
        Pneumothorax
        Pleural effusion
    "Bellows" disease
        Neuromuscular disease (e.g., polymyositis, myasthenia gravis, Guillain-Barré syndrome)
        Chest wall disease (e.g., kyphoscoliosis)
Cardiovascular
    Elevated pulmonary venous pressure
        Left ventricular failure
        Mitral stenosis
    Decreased cardiac output
    Severe anemia
Anxiety/Psychosomatic

psychosomatic. Disorders at many levels of the respiratory system—airways, pulmonary parenchyma, pulmonary vasculature, pleura, and bellows—cause dyspnea; it is primarily on these clinical problems that we will focus our attention.

Airway diseases causing dyspnea result primarily from obstruction to airflow, occurring anywhere from the upper airway to large, medium, or small intrathoracic bronchi and bronchioles. Upper airway obstruction, which we define for our purposes here as obstruction above or including the level of the vocal cords, is caused primarily by foreign bodies, tumors, edema (e.g., with anaphylaxis), or stenosis. A clue to upper airway obstruction may be the presence of disproportionate difficulty with inspiration and an audible, prolonged gasping sound called inspiratory stridor. The reason for the inspiratory problem will be considered further in Chapter 7, in which the pathophysiology of upper airway obstruction is discussed.

Airways below the level of the vocal cords, from the trachea down to the small bronchioles, are the ones more commonly involved with disorders that produce dyspnea. An isolated problem, such as an airway tumor, usually does not by itself make the patient dyspneic, unless it occurs in the trachea or in a major bronchus. In contrast, diseases such as asthma or chronic obstructive pulmonary disease have widespread effects throughout the tracheobronchial tree, which may have narrowing due to airway spasm, edema, secretions, or loss of radial support (see Chapter 4). With this type of obstruction, difficulty with expiration generally predominates over that with inspiration, and the physical findings associated with obstruction (wheezing, prolongation of airflow) are more prominent on expiration.

The category of pulmonary parenchymal disease includes disorders causing inflammation, infiltration, fluid accumulation, or scarring of the alveolar structures. Such disorders may be diffuse in nature, as with the many causes of pulmonary fibrosis, or they may be more localized, as occurs with a bacterial pneumonia.

Pulmonary vascular disease refers to those problems that result in blockage or loss of vessels in the lung. The most common acute disorder within this category is pulmonary embolism, in which one or many pulmonary vessels are occluded by thrombi originating in systemic veins. Chronically, vessels may be blocked by recurrent pulmonary emboli or by inflammatory or scarring processes that result in thickening of vessel walls or obliteration of the vascular lumen.

Two major disorders affecting the pleura may result in dyspnea—pneumothorax (air in the pleural space) or pleural effusion (liquid in the pleural space). With pleural effusions, there generally must be a substantial amount of fluid in the pleural space to result in dyspnea, unless the patient also has significant underlying cardiopulmonary disease or there are additional complicating features.

In using the term "bellows" for the final category of respiratory-related disorders causing dyspnea we are referring to the pump system that works under the control of a central nervous system generator to expand the lungs and allow airflow. This pump system includes a variety of muscles (primarily but not exclusively diaphragm and intercostals) and the chest wall. Primary disease affecting the muscles, their nerve supply, or neuromuscular interaction, including polymyositis, myasthenia gravis, or Guillain-Barré syndrome, may result in dyspnea. Deformity of the chest wall, particularly kyphoscoliosis, produces dyspnea by several pathophysiologic mechanisms, not the least of which is the increased work of breathing. These disorders of the respiratory bellows will be covered in Chapter 19.

The second major category of disorders producing dyspnea is cardiovascular. In the large majority of cases, the feature that such patients have in common is an elevated pressure in the pulmonary veins and capillaries, which leads to a transudation or leakage of fluid into the pulmonary interstitium and the alveoli. Left ventricular failure, from either ischemic or valvular heart disease, is the most common example. Additionally, mitral stenosis, with elevated left atrial pressure, produces elevated pulmonary venous and capillary pressures even though left ventricular function and pressure are normal. A frequent accompaniment of the dyspnea associated with these forms of cardiac disease is orthopnea and/or paroxysmal nocturnal dyspnea. Though a worsening of dyspnea in the supine position is not specific to pulmonary venous hypertension and can also be found in some patients with pulmonary disease, improvement of dyspnea in the supine position is a point against left ventricular failure as the etiology.

Finally, dyspnea may be due to anxiety or to other psychosomatic problems. Since the sensation of dyspnea is such a subjective one, any awareness of one's breathing may start a self-perpetuating problem; the patient breathes faster, becomes more aware of breathing, and finally has a sensation of frank dyspnea. At the extreme, one can hyperventilate and lower the arterial P_{CO_2} sufficiently to cause additional symptoms of lightheadedness and tingling, particularly of the fingers and around the mouth. It is important to remember, however, that patients who may seem anxious or have a history of psychologic problems can certainly also have lung disease. Similarly, patients with lung or heart disease can also at times have dyspnea with a functional etiology unrelated to their underlying disease process.

COUGH

Unlike dyspnea, cough is a symptom that everyone has experienced at some point, mainly because it is a physiologic mechanism for clearing and protecting the airway and does not necessarily imply disease. Normally cough is protective against food or other foreign material entering the airway, and it is also responsible for aiding in clearance of secretions produced within the tracheobronchial tree. Generally, mucociliary clearance is adequate to propel secretions upward through the trachea and into the larynx, so that they can be removed from the airway and swallowed. However, if the mucociliary clearance mechanism is temporarily damaged or not functioning well, or if it is overwhelmed by excessive production of secretions, then cough becomes an important additional mechanism for clearing the tracheobronchial tree.

Cough is usually initiated by stimulation of receptors (called irritant receptors) at any of a number of locations. These irritant receptor nerve endings are found primarily in the larynx, trachea, and major bronchi, particularly at points of bifurcation. However, there are also sensory receptors located in other parts of the upper airway as well as on the pleura, the diaphragm, and even the pericardium. Irritation of these nerve endings initiates an impulse that travels via afferent nerves (primarily the vagus but also trigeminal, glossopharyngeal, and phrenic) to a poorly defined cough center in the medulla. The efferent signal is then carried in the recurrent laryngeal nerve (a branch of the vagus), which controls closure of the glottis, and in phrenic and spinal nerves, which effect contraction of the diaphragm and the expiratory muscles of the chest and abdominal walls. The initial part of the cough sequence is a deep inspiration to a high lung volume, followed by closure of the glottis, contraction of the expiratory muscles, and finally opening of the glottis. When the glottis suddenly opens, contraction of the expiratory muscles and relaxation of the diaphragm produce an explosive rush of air at high velocity, which transports airway secretions or foreign material out of the tracheobronchial tree.

The major causes of coughing are outlined in Table 2–2. Cough commonly results from an external inhaled irritant, regardless of whether the subject is normal or has respiratory system disease. The most common inhaled irritant is clearly cigarette smoke; noxious fumes, dusts, or chemicals also stimulate irritant receptors and result in cough. Aspiration of gastric contents or upper airway secretions, which amounts to "inhalation" of liquid or solid material, can also result in cough, the cause of which may be unrecognized if the aspiration has not been clinically apparent.

Cough caused by respiratory system disease comes mainly but not exclusively from disorders affecting the airway. Most commonly, viruses producing upper respiratory tract infections also affect parts of the tracheobronchial tree, and the airway inflammation results in a bothersome cough lasting sometimes from weeks to months. Bacterial infections of the lung, either acute (pneumonia, acute bronchitis) or chronic (bronchiectasis, chronic bronchitis, lung abscess), generally have an airways component and an impressive amount of associated coughing. Space-occupying lesions in the tracheobronchial tree (tumors, foreign

Table 2–2. DIFFERENTIAL DIAGNOSIS OF COUGH

External inhaled irritant (smoke, dusts, fumes)
Aspiration
    Gastric contents
    Oral secretions
    Foreign body
Airways disease
    Upper respiratory tract infection
    Acute or chronic bronchitis
    Bronchiectasis
    Neoplasm
    External compression by a node or mass lesion
    Reactive airways disease (asthma)
Parenchymal disease
    Pneumonia
    Lung abscess
    Interstitial lung disease
Congestive heart failure
Miscellaneous

bodies, granulomas) or external lesions compressing the airway (mediastinal masses, lymph nodes, other tumors) commonly present with cough secondary to airway irritation. Hyperirritable airways with airway constriction, as seen in asthma, are frequently associated with cough, even when a specific inhaled irritant is not identified. The more readily recognized manifestations of asthma, wheezing and dyspnea, may not be apparent, so that cough may be the sole presenting symptom. Patients with pulmonary interstitial disease may also have cough, probably owing more to secondary airway or pleural involvement, since few irritant receptors are in the lung itself. In congestive heart failure, cough may be related to the same unclear mechanism operative in patients with interstitial lung disease, or may be secondary to bronchial edema.

A variety of miscellaneous causes of cough, such as irritation of the tympanic membrane by wax or a hair, or of one of the afferent nerves by osteophytes or neural tumors, have been identified but will not be discussed in further detail here. Finally, coughing may be a nervous habit that can be especially prominent when the patient is anxious, though the physician must not neglect the possibility that an organic cause may also be present.

Yellow or green sputum reflects the presence of numerous leukocytes, either neutrophils or eosinophils.

The symptom of cough is generally characterized by whether it is productive or nonproductive of sputum. Virtually any cause of cough may be productive at times of small amounts of clear or mucoid sputum. However, the presence of thick yellow or green sputum is indicative of the presence of numerous leukocytes in the sputum, either neutrophils or eosinophils. Neutrophils may be present with just an inflammatory process of the airways or parenchyma, but they also frequently reflect the presence of a bacterial infection. Specific examples include bacterial bronchitis, bronchiectasis, lung abscess, or pneumonia. Eosinophils, which can be seen after special preparation of the sputum, often occur with bronchial asthma, whether or not an allergic component plays a role.

HEMOPTYSIS

Hemoptysis is defined as coughing or spitting up of blood derived from airways or the lung itself. When the patient presents with this symptom, it is not always apparent whether the blood has in fact originated from the respiratory system, and it is incumbent upon the physician to give this question priority. Other sources of blood include the nasopharynx (particularly with the common nosebleed), the mouth (even lip or tongue biting can be mistaken for hemoptysis), and the upper gastrointestinal tract (esophagus, stomach, or duodenum). The patient often is able to distinguish some of these causes of "pseudo-hemoptysis," but the physician also should search by exam for a mouth or nasopharyngeal source.

The major etiologies of hemoptysis fall into three categories by location—airways, pulmonary parenchyma, and vasculature (Table 2–3). Airways disease is the most common cause, with bronchitis, bronchiectasis, and bronchogenic carcinoma heading the list. Bronchial

Table 2–3. DIFFERENTIAL DIAGNOSIS OF HEMOPTYSIS

Airways disease
    Acute or chronic bronchitis
    Bronchiectasis
    Bronchogenic carcinoma
    Bronchial carcinoid tumor (bronchial adenoma)

Parenchymal disease
    Tuberculosis
    Lung abscess
    Pneumonia
    Mycetoma ("fungus ball")
    Miscellaneous
        Goodpasture's syndrome
        Idiopathic pulmonary hemosiderosis

Vascular disease
    Pulmonary embolism
    Elevated pulmonary venous pressure
        Left ventricular failure
        Mitral stenosis
    Vascular malformation

carcinoid tumor (bronchial adenoma), a less common neoplasm with variable malignant potential, also originates in the airway and falls within this category.

Parenchymal causes of hemoptysis are frequently infectious in nature—tuberculosis, lung abscess, pneumonia, and a localized fungal infection (generally due to *Aspergillus*) termed a mycetoma ("fungus ball") or aspergilloma. Rarer etiologies of parenchymal hemorrhage are Goodpasture's syndrome or idiopathic pulmonary hemosiderosis, both of which will be discussed in Chapter 11.

Vascular lesions resulting in hemoptysis are generally related to problems with the pulmonary circulation. Pulmonary embolism, either with frank infarction or a picture of reversible bleeding in the lung termed "congestive atelectasis," is often a cause of hemoptysis. Elevated pressure in the pulmonary venous and capillary bed may also be associated with hemoptysis. Acutely, elevated pressure as in pulmonary edema may have associated hemoptysis, commonly seen as pink or red-tinged frothy sputum. Chronically, pulmonary venous pressure may be elevated with mitral stenosis, but this valvular lesion is relatively infrequent today as a cause of significant hemoptysis. Vascular malformations, such as an arteriovenous malformation, may also be associated with the coughing of blood.

Finally, a host of miscellaneous etiologies of hemoptysis should be considered. Some of these can fall into more than one of the above categories but others are included here because of their rarity. Cystic fibrosis involves both airways and parenchymal disease, and either component can be responsible for hemoptysis. Another interesting lesion is that of pulmonary endometriosis, in which implants of endometrial tissue in the lung can bleed coincident with the time of the menstrual cycle. Other causes are even more rare, and further discussion of them is beyond the scope of this chapter.

Diseases of the airways, e.g., bronchitis, are the most common causes of hemoptysis.

CHEST PAIN

Chest pain as a reflection of respiratory system disease does not originate in the lung itself, which is free of sensory pain fibers. When chest pain does occur in this setting, its origin is usually either the parietal pleura (lining the inside of the chest wall), the diaphragm, or the mediastinum, each of which has extensive innervation by nerve fibers capable of pain sensation.

For the parietal pleura or the diaphragm, an inflammatory process of some sort generally produces the pain. When the diaphragm is involved, the pain is commonly referred to the shoulder. Pain from the parietal pleura, in contrast, is usually relatively well localized over the area of involvement. Pain involving the pleura or the diaphragm is often worsened on inspiration; in fact, chest pain that is particularly pronounced on inspiration is described as being "pleuritic" in nature.

Inflammation of the parietal pleura producing pain is often secondary to pulmonary embolism or to pneumonia extending to the pleural surface. A pneumothorax may result in the acute onset of pleuritic pain, though the mechanism is not clear, since an acute inflammatory process is unlikely to be involved. Finally, some viruses, such as Coxsackie, affect the pleura to produce pain; and some diseases, particularly connective tissue disorders such as lupus, may result in episodes of pleuritic chest pain from a primary inflammatory process.

A variety of disorders originating in the mediastinum may eventuate in pain; they may or may not be associated with additional problems in the lung itself. These disorders of the mediastinum will be discussed in more detail in Chapter 16.

REFERENCES

Dyspnea

Raffin, T. A., and Theodore, J.: Separating cardiac from pulmonary dyspnea. JAMA 238:2066–2067, 1977.
Rapaport, E.: Dyspnea: pathophysiology and differential diagnosis. Prog. Cardiovasc. Dis. 13:532–545, 1971.
Wasserman, K.: Dyspnea on exertion: is it the heart or the lungs? JAMA 248:2039–2043, 1982.

Cough

Corrao, W. M., Braman, S. S., and Irwin, R. S.: Chronic cough as the sole presenting manifestation of bronchial asthma. N. Engl. J. Med. 300:633–637, 1979.
Irwin, R. S., Corrao, W. M., and Pratter, M. R.: Chronic persistent cough in the adult: the spectrum and frequency of causes and successful outcome of specific therapy. Am. Rev. Respir. Dis. 123:413–417, 1981.
Irwin, R. S., Rosen, M. J., and Braman, S. S.: Cough: a comprehensive review. Arch. Intern. Med. 137:1186–1191, 1977.
Poe, R. H., Israel, R. H., Utell, M. J., and Hall, W. J.: Chronic cough: bronchoscopy or pulmonary function testing? Am. Rev. Respir. Dis. 126:160–162, 1982.

Hemoptysis

Weaver, L. J., Solliday, N., and Cugell, D. W.: Selection of patients with hemoptysis for fiberoptic bronchoscopy. Chest 76:7–10, 1979.
Wolfe, J. D., and Simmons, D. H.: Hemoptysis: diagnosis and management. West. J. Med. 127:383–390, 1977.

Chest Pain

Branch, W. T., Jr., and McNeil, B. J.: Analysis of the differential diagnosis and assessment of pleuritic chest pain in young adults. Am. J. Med. 75:671–679, 1983.

3

Evaluation of the Patient with Pulmonary Disease

Evaluation on a Macroscopic Level
  Physical Examination
  Chest Roentgenography
  Computed Tomography
  Lung Scanning
  Pulmonary Angiography
  Ultrasonography
  Bronchoscopy
Evaluation on a Microscopic Level
  Obtaining Specimens
  Processing Specimens
Assessment on a Functional Level
  Pulmonary Function Tests
    Interpretation of Normality in Pulmonary Function Testing
    Patterns of Pulmonary Function Impairment
    Other Tests
  Arterial Blood Gases
  Exercise Testing

We can evaluate the respiratory system in many ways. Ultimately, the physician is concerned with three levels of evaluation—the macroscopic level, the microscopic level, and the functional level. The methods that are available to assess each of these range from simple and readily available studies to very sophisticated and elaborate techniques requiring state-of-the-art technology.

We will consider each level in turn, emphasizing the basic principles and utility of the studies. In subsequent chapters, we will repeatedly refer to these methods, since they form the backbone of the physician's approach to the patient.

EVALUATION ON A MACROSCOPIC LEVEL

Physical Examination

The most accessible method for evaluating the patient with respiratory disease is the physical examination, which requires only a stethoscope, the eyes, ears, and hands of the examiner, and his or her skill in eliciting and recognizing abnormal findings. Because the purpose of this section is not to elaborate the details of a chest examination, but rather to examine a few of the basic principles, we will focus primarily on selected aspects of the examination and what is known about mechanisms producing abnormalities.

Apart from general observation of the patient, the respiratory rate, and the pattern and difficulty of breathing, the examiner relies primarily on percussion of the chest and auscultation with a stethoscope. In percussing, the physician notes the quality of sound produced by tapping a finger of one hand against a finger of the opposite hand pressed closely to the patient's chest wall. The principle is similar to that of tapping a surface and judging whether what is underneath is solid or hollow. Normally, percussion of the chest wall overlying air-containing lung gives a resonant sound; in contrast, percussion over a solid organ such as the liver produces a dull sound. This contrast allows the examiner to detect areas with something other than air-containing lung beneath the chest wall, such as fluid in the pleural space (pleural effusion) or airless (consolidated) lung, each of which sounds dull to percussion. At the other extreme, air in the pleural space (pneumothorax) or a hyperinflated lung (as in emphysema) may produce a hyperresonant or more "hollow" sound, approaching what one hears when percussing over a hollow viscus, such as the stomach. Additionally, the examiner can locate the approximate position of the diaphragm by a change in the quality of the percussed note, from resonant to dull, toward the bottom of the lung. A convenient aspect of this and the other parts of the chest examination is the basically symmetric nature of the two sides of the chest; a difference in the findings between the two sides suggests a localized abnormality.

Goals of auscultation:
(1) assessment of breath sounds
(2) detection of adventitious sounds

When auscultating the lungs with a stethoscope, the examiner is actually concerned about two features—the quality of the breath sounds and the presence of any abnormal (commonly called *adventitious*) sounds. When the patient takes a deep breath, the sound of airflow can be heard through the stethoscope. Exactly what the examiner hears, though, depends on where he or she is listening. If the stethoscope is placed directly over the trachea, for example, the sound is fairly loud and harsh, and expiration is at least as loud and as long as inspiration. In contrast, when the stethoscope is placed over the lower parts of normal lungs, sound is heard almost exclusively during inspiration, and the quality of the sound is much softer and smoother.

Why the quality of the sound is different at these locations is not intuitively obvious. It is currently thought that sound is produced by turbulent airflow in the upper respiratory tract, trachea, and large bronchi. When listening over the trachea, the examiner hears the sound directly at its site of production. When the sound passes peripherally, lung tissue acts as a filter, and the quality and intensity of the sound change considerably. If an area of lung is consolidated, sound passing through it is not subjected to the same filtering process, and the listener hears an unfiltered sound approaching the quality of what would be heard over the trachea.

Therefore, the sound generated by airflow is transmitted better through consolidated than through air-containing lung. Such breath sounds are called *bronchial*, as opposed to the normal, or *vesicular*, breath sounds heard over the lung bases. The difference is not only in the quality of sound, but also in the relative duration of inspiration and expiration—with vesicular sounds expiration is nearly silent, while bronchial breath sounds are characterized by expiration at least as audible and as long as inspiration. When the stethoscope is placed closer to the trachea, such as over larger bronchi, or over an area of partially consolidated lung, the breath sounds are intermediate between bronchial and vesicular and logically are termed *bronchovesicular*.

Consolidated lung does not filter sound as the air-containing lung does.

Better transmission of sound through consolidated rather than normal lung is also true when the patient whispers or speaks. The enhanced transmission of whispered sound results in more distinctly heard syllables and is termed *whispered pectoriloquy*. The sound of spoken words is also more distinctly heard through the stethoscope placed over the involved area and is called *bronchophony*. When the patient says the vowel "E," the resulting sound through consolidated lung has a nasal "A" quality; this "E to A change" is termed *egophony*. All of these findings are variations on the same theme—an altered transmission of sound through airless lung—and basically have the same significance.

Two qualifications are important when interpreting the quality of breath sounds. First, normal transmission of sound depends on patency of the airway. If a relatively large bronchus is occluded, such as by tumor, secretions, or a foreign body, transmission of sounds is decreased, and the examiner hears decreased or absent breath sounds when listening over the affected area. A blocked airway proximal to consolidated or airless lung also eliminates the increased transmission described above. Second, either air or fluid in the pleural space acts as a barrier to sound, so that either a pneumothorax or a pleural effusion causes a diminution of breath sounds.

The second major task of the examiner is to listen for adventitious sounds. Unfortunately, the terminology for these adventitious sounds varies considerably from examiner to examiner, and we will therefore consider only the most commonly used terms. The major types of adventitious sounds that we will discuss are crackles, wheezes, and friction rubs. A fourth category, rhonchi, is used inconsistently by different examiners, thus decreasing its clinical usefulness for communicating abnormal findings.

Crackles, also called *rales*, are a series of individual clicking or popping noises heard with the stethoscope over an involved area of lung. Their quality can range from the sound produced by rubbing hairs together to that generated by opening a Velcro fastener or crumpling a piece of cellophane. These sounds are "opening" sounds of small airways or alveoli that have been collapsed or decreased in volume during expiration because of fluid, inflammatory exudate, or poor aeration. On each subsequent inspiration, opening of the airways

Crackles, heard during inspiration, are "opening" sounds of alveoli and small airways.

and alveoli creates the series of clicking or popping sounds heard either throughout or at the latter part of inspiration. The most common disorders producing rales are pulmonary edema, pneumonia, interstitial lung disease, and atelectasis. Though some clinicians feel that the quality of the crackles helps to distinguish the different disorders, others feel that such distinctions in quality are of little clinical value.

Wheezes reflect airflow through narrowed airways.

Wheezes are high-pitched, continuous sounds that are generated by airflow through narrowed airways. The causes of such narrowing include airway smooth muscle constriction, edema, secretions, or collapse due to poorly supported walls. These individual pathophysiologic features will be discussed in more detail in the subsequent chapters on obstructive lung disease. For reasons that will also be described later, the diameter of intrathoracic airways is less during expiration than inspiration, and wheezing is generally more pronounced or exclusively heard in expiration. However, at least a certain minimum amount of airflow is necessary to generate wheezing; if airway narrowing becomes sufficiently severe, wheezing may no longer be heard.

Though there is general agreement that the term *rhonchi* refers to sounds generated by secretions in airways, different examiners use the term to describe different sounds. On the one hand, the term is used to describe low-pitched continuous sounds that are somewhat coarser than high-pitched wheezing; on the other hand, the very coarse crackles that often result from airway secretions are also termed rhonchi by some examiners. The end result is that the term is frequently used to describe the variety of noises, squeaks, and clicks that cannot be readily classified within the more generally accepted categories of crackles and wheezes, but which all appear to have airway secretions as their common underlying cause.

A *friction rub* is the term for the sounds generated by inflamed or roughened pleural surfaces rubbing against each other during respiration. A rub is a series of creaky or rasping sounds heard during both inspiration and expiration. The most common etiologies are primary inflammatory diseases of the pleura or parenchymal processes that extend out to the pleural surface, such as pneumonia or pulmonary infarction.

Though we have focused on the chest examination itself as a reflection of pulmonary disease, it is important to realize that other nonthoracic manifestations of primary pulmonary disease may be detected on physical examination. The two that we will discuss briefly are clubbing (with or without hypertrophic pulmonary osteoarthropathy) and cyanosis.

Clubbing is a change in the normal configuration of the nails and the distal phalanx of the fingers and/or toes (Fig. 3–1). Several features may be seen: (1) loss of the normal angle between the nail and the skin; (2) increased curvature of the nail; (3) increased sponginess of the tissue below the proximal part of the nail; and (4) flaring or widening of the terminal phalanx. Though several nonpulmonary disorders can result in clubbing (such as congenital heart disease with right-to-left shunting, endocarditis, chronic liver disease, or inflammatory bowel disease), the most common causes are clearly pulmonary. Carcinoma of the lung (or the pleura) is the single leading etiologic factor; other pulmonary causes include chronic pulmonary infection with suppuration (such as bronchiectasis or lung abscess) and interstitial lung disease.

Clubbing occurs with:
(1) carcinoma of the lung (or pleura)
(2) chronic pulmonary infection
(3) interstitial lung disease

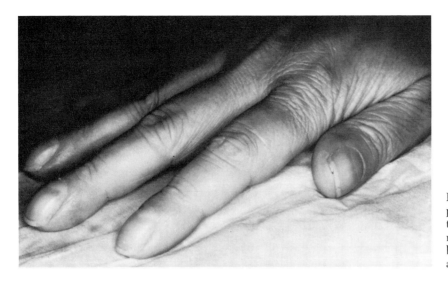

Figure 3–1. Clubbing in a patient with carcinoma of the lung. Curvature of the nail and loss of the angle between the nail and the adjacent skin can be seen.

Uncomplicated chronic obstructive lung disease is not associated with clubbing, and its presence in such a patient should suggest unsuspected malignancy or suppurative disease.

Clubbing may also be accompanied by *hypertrophic pulmonary osteoarthropathy*, characterized by subperiosteal bone formation, particularly in the long bones, and arthralgias and arthritis of any of several joints. When there is coexistent pulmonary osteoarthropathy, either pulmonary or pleural malignancy is the overwhelmingly likely cause of the clubbing, since pulmonary osteoarthropathy is exceedingly rare with the other causes of clubbing.

The mechanism of clubbing and hypertrophic pulmonary osteoarthropathy is not at all clear. It has been observed that clubbing is associated with an increase in digital blood flow, while the osteoarthropathy is characterized by an overgrowth of highly vascular connective tissue. Why these changes occur, however, is a mystery. One interesting theory suggests an important role for nerve stimuli coming through the vagus nerve, because vagotomy frequently ameliorates some of the bone and nail changes.

Cyanosis, the second extrapulmonary physical finding arising from lung disease, is a bluish discoloration of the skin (particularly under the nails) and mucous membranes. Whereas saturated hemoglobin gives the skin its usual pink color, a sufficient amount of unsaturated hemoglobin produces cyanosis. Cyanosis may be either generalized, owing to a low P_{O_2} or very low systemic blood flow resulting in increased extraction of oxygen from the blood, or localized, owing to low blood flow and increased oxygen extraction within the localized area. With lung disease, the common factor resulting in cyanosis is a low P_{O_2}, and several different types of lung disease may be responsible. It is also important to remember that the total amount of hemoglobin affects the likelihood of detecting cyanosis. In the anemic patient, if the total quantity of desaturated hemoglobin is less than the amount needed to produce the bluish discoloration, even a very low P_{O_2} may not be associated with cyanosis. In the polycythemic patient, in contrast, much less depression of the P_{O_2} is necessary before sufficient unsaturated hemoglobin exists to produce cyanosis.

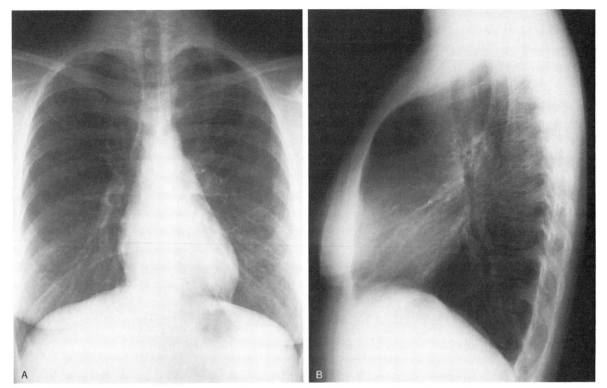

Figure 3–2. Normal chest roentgenogram. *A*, Posteroanterior (PA) view. *B*, Lateral view. Compare with Figure 3–3 for position of each lobe.

Chest Roentgenography

The chest roentgenogram, which is largely taken for granted in the practice of medicine today, is used not only in evaluating patients with suspected respiratory disease, but also frequently in the routine evaluation of asymptomatic patients. Of all the viscera, the lungs are clearly the best suited for radiographic examination. The reason is straightforward—air in the lungs provides an excellent background against which abnormalities can stand out. Additionally, the presence of two lungs allows each to serve as a control for the other, so that unilateral abnormalities can be more easily recognized.

A detailed description of interpretation of the chest radiograph is beyond the scope of this text. However, we will mention a few principles to aid the reader in viewing films presented in this and subsequent chapters.

First, the appearance of any structure on a radiograph depends on its density; the denser it is, the whiter it appears on the film. At one extreme is air, which is radiolucent and appears black on the film. At the other extreme are metallic densities, which appear white. In between, there is a spectrum of increasing density from fat to water to bone. The viscera and muscles fall within the realm of water density tissues and cannot be distinguished in their radiographic density from water or blood.

Second, in order for a line or an interface to appear between two adjacent structures on a radiograph, the two structures must differ in density. For example, within the cardiac shadow, the heart muscle cannot be distinguished from the blood coursing within the chambers, as they are both of water density. In contrast, the borders of the heart are visible against the lungs, since the water density of the heart contrasts with the density of the lungs, which is closer to that of air. However, if the lung adjacent to a normally denser structure (such as the heart or diaphragm) is airless, either because of collapse or consolidation, the neighboring structures are now both of the same density, and no visible interface or boundary separates them. This principle is the basis of the very useful *silhouette sign*; if an expected border with an area of lung is not visualized or is not distinct, the adjacent lung is abnormal and lacks full aeration.

Chest roentgenograms are usually taken in two standard views—posteroanterior (PA) and lateral (Fig. 3–2). For a PA film, the roentgen beam goes from the back to the front of the patient, and the patient's chest is adjacent to the film. The lateral view is taken with

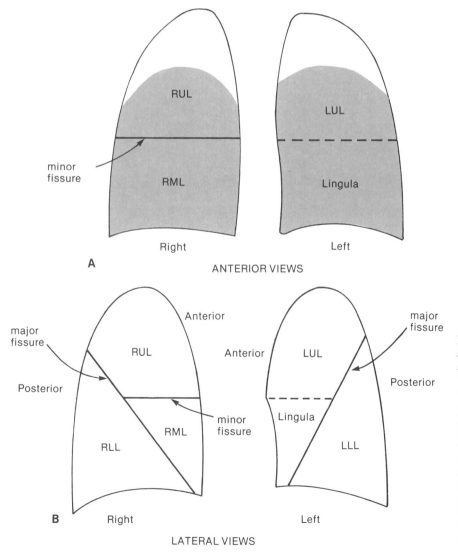

Figure 3–3. Lobar anatomy as seen from anterior (*A*) and lateral (*B*) views. RUL = right upper lobe; RML = right middle lobe; RLL = right lower lobe; LUL = left upper lobe; LLL = left lower lobe. In the anterior views, the shaded regions represent the lower lobes and are behind the upper and middle lobes. The lingula is part of the LUL, and the dotted line between the two does not represent an actual fissure.

the patient's side against the film, and the beam is directed through the patient to the film. If a film cannot be taken with the patient standing and with his chest to the film, as in the case of a bedridden patient, then an anteroposterior (AP) view is taken. For this view, which is generally used with portable chest radiographs in a patient's hospital room, the film is placed behind the patient (generally between his back and the bed), and the beam is directed through the patient from front to back. Lateral decubitus views, either right or left, are done with the patient lying on his side, and with the beam directed horizontally. Decubitus views are particularly useful for detecting fluid that is free-flowing within the pleural space and are therefore often used when there is suspicion of a pleural effusion.

Posteroanterior (PA) and lateral radiographs are often both necessary for localization of an abnormality.

Knowledge of radiographic anatomy is fundamental for the interpretation of consolidation or collapse (atelectasis) and for localization of other abnormalities on the chest film. Lobar anatomy and the locations of fissures separating the lobes are shown in Figure 3–3. It is important to realize that localization of an abnormality often requires information from both the PA and lateral views, which should both be taken when an abnormality is being evaluated. As can be seen from Figure 3–3, the major fissure separating the upper (and middle) lobes from the lower lobe runs obliquely through the chest. Hence it is easy to be fooled about location on the PA film alone—a lower lobe lesion may appear in the upper part of the chest, while an upper lobe lesion may appear much lower in position.

When a lobe becomes filled with fluid or inflammatory exudate, as can be seen with pneumonia, it has water rather than air density and therefore is easily delineated on the chest roentgenogram. With pure consolidation, the lobe does not lose volume, and it therefore occupies its usual position and has its usual size. An example of lobar consolidation on PA and lateral roentgenograms is shown in Figure 3–4.

In contrast, when a lobe has airless alveoli and collapses, it not only becomes more dense, but also has features of volume loss characteristic for each individual lobe. Such features of volume loss include change in position of a fissure or the indirect signs of displacement of the hilum, diaphragm, trachea, or mediastinum in the direction of the volume loss (Fig. 3–5). A common cause for atelectasis is occlusion of the airway leading to the collapsed region of lung, e.g., by a tumor, an aspirated foreign body, or a mucous plug. So far, we have given examples of either pure consolidation or pure collapse. In practice, however, a combination of these processes often occurs, leading to consolidation accompanied by partial volume loss.

Diffuse increase in density on the radiograph can often be categorized as either alveolar or interstitial.

With relatively diffuse abnormalities on the chest film, it is necessary to determine whether the process is primarily *interstitial*, i.e., affecting the alveolar walls and interstitial tissue, or *alveolar*, i.e., filling the alveolar spaces. This distinction is frequently important because of the clues it gives about etiology—many diffuse disorders of the lung are characterized by one or the other roentgenographic pattern. An interstitial pattern generally is described as *reticulonodular*, consisting of an interlacing network of linear and small nodular densities. In contrast, an alveolar pattern appears more fluffy, and the outlines of air-filled bronchi coursing through the alveolar densities are often seen. This latter finding is called an *air bronchogram* and is due

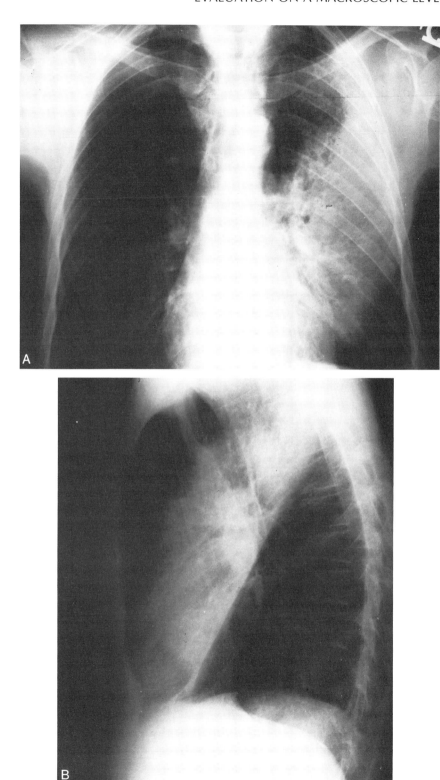

Figure 3–4. Posteroanterior *(A)* and lateral *(B)* chest radiographs in a patient with left upper lobe (LUL) consolidation due to pneumonia. The anatomic boundary is best appreciated on the lateral view, where it is easily seen that the normally positioned major fissure defines the lower border of the consolidation (compare with Fig. 3–3). Part of the LUL is spared. (Courtesy of Dr. T. Scott Johnson.)

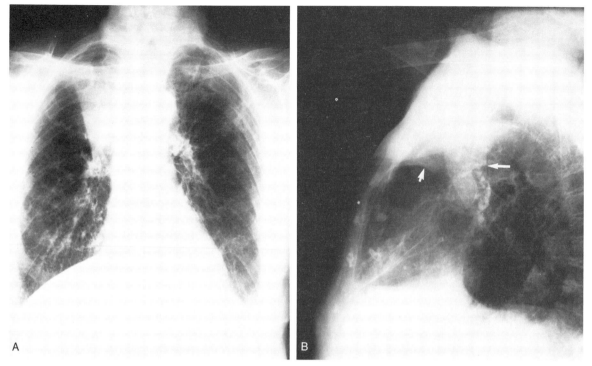

Figure 3–5. Posteroanterior *(A)* and lateral *(B)* chest radiographs demonstrating right upper lobe (RUL) collapse. In *A*, the displaced minor fissure outlines the airless (dense) RUL. In *B*, the RUL is outlined by an elevated minor fissure (short arrow) and an anteriorly displaced major fissure (long arrow).

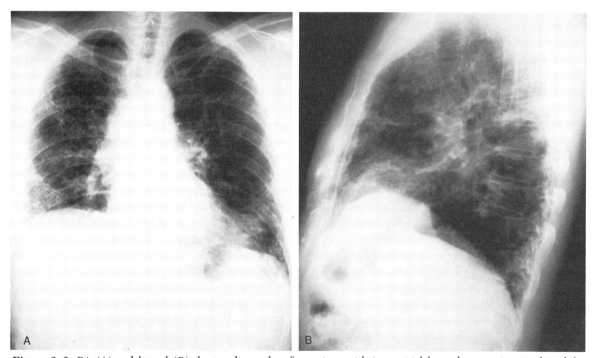

Figure 3–6. PA *(A)* and lateral *(B)* chest radiographs of a patient with interstitial lung disease. A reticulonodular pattern is present throughout but is most prominent in the right lung and at the base of the left lung.

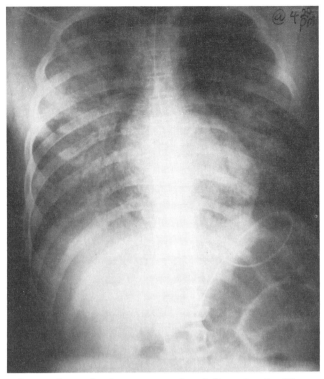

Figure 3–7. Chest radiograph of a patient with a diffuse alveolar filling process. Air bronchograms, representing air-filled bronchi adjacent to fluid-filled lung parenchyma, can be seen, most prominently in the right mid and lower lung zones.

to air in the bronchi being surrounded and outlined by alveoli that are filled with fluid; this finding does not occur with a purely interstitial pattern. Examples of diffusely abnormal chest radiographs due to interstitial disease and to alveolar filling are presented in Figures 3–6 and 3–7, respectively.

Though we have mentioned and shown some of the typical abnormalities as an introduction to pattern recognition on a chest roentgenogram, the careful physician uses a systematic approach in analyzing the film. We perform a chest roentgenogram not merely to see the lungs alone; roentgenographic examination may also detect changes in bones, soft tissues, the heart, other mediastinal structures, and the pleural space. We will not go into further detail about the approach to the chest film, as this is a topic for much more extensive discussion.

Though the standard PA and lateral views are the most commonly performed chest films, other views and roentgenographic techniques often provide additional information. Perhaps the most important to mention here is tomography, a technique that provides views at different planes through the lung, rather than a summation of all areas that the beam passes through (Fig. 3–8). This method may be used to give better definition of small or questionable lesions, and it is particularly useful for determining if a lesion has calcification within it.

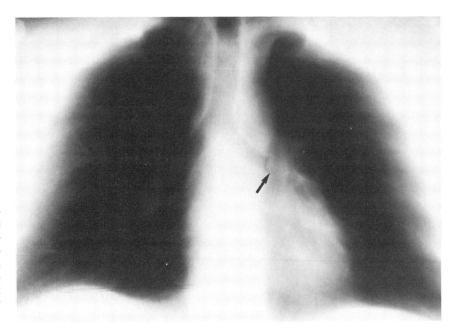

Figure 3–8. Lung tomogram showing an oval mass (arrow) within the left mainstem bronchus. In this relatively anterior section through the lung, the trachea and mainstem bronchi are well outlined. (Courtesy of Dr. T. Scott Johnson.)

However, with the advent of computed tomography, plain tomograms are now done much less frequently than they were in the past.

Computed Tomography

A recently available technique now revolutionizing the field of diagnostic radiology is computed tomography (computerized axial tomography), commonly referred to as CT or CAT scanning. It has now been widely used for evaluation of the brain and abdomen, but we will limit our discussion to computed tomography of the chest. With this technique, a narrow beam of x-rays is passed through the body and sensed by a rotating detector on the other side of the patient. The beam is partially absorbed within the patient, depending on the density of the intervening tissues. Computerized analysis of the information received by the detector allows a series of cross-sectional images to be constructed (Fig. 3–9).

The CT scan is particularly useful in detecting subtle differences in tissue density that cannot be distinguished by conventional radiography. In addition, the cross-sectional views obtained from the slices provide very different information from that provided by the vertical orientation of plain films or conventional tomographic techniques. So far, the greatest utility of CT has been in evaluating pulmonary nodules, chest wall and pleural disease, pulmonary cavities, and the mediastinum. It has also frequently been used for defining a variety of pulmonary parenchymal lesions that are best seen on cross-sectional views. Exactly how useful CT scanning will be for certain other purposes, such as staging of lung cancer and evaluation of overall pulmonary density (for early detection of emphysema or interstitial lung disease), remains to be seen.

CT scanning provides cross-sectional views of the chest and detects subtle differences in tissue density.

It is fair to say that even though computed tomography appears to be here to stay, we are still gaining experience and learning about its usefulness and limitations. Because of this fact as well as its expense, it is not a screening procedure and should be used only when it can provide other information not available by simpler, less expensive, but equally noninvasive techniques.

Lung Scanning

With the use of injected or inhaled radioisotopes, information about pulmonary blood flow and ventilation may be readily obtained.

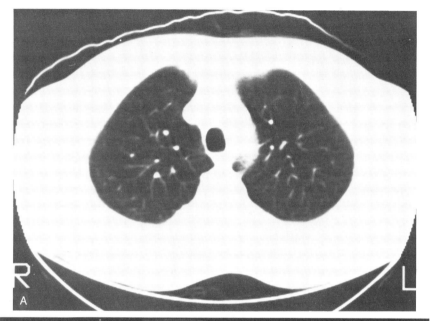

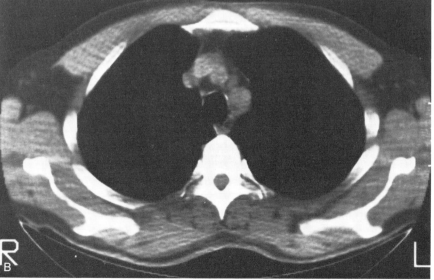

Figure 3–9. Representative cross-sectional "slice" from a normal computed tomographic (CT) scan. The two images were taken using different "windows" at the same cross-sectional level. On the top view (A), settings were chosen to optimize visualization of the lung parenchyma. On the bottom view (B), the settings were chosen to distinguish different densities of soft tissues, such as the structures within the mediastinum.

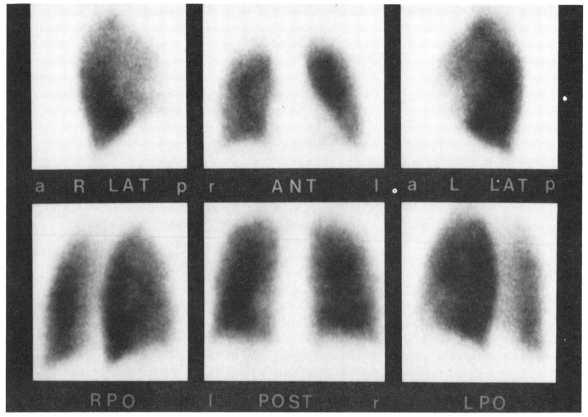

Figure 3–10. Normal perfusion lung scan. Six views are shown. LAT = lateral; ANT = anterior; POST = posterior; RPO = right posterior oblique; LPO = left posterior oblique; a = anterior; p = posterior; r = right; l = left. (Courtesy of Dr. Henry Royal.)

Imaging of the gamma radiation produced by these isotopes results in a picture showing the distribution of blood flow and ventilation throughout both lungs (Fig. 3–10).

For lung perfusion scanning, the most common technique involves injecting aggregates of human albumin labeled with a radionuclide, usually technetium-99m, into a peripheral vein. These aggregates, which are approximately 10 to 50 microns in diameter, travel through the right side of the heart, enter the pulmonary vasculature, and become lodged in small pulmonary vessels. Only areas of the lung receiving perfusion from the pulmonary arterial system demonstrate uptake of tracer, while nonperfused regions show no uptake of the labeled albumin.

For ventilation scanning, a gaseous radioisotope, usually xenon-133, is inhaled, and sequential pictures are obtained showing how the gas distributes within the lung. Pictures at different times after inhalation reveal information about gas distribution after the first breath (wash-in phase), after a longer time of breathing the gas (equilibrium phase), and after the patient again breathes air to eliminate the radioisotope (wash-out phase). Ventilation scanning shows which regions of the lungs are being ventilated, and whether there are significant localized problems with expiratory airflow and "gas trapping" of the radioisotope during the wash-out phase.

Perfusion and ventilation scans are performed for two major reasons—detection of pulmonary emboli and assessment of regional lung function. When a pulmonary embolus occludes a pulmonary artery, blood flow ceases to the lung region normally supplied by that vessel, and a corresponding "perfusion defect" results. Generally, ventilation is preserved, and a ventilation scan does not show a corresponding "ventilation defect." In practice, many pieces of information are considered in the interpretation of the scan, including the appearance of the chest radiograph and the size and distribution of the defects on the perfusion scan. These issues will be discussed in more detail in Chapter 13.

Perfusion and ventilation lung scans are useful for detection of pulmonary emboli and evaluation of regional lung function.

Ventilation and perfusion lung scanning to assess regional lung function is often performed before surgery involving resection of a part of the lung, usually one or more lobes. By visualizing which areas of lung receive ventilation and perfusion, the physician can determine how much the area to be resected is contributing to overall lung function. When the scanning techniques are used in conjunction with pulmonary function testing, the physician can also predict postoperative pulmonary function, which is a guide to postoperative respiratory problems and impairment.

Pulmonary Angiography

Though the perfusion lung scan provides useful information about pulmonary blood flow and is usually the first procedure performed to diagnose pulmonary embolism, it has limitations, particularly in patients with other forms of underlying lung disease. For this reason, the physician must frequently turn to pulmonary angiography, a radiographic technique in which a catheter is guided from a peripheral vein through the right atrium and ventricle, and into the main pulmonary artery or one of its branches. A radio-opaque dye is then injected, and the pulmonary arterial tree is visualized on a series of rapidly exposed chest films (Fig. 3–11). A clot in a pulmonary vessel appears either as

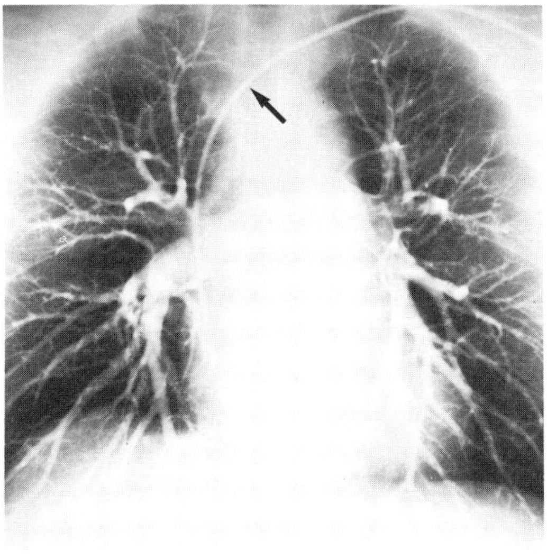

Figure 3–11. Normal pulmonary angiogram. The radio-opaque dye was injected directly into the pulmonary artery, and the pulmonary arterial tree is well visualized. The catheter used for injecting the dye is marked with an arrow. (Courtesy of Dr. Morris Simon.)

an abrupt termination ("cut-off") of the vessel or as a filling defect within its lumen.

The pulmonary angiogram also has a variety of other possible indications, including investigation of congenital vascular anomalies or invasion of a vessel by tumor. However, use of the angiogram in these situations is much less frequent than its use for diagnosis of pulmonary emboli.

Ultrasonography

The ability of different types of tissue to transmit sound and of tissue interfaces to reflect sound has made ultrasonography useful for evaluating a variety of body structures. A piezoelectric crystal generates sound waves, and the reflected echoes are detected and recorded by the same crystal. Images are displayed on a screen and can be photographed for a permanent record.

The heart is certainly the intrathoracic structure most frequently studied by ultrasonography, but the technique is also useful in the evaluation of pleural disease. In particular, ultrasonography is capable of detecting small amounts of pleural fluid and is often used to guide placement of a needle for sampling a small amount of this fluid. Additionally, it can detect walled-off compartments (loculations) within pleural effusions and distinguish fluid from pleural thickening.

Ultrasound is also capable of localizing the diaphragm and detecting disease immediately below the diaphragm, such as a subphrenic abscess. In contrast, ultrasound is not useful for defining structures or lesions within the pulmonary parenchyma, since the ultrasound beam penetrates air poorly.

Bronchoscopy

Direct visualization of the airways is possible by a procedure known as bronchoscopy, performed originally with a hollow, rigid metal tube and more recently (and now also much more commonly) with a flexible instrument (Fig. 3–12). The flexible instrument has fiberoptic bundles, the fibers of which transmit light even when they are bent or curved. Because of the flexible nature of the scope, the bronchoscopist can bend the tip at will with a control lever and maneuver into airways at least down to the subsegmental level.

With the fiberoptic bronchoscope, airways are visualized and laboratory samples obtained.

Not only can the bronchoscopist obtain an excellent view of the airways (Fig. 3–13), but he or she can also obtain a variety of samples for cytologic, pathologic, and microbiologic examination. Sterile saline can be injected through the scope and suctioned back into a collection chamber. This technique, called *bronchial washing*, samples cells and, if present, microorganisms from the lower respiratory tract. When the bronchoscope is passed as far as possible before saline is injected, the washings are actually able to sample the contents of the alveolar spaces.

A long, flexible wire instrument with a small brush at the tip may also be passed through the bronchoscope. The surface of a lesion within a bronchus can be brushed, and the cells collected or smeared onto a

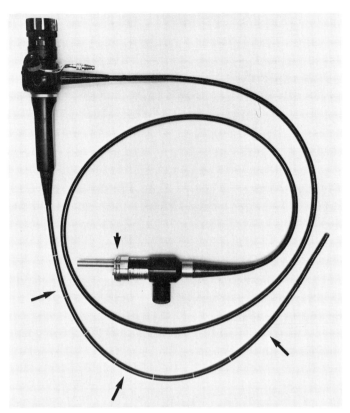

Figure 3–12. Photograph of a fiberoptic bronchoscope. The long arrows point to the flexible part passed into the patient's airways. The short arrow points to the portion of the bronchoscope connected to the light source. The eyepiece and the controls for the person performing the procedure are shown at the upper left.

slide for cytologic examination. Brushes are also frequently passed into diseased areas of the lung parenchyma; the material collected by the bristles is then subjected to cytologic and microbiologic analysis.

A small biopsy forceps, when passed through the bronchoscope, can biopsy a lesion visualized on the bronchial wall (*endobronchial biopsy*). When a fluoroscope is used to aid in passage of the forceps, the lung parenchyma is quite accessible after the forceps punctures a small bronchus and moves out into the distal parenchyma. This latter procedure, known as a *transbronchial biopsy*, yields a piece of tissue that is small but has a sizable number of alveoli.

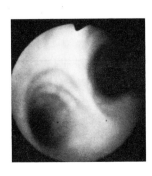

Figure 3–13. Photograph of normal airways as seen through a fiberoptic bronchoscope. At this level, the carina can be seen separating the right and left mainstem bronchi.

There are now many indications for bronchoscopy, usually with a fiberoptic instrument, though there are occasional circumstances in which the rigid instrument is preferred. Some of the indications for bronchoscopy include the following: (1) evaluation of a suspected endobronchial malignancy; (2) sampling of an area of parenchymal disease either by washings, brushings, or biopsy; (3) evaluation of hemoptysis; and (4) removal of a foreign body (with special instruments that can be passed through the scope and are capable of snagging objects).

This procedure has become a very common and useful technique in the evaluation of pulmonary pathology. Even though the physician who first suggested placing a tube into the larynx and bronchi was censured in 1847 for proposing a technique that is "an anatomical impossibility and an unwarrantable innovation in practical medicine," bronchoscopy is generally well tolerated and complications are infrequent.

EVALUATION ON A MICROSCOPIC LEVEL

Microscopy often provides the definitive diagnosis of pulmonary pathology suggested by the history, physical examination, or chest roentgenogram. Several types of disorders are particularly amenable to diagnosis by microscopy—lung tumors (by either histology or cytology), pulmonary infection (by microscopic identification of a specific organism), and a variety of miscellaneous pulmonary diseases, particularly those affecting the interstitium of the lung (by histology). Frequently, when a diagnosis is uncertain, the same techniques are utilized to obtain samples that are processed both for histologic (or cytologic) examination and for identification of microorganisms. In this section we will first discuss how specimens are obtained and then consider how the specimens are processed.

Obtaining Specimens

There are three main types of specimens that the physician uses for microscopic analysis in diagnosing the patient with lung disease: (1) tracheobronchial secretions, (2) tissue, and (3) fluid from the pleural space. For tracheobronchial secretions and tissue, a number of methods are available for obtaining specimens; here knowledge of the yield and the complications determines the most appropriate method.

The easiest way to obtain a specimen of tracheobronchial secretions is to collect sputum spontaneously expectorated by the patient. The sample can be used for identification of inflammatory or malignant cells, and for staining (and culturing) of microorganisms. Though collecting sputum sounds simple, it presents several potential problems. First, the patient may not have any spontaneous cough and sputum production. If this is the case, sputum can frequently be induced by having the patient inhale an irritating aerosol, such as hypertonic saline. Second, what is thought to be sputum originating from the tracheobronchial tree is frequently either nasal secretions or "spit" expectorated from the mouth or the back of the throat. Finally, as a result of passage through the mouth, even a good, deep sputum specimen is contaminated by microorganisms from the mouth. Because of this contamination, care is required in interpreting the results of sputum culture, particularly with regard to the normal flora of the upper respiratory tract. Despite these limitations, collection of sputum remains an important and valuable technique in looking for malignancy and infectious processes, such as bacterial pneumonia and tuberculosis.

Tracheobronchial secretions can also be obtained by two other routes—transtracheal aspiration and bronchoscopy. With transtracheal aspiration, a small plastic catheter is passed inside (or over) a needle inserted through the cricothyroid membrane and into the trachea. The catheter induces coughing, and secretions are collected either with or without the additional instillation of saline through the catheter. This technique avoids the problem of contamination by upper airway flora, and it also allows collection of a sample even when the patient has no spontaneous sputum production. However, it is not without risk—bleeding complications and, to a lesser extent, subcutaneous emphysema (air dissecting through tissues in the neck) are potentially serious sequelae. The extent to which transtracheal aspiration is used varies tremendously from institution to institution, depending on the experience (and fear of complications) of individual physicians.

Tracheobronchial secretions are provided by
(1) expectorated sputum
(2) transtracheal aspiration
(3) fiberoptic bronchoscopy

Bronchoscopy, generally with a fiberoptic instrument, is also a suitable way to obtain tracheobronchial secretions. It has the additional advantage of allowing visualization of the airways as well as collection of secretions. However, since the instrument does pass through the upper respiratory tract, it is also subject to the same problem of contamination by upper airway flora. It has distinct advantages in collecting material for cytologic analysis, since specimens may be collected from a localized area directly visualized with the scope.

As is true of tracheobronchial secretions, tissue specimens for microscopic examination can be collected in numerous ways. Through a bronchoscope, one can pass a brush or a biopsy forceps. The brush is often used to scrape cells from the surface of an airway lesion, but it can also be passed more distally into the lung parenchyma to obtain specimens directly from a diseased area. The biopsy forceps are used in a similar fashion, to sample tissue either from a lesion in the airway (endobronchial biopsy) or from an area of disease in the parenchyma (transbronchial biopsy, so named because the forceps must puncture a small bronchus to sample the parenchyma). In the case of bronchial brushing, the specimen adherent to the brush is smeared onto a slide for staining and microscopic examination. For both endobronchial and transbronchial biopsies, the tissue obtained can be fixed and sectioned, and slides made for subsequent microscopic examination.

Rather than approach the lung parenchyma from the airway, a lesion or diseased area may also be reached with a needle through the chest wall. Depending on the type of needle used, a small sample may be either aspirated or biopsied. Bleeding and pneumothorax are potential complications, just as they are for a transbronchial biopsy with a bronchoscope.

Tissue is also frequently obtained by an actual surgical procedure, such as an open lung biopsy, during which the surgeon removes a

Lung biopsies can be obtained by
(1) fiberoptic bronchoscopy
(2) percutaneous needle aspiration or biopsy
(3) an open surgical procedure

small piece of lung through an incision in the chest. Though the specimens obtained are generally excellent, a less invasive way of making a diagnosis is desirable if possible.

Finally, fluid in the pleural space is frequently sampled in the evaluation of a patient with a pleural effusion. A small needle is inserted through the chest wall and into the pleural space, and fluid is withdrawn. The fluid can be examined for malignant cells and microorganisms, but chemical analysis of the fluid (see Chapter 15) often provides additional useful diagnostic information. Frequently, a biopsy of the parietal pleural surface (the tissue layer lining the pleural space) is also performed with a special needle, and the tissue examined by microscopy.

Processing Specimens

Once the specimens are obtained, the techniques of processing and the types of examination performed are not unique, but rather are common to many other types of tissue and fluid specimens.

Specimens can be processed for staining, culture, cytology, and histopathology.

Diagnosis of pulmonary infections depends upon smears and cultures of the material obtained, such as sputum, other samples of tracheobronchial secretions, or pleural fluid. The standard Gram stain technique often allows initial identification of organisms, and inspection may also reveal inflammatory cells (particularly polymorphonuclear leukocytes) and upper airway (squamous epithelial) cells, the latter indicating contamination of sputum by upper airway secretions. Final culture results give definitive identification of an organism, but the results must always be interpreted with the knowledge that the specimen may be contaminated and that what is grown is not necessarily causally related to the clinical problem.

Identification of mycobacteria, the causative agent for tuberculosis, requires special staining and culturing techniques. Mycobacteria are stained by agents such as carbolfuchsin or auramine-rhodamine, and the organisms are almost unique in their ability to retain the stain after acid is added. Hence the expression *acid-fast bacilli* or *AFB* is used commonly in referring to mycobacteria. Frequently used staining methods are the Ziehl-Neelson stain or a modification called the Kinyoun stain. A more sensitive (and faster) way to detect mycobacteria involves use of a fluorescent dye such as auramine-rhodamine; mycobacteria take up the dye and fluoresce, and they can be detected relatively easily even when present in small numbers. Since mycobacteria are slow-growing, the organism usually requires six weeks or so for growth and identification on culture media.

Organisms other than the common bacterial pathogens and mycobacteria often require other specialized staining and culture techniques. Fungi may be diagnosed by special stains performed on tissue specimens, such as methenamine silver or periodic acid–Schiff (PAS) stains. They may also be cultured on special culture media favorable to the growth of fungi. *Pneumocystis carinii*, a protozoon pathogen that is most common in patients with impaired defense mechanisms, is also stained in tissue (and sometimes tracheobronchial secretions) by the methenamine silver stain. The recently identified organism *Legionella pneumophila*, the causative agent of Legionnaires' disease, can be diagnosed by silver impregnation or immunofluorescence staining; it can also be grown with difficulty on some special media.

Cytologic examination for malignant cells is available for expectorated sputum, bronchial washings or brushings obtained with a bronchoscope, and pleural fluid. A specimen can be directly smeared onto a slide (as with a bronchial brushing), subjected to concentration (bronchial washings, pleural fluid), or digested (sputum) prior to smearing on the slide. The slide is then stained by the Papanicolaou technique, and the cells are examined for findings suggestive or diagnostic of malignancy.

Pathologic examination of tissue sections obtained by biopsy is most useful for diagnosis of malignancy or infection (with either affecting the lung or the pleura) as well as a wide variety of other processes affecting the pulmonary parenchyma. In many circumstances, examination of tissue obtained by biopsy is the "gold standard" for diagnosis, though it must be remembered that even biopsies may be falsely negative or may give misleading information.

Tissue obtained by biopsy is routinely stained with hematoxylin and eosin (H and E) for histologic examination. A wide assortment of other stains are available that more or less specifically stain collagen, elastin, and a variety of microorganisms. Further discussion of the specific techniques and stains are beyond the scope of this chapter but can be found in standard textbooks of pathology.

ASSESSMENT ON A FUNCTIONAL LEVEL

Pulmonary evaluation on either a macroscopic or a microscopic level aims at a diagnosis of lung disease, but neither is able to determine the extent to which normal functions of the lung are impaired. This final aspect of evaluation adds an important dimension to overall assessment of the patient, since it reflects how much the disease may limit a patient's daily activities. The two most common ways that we look at a patient's functional status are by pulmonary function tests and measurement of arterial blood gases, each of which will be discussed in some detail. In addition, it is also possible to perform a variety of measurements during exercise that help us determine how much exercise a patient can perform, and what factors contribute to any limitation of exercise. Many other types of functional studies are useful for either clinical or research purposes, but they will not be discussed in this chapter.

Pulmonary Function Tests

Pulmonary function testing provides an objective method for assessing functional changes in a patient with known or suspected lung disease. With the results of screening tests that are available at most hospitals, the physician is able to answer several questions, such as the following: (1) Does the patient have significant lung disease sufficient to cause respiratory impairment and to account for his or her symptoms?

(2) What functional pattern of lung disease does the patient have, i.e., restrictive versus obstructive disease?

In addition, serial evaluation of pulmonary function allows the physician to quantitate any improvement or deterioration in a patient's functional status. Information obtained from such objective evaluation may be essential in deciding when to treat a patient with lung disease and in assessing whether a patient has responded to therapy. Evaluation of patients preoperatively can also be useful in predicting which patients are likely to have significant postoperative respiratory problems and which are likely to have adequate pulmonary function after lung resection.

Three main categories of information can be obtained with "screening" or routine pulmonary function testing:

1. Lung volumes, which provide a measurement of the size of the various compartments within the lung

2. Flow rates, which measure maximal flow within the airways

3. Diffusing capacity, which indicates how readily gas transfer occurs from the alveolus to the pulmonary capillary blood

Before examining how these tests indicate what type of functional lung disease a patient has, we will first discuss the tests within each category and describe how they are performed.

Lung Volumes. Although the lung can be subdivided into compartments in different ways, four volumes in particular need to be remembered (Fig. 3–14):

1. Total lung capacity (TLC)—the total volume of gas within the lungs after a maximal inspiration

2. Residual volume (RV)—the volume of gas remaining within the lungs after a maximal expiration

3. Vital capacity (VC)—the volume of gas expired when going from TLC to RV

4. Functional residual capacity (FRC)—the volume of gas within the lungs at the resting state, i.e., at the end of expiration during the normal tidal breathing pattern

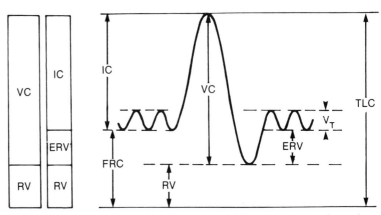

Figure 3–14. Subcompartments of the lung, i.e., lung volumes. On the right side of the figure, lung volumes are labeled on a spirographic tracing. On the left side of the figure are block diagrams showing two ways that the total lung capacity can be subdivided. TLC = total lung capacity; VC = vital capacity; RV = residual volume; IC = inspiratory capacity; ERV = expiratory reserve volume; FRC = functional residual capacity; V_T = tidal volume.

The vital capacity can be easily measured by having the patient breathe into a spirometer from total lung capacity down to residual volume; by definition, the volume expired in this manner is the vital capacity. However, since residual volume, functional residual capacity, and total lung capacity all include the amount of gas left within the lungs even after a maximal expiration, these volumes cannot be determined simply by having the patient breathe into a spirometer. In order to quantitate these volumes, a variety of methods are available that can measure one of the three parameters (RV, FRC, or TLC), and the other two can then be calculated or derived from the spirometric tracing. Several categories of tests are available to quantitate these volumes, two of which are described here:

1. Dilution tests—a known volume of an inert gas (usually helium) at a known concentration is inhaled into the lungs. This gas is diluted by the volume of gas already present within the lungs, and the concentration of expired gas (relative to inspired) therefore reflects the initial volume of gas in the lungs.

2. Body plethysmography—the patient, sitting inside an airtight box, performs a maneuver that causes expansion and compression of gas within the thorax. By quantitating volumes and pressure changes and by applying Boyle's law, one can calculate the volume of gas present in the thorax.

Under most circumstances, dilution methods are adequate for determination of lung volumes and are preferred for routine use. However, in those patients who have airspaces within the lung that do not communicate with the bronchial tree, e.g., bullae, the inhaled gas is not diluted in these noncommunicating areas, and the measured lung volumes determined by dilution methods are falsely low. In such a situation, body plethysmography gives a more accurate reflection of intrathoracic gas volume as it does not depend upon ready communication of all peripheral airspaces with the bronchial tree.

Lung volumes are determined by spirometry and either gas dilution or body plethysmography.

Flow Rates. The measurement of flow rates on routine pulmonary function testing involves assessing airflow during maximal forced expiration, i.e., with the patient breathing as hard and as fast as possible from TLC down to RV. The volume expired during this maneuver is the *forced vital capacity* or *FVC*, while the amount expired during the first second is the *forced expiratory volume in 1 second* or *FEV_1* (Fig. 3–15). When interpreting flow rates, it is common to use the ratio between these two parameters (i.e., FEV_1/FVC) as a measure of obstruction to airflow. Another parameter often calculated from the forced expiratory maneuver is the maximal mid-expiratory flow rate (MMEFR or MMFR), which is the rate of airflow during the middle one-half of the expiration (i.e., between 25 and 75 percent of the volume expired during the forced vital capacity). It is also frequently called the forced expiratory flow between 25 and 75 percent of vital capacity, or the $FEF_{25-75\%}$. The MMFR or $FEF_{25-75\%}$ is a relatively sensitive index of airflow obstruction and may be abnormal when the FEV_1/FVC ratio is still preserved.

Maximal expiratory airflow is assessed by the FEV_1/FVC ratio and the MMFR.

Diffusing Capacity. The diffusing capacity is a measurement of the rate of transfer of gas from the alveolus to the capillary measured in relation to the driving pressure of the gas across the alveolar-capillary membrane. Small concentrations of carbon monoxide are generally used for this purpose. Carbon monoxide combines readily with hemo-

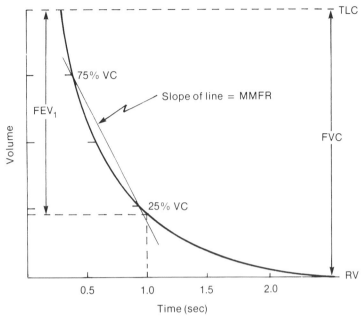

Figure 3–15. Forced expiratory spirogram. Volume is plotted against time, while the patient breathes out as hard and as fast as possible from total lung capacity to residual volume. FVC = forced vital capacity; FEV_1 = forced expiratory volume in 1 second; TLC = total lung capacity; RV = residual volume; MMFR = maximal mid-expiratory flow rate (also called forced expiratory flow from 25-75%, or $FEF_{25-75\%}$).

globin, and the rate of transfer of gas from the alveolus to the capillary depends on movement through the alveolar-capillary membrane and the amount of hemoglobin available for binding the carbon monoxide.

Diffusing capacity for carbon monoxide is largely dependent upon the surface area for gas exchange and the pulmonary capillary blood volume.

Although the diffusing capacity to some extent reflects the "thickness" of the alveolar-capillary membrane, it is probably most dependent on the number of functioning "alveolar-capillary units" and may be depressed in emphysema, interstitial lung disease, or pulmonary vascular disease because of loss of surface area available for gas exchange. Other factors that also influence the diffusing capacity for carbon monoxide include significant ventilation-perfusion inequality, pulmonary capillary blood volume, and hematocrit. Since diffusing capacity may be depressed if a patient is anemic (due to less available hemoglobin to bind carbon monoxide), the observed value is generally corrected for the patient's hemoglobin level.

Interpretation of Normality in Pulmonary Function Testing

Interpretation of pulmonary function tests necessarily involves a qualitative judgment about normality or abnormality using the quantitative data obtained from these tests. In order to arrive at a relatively objective way to make such judgments, normal standards have been established for each test using large numbers of normal, nonsmoking controls. Regression lines have been constructed to fit the data obtained from these normal controls. A "normal" value for a test in a given patient can then be found by putting the patient's age and height into the regression equation. For most tests, an arbitrary cutoff for normality has been established: an observed value is considered normal if it is greater than 80 percent of the predicted value. Since this is clearly an arbitrary cutoff, it is important to take all the data into consideration to see if certain patterns are consistently present. Interpretation of a single test in this manner, with the assumption that a patient with a value of 79 percent has lung disease while one with a value of 81 percent is normal, is obviously fraught with danger.

Interpretation of the FEV_1/FVC ratio is the only exception to the general rule that a normal value is greater than 80 percent predicted. If this ratio is compared with the predicted ratio (the latter often approximately 75 to 80 percent), this "ratio of the ratios" should be greater than about 95 percent. It is important to emphasize that this 95 percent value does not refer to the actual FEV_1/FVC ratio, but rather to the comparison of this observed ratio with the predicted ratio.

Patterns of Pulmonary Function Impairment

When analyzing pulmonary function tests, abnormalities are usually categorized into one of two patterns (or a combination of the two): (1) an obstructive pattern, characterized mainly by obstruction to airflow, and (2) a restrictive pattern, with evidence of decreased lung volumes but no airflow obstruction.

Patterns of impairment: (1) obstructive—diminished rates of expiratory airflow ($\downarrow FEV_1/FVC$, $\downarrow MMFR$); (2) restrictive—diminished lung volumes (especially $\downarrow TLC$); preserved expiratory airflow.

An obstructive pattern, as seen in patients with asthma, chronic bronchitis, or emphysema, consists of a decrease in rates of expiratory airflow and is usually manifest as a decrease in MMFR and the FEV_1/FVC ratio (Fig. 3–16). There is generally a high residual volume

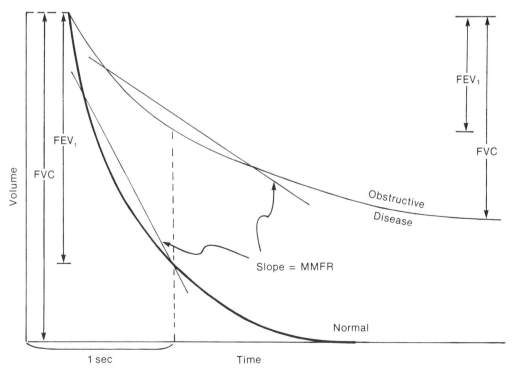

Figure 3–16. Forced expiratory spirograms in a normal individual and in a patient with airflow obstruction. Note the prolonged expiration and the changes in FEV_1 and FVC in the patient with obstructive disease.

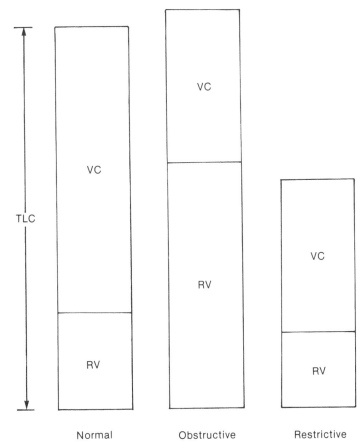

Figure 3–17. Diagram of lung volumes (TLC and subcompartments VC and RV) in a normal individual and in patients with obstructive and restrictive disease.

and increased RV/TLC ratio, indicating "air trapping" due to closure of airways during forced expiration (Fig. 3–17). "Hyperinflation," reflected by an increased TLC, is often found, particularly in patients with either asthma or emphysema. Diffusing capacity tends to be decreased in those patients who have loss of alveolar-capillary bed (i.e., emphysema) but not in those without loss of available surface area for gas exchange (i.e., chronic bronchitis or asthma).

The hallmark of restrictive disease, on the other hand, is a reduction in lung volumes, while expiratory airflow is normal (Fig. 3–17). Therefore, TLC, RV, VC, and FRC all tend to be reduced, while MMFR and FEV_1/FVC are preserved. In some patients with significant loss of volume from restrictive disease, the MMFR is decreased because of less volume available to generate a high flow rate. It is therefore difficult to interpret a low MMFR in the face of significant restrictive disease unless it is clearly decreased out of proportion to the decrease in lung volumes. A wide variety of parenchymal, pleural, and neuromuscular diseases can demonstrate a restrictive pattern. Patients with interstitial disease affecting the lung parenchyma generally show loss of alveolar-capillary units and a decrease in the diffusing capacity for carbon monoxide.

Although lung diseases often present with one or the other of these patterns, a mixed picture of obstructive and restrictive disease can be present, making interpretation of the tests much more complex. It should also be noted that these tests do not directly reflect a patient's overall capability for O_2 and CO_2 exchange, which are assessed by measurement of arterial blood gases.

Other Tests

A significant amount of work has been done in recent years to develop tests that detect "early" obstruction to airflow, particularly that due to small or peripheral airways obstruction. Such tests include maximal expiratory flow-volume loops, analysis of closing volume, and frequency dependent dynamic compliance. The latter two tests are generally reserved for research laboratories, but the maximal expiratory flow-volume loop has sufficient routine clinical applicability to warrant a short discussion here.

The flow-volume loop is a graphic record of maximal inspiratory and maximal expiratory maneuvers. However, rather than the graph of volume versus time that is given with usual spirometric testing, the flow-volume loop has a plot of flow (on the Y axis) versus volume (on the X axis). Although the initial flows obtained during the early part of a forced expiratory maneuver are effort dependent, the flows during the latter part of the maneuver are effort independent and primarily reflect the mechanical properties of the lungs and the resistance to airflow.

In those patients with evidence of airflow obstruction, flow rates at a given volume are decreased, often giving the curve a "scooped" or "coved" appearance. The flow data obtained from maximal expiratory flow volume loops can be interpreted quantitatively (comparing observed flow rates at specified volumes with predicted values) or qualitatively (by visually analyzing the shape and concavity of the expiratory portion of the curve). When routine spirometric parameters reflecting airflow obstruction (MMFR, FEV_1/FVC) are abnormal, the flow-volume loop is generally abnormal. In addition, however, in patients with "small-airways disease" without involvement of larger bronchi, the contour of the flow-volume loop is often abnormal even when the FEV_1/FVC ratio is normal. Examples of flow-volume loops in a normal patient and in a patient with obstructive lung disease are shown in Figure 3–18.

In obstructive lung disease, the expiratory portion of the flow-volume curve has a "scooped out" or "coved" appearance.

Another important application of flow-volume loops is the diagnosis and localization of upper airway obstruction. By analyzing the contour of both the inspiratory and expiratory portions of the curve, one can categorize the obstruction as *fixed* versus *variable* as well as *intrathoracic* versus *extrathoracic*. With a fixed lesion, changes in pleural pressure do not affect the degree of obstruction, and a limitation in peak airflow, i.e., a plateau, is seen on both the inspiratory and expiratory portions of the curve. In a variable lesion, the amount of obstruction is determined by the location of the lesion and by the effect of alterations in pleural and airway pressure with inspiration and expiration (see Fig. 3–19). A variable intrathoracic lesion is characterized by expiratory limitation of airflow and a plateau on the expiratory portion of the flow-volume curve, while a variable extrathoracic lesion demonstrates inspiratory limitation of airflow and a plateau on the inspiratory portion of the flow-volume curve (Fig. 3–20).

Upper airway obstruction is characterized by maximal inspiratory and expiratory flow-volume curves.

Figure 3–18. Flow-volume loops in a normal individual and in a patient with airflow obstruction. Expiratory "coving" is apparent on the tracing of the patient with airflow obstruction. RV (N) = residual volume in the normal individual; RV (O) = residual volume in the patient with obstructive disease.

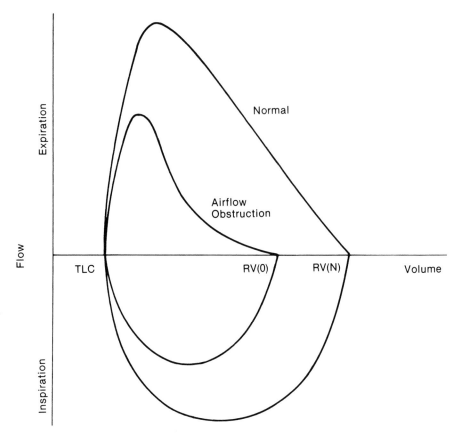

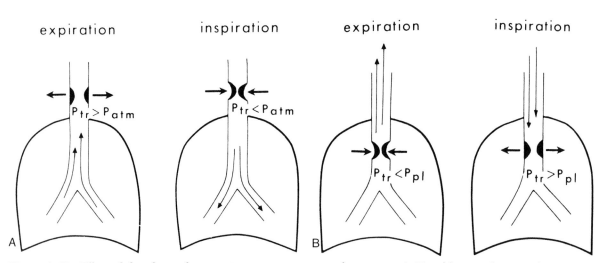

Figure 3–19. Effect of the phase of respiration on upper airway obstruction. *A*, Variable extrathoracic obstruction. During forced inspiration, airway or tracheal pressure (P_{tr}) becomes more negative than surrounding atmospheric pressure (P_{atm}), and airway diameter decreases. During forced expiration, more positive intratracheal pressure distends the airway and decreases the magnitude of the obstruction. *B*, Variable intrathoracic obstruction. Pleural pressure surrounds and acts on the large intrathoracic airways, affecting airway diameter. During forced expiration, pleural pressure is markedly positive, and airway diameter is decreased. During forced inspiration, negative pleural pressure causes intrathoracic airways to be increased in size, and the obstruction is decreased. (From Kryger, M., Bode, F., Antic, R., and Anthonisen, N.: Am. J. Med. 61:85–93, 1976. Reproduced with permission.)

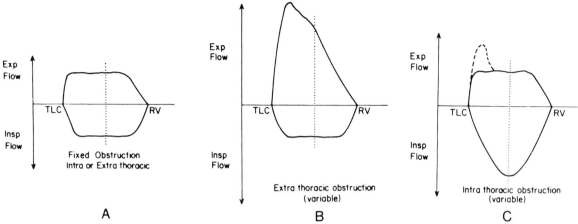

Figure 3–20. Maximal inspiratory and expiratory flow-volume curves in the three types of upper airway obstruction. *A*, Fixed obstruction, either intrathoracic or extrathoracic. The obstruction is equivalent during inspiration and expiration, so that maximal inspiratory and expiratory flows are limited to the same extent. *B*, Variable extrathoracic obstruction. Obstruction is more marked during inspiration, and only the inspiratory part of the curve demonstrates a plateau. *C*, Variable intrathoracic obstruction. Obstruction is more marked during expiration, and only the expiratory part of the curve demonstrates a plateau. The dashed line represents a higher initial flow that is occasionally observed before the plateau in intrathoracic obstruction. (From Kryger, M., Bode, F., Antic, R., and Anthonisen, N.: Am. J. Med. 61:85–93, 1976. Reproduced with permission.)

Maximal expiratory flow-volume loops have also been recently performed with helium-oxygen mixtures in order to localize intrathoracic obstruction within central versus peripheral airways. A description of this technique, which is beyond the scope of this discussion, can be found in the references listed at the end of this chapter.

Arterial Blood Gases

Despite the extensive information that pulmonary function tests provide, they do not show the net effect of lung disease on gas exchange, which is easily assessed by studies performed on arterial blood. Arterial blood can be conveniently sampled by needle puncture of a radial artery or, less commonly and with more potential risk, of a brachial or femoral artery. The blood is collected into a heparinized syringe (to prevent clotting), and care is taken to expel air bubbles from the syringe and to analyze the sample quickly (or to keep it on ice until analyzed). Three measurements are routinely obtained—arterial P_{O_2}, P_{CO_2}, and pH.

Arterial P_{O_2} is normally between approximately 80 and 100 torr, but the expected value depends significantly on the patient's age and the simultaneous level of P_{CO_2} (reflecting alveolar ventilation, an important determinant of alveolar and, secondarily, arterial P_{O_2}). From the arterial blood gases, the alveolar-arterial oxygen gradient (AaD$_{O_2}$) can be calculated, as was discussed in Chapter 1. Normally, the difference between alveolar and arterial P_{O_2} is less than 10 to 15 torr, but again this depends on the patient's age. As we also saw in Chapter 1, the actual oxygen content of the blood does not begin to fall significantly until the arterial P_{O_2} drops below approximately 60 torr.

Therefore, an abnormally low P_{O_2} generally does not affect oxygen transport to the tissues until it drops below this level and the saturation falls.

The range of normal arterial P_{CO_2} is approximately 35 to 45 torr, with a corresponding pH between 7.45 and 7.35. Respiratory and metabolic factors interact closely in determining these numbers and a patient's acid-base status. Interpretation of the P_{CO_2} and pH should be done simultaneously, as both pieces of information are necessary to distinguish respiratory from metabolic abnormalities.

When the P_{CO_2} rises acutely, the concentration of H^+ also rises, and the pH therefore falls. As a general rule, the pH falls approximately 0.08 (or, rounded off, about 0.1) for each 10 torr increase in P_{CO_2}. Such a rise in P_{CO_2} with an appropriate decrease in pH is termed an *acute respiratory acidosis.* Conversely, a drop in P_{CO_2} due to hyperventilation, with the attendant increase in pH, is termed an *acute respiratory alkalosis.* With time (hours to days), the kidneys attempt to compensate for a prolonged respiratory acidosis by retaining bicarbonate (HCO_3^-), or by excreting bicarbonate in the case of a prolonged respiratory alkalosis. In either case, the compensation returns the pH toward but not entirely to normal, and the disturbance is termed a chronic (i.e., compensated) respiratory acidosis or alkalosis.

If, on the other hand, a patient is producing too much (or excreting too little) acid, he is said to have a *primary metabolic acidosis.* Conversely, an excess of HCO_3^- (equivalent to a decrease in H^+) defines a *primary metabolic alkalosis.* In the same way that the kidneys attempt to compensate for a primary respiratory acid-base disturbance, respiratory elimination of CO_2 is adjusted to compensate for metabolic acid-base disturbances. Hence metabolic acidosis stimulates ventilation, CO_2 elimination, and a rise in the pH towards the normal level, while metabolic alkalosis suppresses ventilation and CO_2 elimination, and the pH falls towards the normal range.

In practice, the clinician considers three fundamental questions in defining all acid-base disturbances: (1) Is there an acidosis or alkalosis? (2) Is the primary disorder of respiratory or metabolic origin? (3) Is there evidence for respiratory or metabolic compensation? Table 3–1

Table 3–1. ACID-BASE DISTURBANCES

Condition	P_{CO_2}	pH	HCO_3^-
Normal	35–45	7.35–7.45	23–30
Respiratory acidosis			
No metabolic compensation	↑	↓	Normal (or ↑)
With metabolic compensation	↑↑	↓	↑
Respiratory alkalosis			
No metabolic compensation	↓	↑	Normal (or ↓)
With metabolic compensation	↓↓	↑	↓
Metabolic acidosis			
No respiratory compensation	Normal	↓	↓
With respiratory compensation	↓	↓	↓↓
Metabolic alkalosis			
No respiratory compensation	Normal	↑	↑
With respiratory compensation	↑	↑	↑↑

summarizes the findings in the major types of acid-base disturbances. Unfortunately, in clinical practice matters are not always so and it is quite common to see complex mixtures of acid-base disturbances in patients who have several diseases and are receiving a variety of medications.

Arterial P_{CO_2} and pH together determine the nature of an acid-base disorder and the presence or absence of compensation.

Exercise Testing

Since limited exercise tolerance is frequently the most prominent symptom in patients with a variety of pulmonary problems, study of patients during exercise may provide valuable information about how much and why they are limited. Adding measurements of arterial blood gases during exercise provides an additional dimension, and shows whether gas exchange problems (either hypoxemia or hypercapnia) contribute to the impairment.

Though any form of exercise is theoretically possible for the testing procedure, the patient usually is studied while exercising on a treadmill or a stationary bicycle. Measurements that can be made at various points during exercise include work output, heart rate, ventilation, O_2 consumption, CO_2 production, expired gas tensions, and arterial blood gases. Analysis of these data can often distinguish whether ventilation, cardiac output, or problems with gas exchange (particularly hypoxemia) provide the major limitation to exercise tolerance. The results may then guide the physician to specific therapy, based on the type of limitation found.

REFERENCES

Physical Examination

Andrews, J. L., and Badger, T. L.: Lung sounds through the ages: from Hippocrates to Laennec to Osler. JAMA 241:2625–2630, 1979.
Forgacs, P.: The functional basis of pulmonary sounds. Chest 73:399–405, 1978.
Loudon, R., and Murphy, R. L. H. Jr.: Lung sounds. Am. Rev. Respir. Dis. 130:663–673, 1984.
Shneerson, J. M.: Digital clubbing and hypertrophic osteoarthropathy: the underlying mechanisms. Br. J. Dis. Chest 75:113–131, 1981.
Snider, G. L.: Physical examination of the chest in adults. *In* Sackner, M. A. (ed.): Diagnostic Techniques in Pulmonary Disease (Part I). New York, Marcel Dekker, Inc., 1980, pp. 19–47.

Chest Roentgenography

Felson, B.: Chest Roentgenology. Philadelphia, W. B. Saunders Co., 1973.
Fraser, R. G., and Paré, J. A. P.: Diagnosis of Diseases of the Chest. 2nd ed. Philadelphia, W. B. Saunders Co., 1977.

Computed Tomography

Brown, L. R., and Muhm, J.R.: Computed tomography of the thorax: current perspectives. Chest 83:806–813, 1983.
Heitzmann, E. R.: Computed tomography of the thorax: current perspectives. AJR. 136:2–12, 1981.
Pugatch, R. D., and Faling, L. J.: Computed tomography of the thorax: a status report. Chest 80:618–626, 1981.

Lung Scanning

Spies, W. G., Spies, S. M., and Mintzer, R. A.: Radionuclide imaging in diseases of the chest. Chest 83:122–127; 250–255, 1983.
Wagner, H. N., Jr.: The use of radioisotope techniques for the evaluation of patients with pulmonary disease. Am. Rev. Respir. Dis. 113:203–218, 1976.

Pulmonary Angiography

Bell, W. R., and Simon, T. L.: A comparative analysis of pulmonary perfusion scans with pulmonary angiograms. Am. Heart J. 92:700–706, 1976.
Dalen, J. E., Brooks, H. L., Johnson, L. W., Meister, S. G., Szucs, M. M., Jr., and Dexter, L.: Pulmonary angiography in acute pulmonary embolism: indications, techniques, and results in 367 patients. Am. Heart J. 81:175–185, 1971.
Wilson, J. E., III.: Pulmonary angiography. In Sackner, M. A. (ed.): Diagnostic Techniques in Pulmonary Disease (Part I). New York, Marcel Dekker, Inc., 1980, pp. 301–325.

Ultrasonography

Matalon, T. A., Neiman, H. L., and Mintzer, R. A.: Noncardiac chest sonography: the state of the art. Chest 83:675–678, 1983.
Rosenberg, E. R.: Ultrasound in the assessment of pleural densities. Chest 84:283–285, 1983.

Bronchoscopy

Fulkerson, W. J.: Fiberoptic bronchoscopy. N. Engl. J. Med. 311:511–515, 1984.
Sackner, M. A.: Bronchofiberscopy. Am. Rev. Respir. Dis. 111:62–88, 1975.
Zavala, D. C.: Diagnostic fiberoptic bronchoscopy: techniques and results of biopsy in 600 patients. Chest 68:12–19, 1975.

Obtaining and Processing Specimens

Ball, W. C., Jr.: Thoracentesis and pleural biopsy. In Sackner, M. A. (ed.): Diagnostic Techniques in Pulmonary Disease (Part II). New York, Marcel Dekker, Inc., 1981, pp. 541–566.
Bartlett, J. G.: Bacteriological diagnosis of pulmonary infections. In Sackner, M. A. (ed.): Diagnostic Techniques in Pulmonary Disease (Part II). New York, Marcel Dekker, Inc., 1981, pp. 707–745.
Bartlett, J. G.: Diagnostic accuracy of transtracheal aspiration bacteriologic studies. Am. Rev. Respir. Dis. 115:777–782, 1977.
Epstein, R. L.: Constituents of sputum: a simple method. Ann. Intern. Med. 77:259–265, 1972.
Gaensler, E. A.: Open and closed lung biopsy. In Sackner, M. A. (ed.): Diagnostic Techniques in Pulmonary Disease (Part II). New York, Marcel Dekker, Inc., 1981, pp. 579–622.
Kuhn, C., III, Askin, F. B., and Katzenstein, A–L. A.: Diagnostic light and electron microscopy. In Sackner, M. A. (ed.): Diagnostic Techniques in Pulmonary Disease (Part I). New York, Marcel Dekker, Inc., 1980, pp. 89–202.
Murray, P. R., and Washington, J. A., II.: Microscopic and bacteriologic analysis of expectorated sputum. Mayo Clin. Proc. 50:339–344, 1975.
Nordenstrom, B. E. W.: Needle biopsy of pulmonary lesions. In Sackner, M. A. (ed.): Diagnostic Techniques in Pulmonary Disease (Part II). New York, Marcel Dekker, Inc., 1981, pp. 623–654.
Ries, K., Levison, M. E., and Kaye, D.: Transtracheal aspiration in pulmonary infection. Arch. Intern. Med. 133:453–458, 1974.
Selawry, O. S., and Ng, A. B. P.: Cytologic examination of bronchopulmonary secretions. In Sackner, M. A. (ed.): Diagnostic Techniques in Pulmonary Disease (Part I). New York, Marcel Dekker, Inc., 1980, pp. 203–214.
Westcott, J. L.: Direct percutaneous needle aspiration of localized pulmonary disease: results in 422 patients. Radiology 137:31–35, 1980.
Zavala, D. C.: Pulmonary biopsy. Adv. Intern. Med. 21:21–45, 1976.

Evaluation on a Functional Level

Cherniack, R. M.: Pulmonary Function Testing. Philadelphia, W. B. Saunders Co., 1977.
Cotes, J. E.: Lung Function: Assessment and Application in Medicine. 4th ed. Oxford, Blackwell Scientific Publications, 1979.
Jones, N. L., and Campbell, E. J. M.: Clinical Exercise Testing. 2nd ed. Philadelphia, W. B. Saunders Co., 1982.
Narins, R. G., and Emmett, M.: Simple and mixed acid-base disorders: a practical approach. Medicine 59:161–187, 1980.
Shapiro, B. A., Harrison, R. A., and Walton, J. R.: Clinical Application of Blood Gases. 3rd ed. Chicago, Year Book Medical Publishers, 1982.
Wanner, A.: Interpretation of pulmonary function tests. In Sackner, M. A. (ed.): Diagnostic Techniques in Pulmonary Disease (Part I). New York, Marcel Dekker, Inc., 1980, pp. 353–426.
Wasserman, K., and Whipp, B. J.: Exercise physiology in health and disease. Am. Rev. Respir. Dis. 112:219–249, 1975.

$$4$$

Anatomic and Physiologic Aspects of Airways

Structure
Function
  Airway Resistance
  Patterns of Airflow
  Maximal Expiratory Effort

In its transit from the nose or mouth to the gas-exchanging region of the lung, air passes through the larynx and then along a series of progressively branching tubes, from the trachea down to the smallest bronchioles. This chapter describes the structure of these airways and then considers how they function, in preparation for our discussion of diseases affecting the airways.

STRUCTURE

The trachea, bronchi, and bronchioles down to the level of the terminal bronchioles constitute the *conducting airways*, since their function is purely one of transport. In contrast, beyond the terminal bronchioles are the *respiratory bronchioles*; they mark the beginning of the *respiratory zone* of the lung, where gas exchange actually takes place. Respiratory bronchioles are considered part of the gas-exchanging region of lung, since alveoli are present along their walls. With successive generations of respiratory bronchioles, more alveoli appear along the walls until one reaches the alveolar ducts, which are entirely "alveolarized" (Fig. 4–1). We will limit our discussion in this chapter to the conducting airways and to those aspects of the more distal airways that affect air movement but not gas exchange. Alveolar structure will be discussed further in Chapter 8.

The airways are composed of several layers of tissue (Fig. 4–2). Adjacent to the airway lumen is the mucosa, beneath which is a basement membrane separating the epithelial cells of the mucosa from the submucosa. Within the submucosa are mucous glands (the contents of which are extruded through the mucosa), smooth muscle, and loose

Conducting airways: trachea, bronchi, bronchioles down to the level of terminal bronchioles.
Respiratory zone: respiratory bronchioles, alveolar ducts, and alveoli.

63

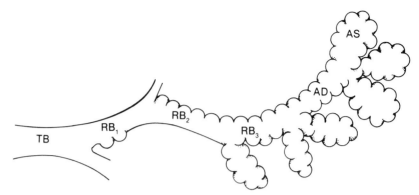

Figure 4–1. Schematic diagram of the most distal portion of the respiratory tree. Each terminal bronchiole (TB) supplies several generations of respiratory bronchioles (RB$_1$ through RB$_3$), which have progressively more respiratory (alveolar) epithelium lining their walls. Alveolar ducts (AD) are entirely lined by alveolar epithelium, as are the alveolar sacs (AS). The region of lung distal to and supplied by a terminal bronchiole is termed an acinus. (From Thurlbeck, W. M.: Chronic obstructive lung disease. In Sommers, S. C., ed.: Pathology Annual. Vol. 3. New York, Appleton-Century-Crofts, 1968. Reproduced with permission.)

connective tissue with some nerves and lymphatics. Surrounding the submucosa is a fibrocartilaginous layer, containing the cartilage rings that support several generations of airways. Finally, a layer of peribronchial tissue, with fat, lymphatics, vessels, and nerves, encircles the rest of the airway wall. We will consider each of these layers in turn, describing the component cells and the way the structure changes as one progresses distally through the tracheobronchial tree.

The surface layer or mucosa consists of pseudostratified, columnar epithelial cells, which appear to be several cells thick in the trachea and large bronchi (Fig. 4–2A). The ciliated cells, which are most

Figure 4–2. Schematic diagram of components of the airway wall. *A* is at the level of large airways (trachea and bronchi), while *B* is at the level of small airways (bronchioles). CC = ciliated columnar epithelial cell; GC = goblet cell; BM = basement membrane; BC = basal cell; SM = smooth muscle; MG = mucous gland; CA = cartilage; CL = Clara cell. (Adapted from Weibel, E. R. and Burri, P. H.: Funktionelle Aspekte der Lungenmorphologie. In Fuchs, W. A. and Voegeli, E., eds.: Aktuelle Probleme der Roentgendiagnostik. Vol. 2. Bern, Huber, 1973. Reproduced with permission.)

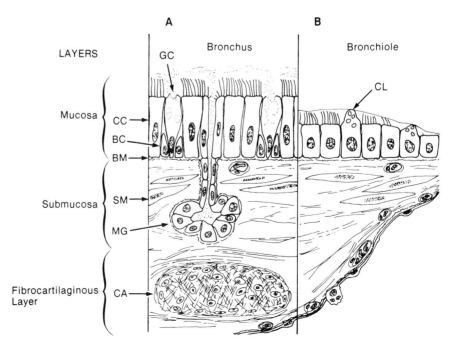

superficial, are responsible for protecting the deeper airways by propelling tracheobronchial secretions (and inhaled particles) toward the pharynx. The cilia have the characteristic ultrastructure seen in other ciliated cells, namely a central pair of microtubules and an outer ring of nine double microtubules (see Fig. 22–1). Small side arms, called dynein arms, are found on the outer double microtubules. Their presence appears to be important for normal functioning of the cilia, since patients with cilia lacking the dynein side arms have impaired ciliary action and recurrent bronchopulmonary infections. Scattered between the ciliated epithelial cells are secretory cells called *goblet cells*, which produce and discharge mucus into the airway lumen. However, as we will see, the goblet cells produce a relatively small proportion of total bronchial mucus, the largest portion of which is made by the bronchial mucous glands in the submucosa.

The mucosal layer of large airways consists of pseudostratified, ciliated columnar epithelial cells.

The deepest layer of epithelial cells, which abuts the basement membrane, includes cells known as *basal cells*. The function of the basal cells is to differentiate into and replenish the more superficial cells of the mucosa, either the ciliated cells or the secretory goblet cells. Another important cell type found in the basal layer of the surface epithelium is the *Kulchitsky* or *K cell*, which is believed to have a neuroendocrine function. These cells are probably part of the APUD (amine precursor uptake and decarboxylation) system and therefore may be capable of producing amine and/or polypeptide products. In addition, K cells have cytoplasmic processes that extend to the luminal surface. As a result of these processes, K cells may be involved in sensing the composition of inspired gas, and it has been postulated that they play a role in the regional control of ventilation and perfusion. As we will see, these different cell types are important not only because of their normal physiologic roles, but also because of the way they respond to airway irritation and their potential for becoming neoplastic.

The submucosal layer has two major components that we will discuss—*bronchial mucous glands* and *bronchial smooth muscle*. The mucous glands are the main source of bronchial secretions; a duct transports the secretions through the mucosa and discharges them into the airway lumen. As we mentioned earlier, superficial goblet cells also produce mucus, which qualitatively appears to be identical to mucus formed by the bronchial mucous glands. However, it is a mystery why both sources of mucus exist and whether both, in fact, are necessary. Airway smooth muscle is present from the trachea down to the level of bronchioles and even appears in the alveolar ducts. Disturbances in the quantity and function of the smooth muscle are very important in disease, particularly in the case of bronchial asthma.

Bronchial secretions are produced by submucosal glands and to a lesser extent by goblet cells in the mucosa.

Finally, the fibrocartilaginous layer is important because of the structural support that cartilage provides to the airways. We will see that the configuration of the cartilage varies significantly at different levels of the tracheobronchial tree, but the function at all levels is probably similar.

What we have described so far is the general structure of the airways. However, this structure varies considerably at different levels of the airway. Some of these differences are illustrated in Figures 4–2A and 4–2B. As one progresses distally through the tracheobronchial tree, the following changes are normally seen:

Airway structure changes considerably as one progresses distally through the tracheobronchial tree.

1. The epithelial layer of cells becomes progressively thinner, until

there is a single layer of cuboidal cells at the level of the terminal bronchioles.

2. Goblet cells decrease in number until they disappear approximately at the level of the terminal bronchiole. In their place are dome-shaped cells that project into the airway lumen, called *Clara cells*. Though the function of the Clara cells is not known with certainty, it is thought that they may be involved in producing a liquid surface layer coating the bronchiolar epithelium.

3. Mucous glands, which are present in the trachea and large bronchi, are actually most numerous in the medium-sized bronchi. They then become progressively fewer in number more distally and are absent from the bronchioles.

4. Smooth muscle changes in configuration at different levels of the tracheobronchial tree. In the trachea and large bronchi, the muscle is found either as bands or as a spiral network, while in the smaller bronchi and bronchioles a continuous layer of smooth muscle encircles the airway. As airway size decreases distally in the tracheobronchial tree, smooth muscle generally occupies a larger portion of the total thickness of the airway wall. This proportion of smooth muscle to airway wall thickness becomes maximal at the level of the terminal bronchiole.

5. Cartilage also changes in configuration. In the trachea, the cartilaginous rings are horseshoe shaped, with the posterior aspect of the trachea being free of cartilage. In the bronchi, there are plates of cartilage, which become smaller and less numerous distally, until cartilage is absent in the bronchioles.

In the preceding discussion, we have described many of the structural features of normal airways. However, with chronic exposure to an irritant, such as cigarette smoke, a variety of changes frequently occur. Some of these changes, particularly in the epithelial cells, are important because of the potential for eventual malignancy, as will be discussed in Chapter 20. Other changes are apparent in the mucus-secreting structures (bronchial mucous glands and goblet cells) and are important features of chronic bronchitis. With chronic irritation, there is hypertrophy of the mucous glands; the goblet cells become more numerous and are found more distally than usual, even in the terminal bronchioles. The implications of these changes in disease states will be discussed in Chapter 6.

FUNCTION

With each breath, air flows from the mouth, through the bronchial tree, to the regions of the lung responsible for gas exchange. In order to generate this flow of air during inspiration, the pressure must be lower in the alveoli than at the mouth, since air flows from a region of higher to one of lower pressure. To this end, the diaphragm and inspiratory muscles of the chest wall cause expansion of the chest and lungs, producing negative pressure in the pleural space and in the alveoli, and hence initiating airflow.

Flow in the airways can be thought of as being analogous to flow of current in an electrical system. However, rather than a voltage drop when electrons flow across a resistance, airways have a pressure difference between two points of airflow, and resistance to flow is provided by the airways themselves. The rate of airflow depends in part on this pressure difference between the two points and in part on the airway resistance. During inspiration, alveolar pressure is negative relative to mouth pressure (which is atmospheric), and air flows inward. In contrast, during expiration, alveolar pressure is positive relative to mouth pressure, and air flows outward from alveoli toward the mouth.

Airway Resistance

Though this model seems comparatively simple, airflow is in fact a much more complex phenomenon. For instance, let's first consider the problem of resistance. Normal airways resistance is approximately 0.5 to 2.0 cm H_2O per liter per second; that is, it requires a pressure difference of 0.5 to 2.0 cm H_2O between mouth and alveoli to get air to flow at a rate of 1 liter per second between these two points. Which airways provide most of the resistance? Although it is obvious that a single smaller airway provides more resistance to airflow than a single larger airway, it does not follow that the aggregate of smaller airways provides the bulk of the resistance. In fact, the opposite is true. For example, even though the trachea is large, there is only one trachea, and the total cross-sectional area of the airways at this level is quite small. In contrast, at the level of small airways (e.g., <2 mm diameter), the enormous number of these airways makes up for the small diameter of each one and results in a very large total cross-sectional area.

Since resistance to airflow in the tracheobronchial tree depends upon the total cross-sectional area of the airways, large and medium-sized airways provide greater resistance than the more numerous small airways.

One can see the total cross-sectional area of the airways at different levels of the tracheobronchial tree in Table 4–1. The major site of resistance (the smallest total cross-sectional area) is at the level of medium-sized bronchi. The small or peripheral airways, generally defined as airways less than 2 mm in diameter, contribute only about 10 to 20 percent of the total resistance. Hence, these airways are frequently called the "silent" zone, since disease in them can affect their size without significantly altering the total airways resistance. For

Table 4–1. AIRWAY NUMBERS AND DIMENSIONS*

Name	Number	Diameter (mm)	Cross-Sectional Area (cm²)
Trachea	1	25	5
Main bronchi	2	11–19	3.2
Lobar bronchi	5	4.5–13.5	2.7
Segmental bronchi	19	4.5–6.5	3.2
Subsegmental bronchi	38	3–6	6.6
Terminal bronchi	1,000	1.0	7.9
Terminal bronchioles	35,000	0.65	116
Terminal respiratory bronchioles	630,000	0.45	1,000
Alveolar ducts and sacs	4×10^6	0.40	17,100
Alveoli	300×10^6	0.25–0.30	700,000 (surface area)

*Adapted from Thurlbeck, W. M.: Chronic obstructive lung disease. *In* Sommers, S. C. (ed.): Pathology Annual. Vol. 3. New York, Appleton-Century-Crofts, 1968.

this reason, physiologists have been interested in techniques for detecting disease of the small airways when total resistance is still normal.

Patterns of Airflow

Discussion of airflow is further complicated by another issue. Different patterns of flow depend on the size of the airway, the flow rate, and the physical properties of the gas. We will briefly consider the two major patterns of flow—laminar and turbulent.

Laminar flow is generally seen in smaller airways with relatively low velocities. It is the type of orderly, linear flow one would expect through a straight tube of small diameter (Fig. 4–3). Under conditions of laminar flow, the resistance of the tube is inversely proportional to the fourth power of the radius; resistance is therefore very sensitive to even small changes in radius. In contrast, turbulent flow, as its name implies, is not linear (Fig. 4–3) and is found in larger airways at higher flow rates. Under conditions of turbulent flow, the pressure drop across the airways is higher than with laminar flow. To be precise, the pressure drop when flow is laminar is directly proportional to the flow rate; when flow is turbulent, the pressure drop is proportional to the square of the flow rate.

Laminar and turbulent flow also differ in the influence of gas density. Changes in gas density do not affect flow or the pressure drop when airflow is laminar. In contrast, when flow is turbulent, an increase in gas density results in a greater pressure drop for any given flow rate. This principle has been used to determine whether flow is limited at the level of small (<2 mm diameter) or larger airways. When flow is limited at the level of the small airways, where flow is laminar, a change in gas density does not affect flow rates. On the other hand, when flow is limited at larger airways, where flow is turbulent, an alteration in the gas density significantly affects flow rates. A helium-oxygen mixture is commonly used to make such distinctions. If expiratory flow rates increase after inhalation of 80 percent helium and 20 percent oxygen, it is likely that flow is limited primarily at the level of larger airways. If no change in expiratory flow is seen with the helium-oxygen mixture, then small airways provide the major site of flow limitation.

Inhalation of a low-density gas, e.g., 80% helium + 20% oxygen, helps determine whether flow is limited in larger airways or smaller airways.

FEATURES

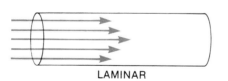

LAMINAR

1. Pressure required is proportional to flow, i.e., resistance is constant as flow is varied.
2. Found in smaller airways.
3. Gas density does not affect flow.

Figure 4–3. Features of laminar and turbulent airflow. (Adapted from Comroe, J. H. et al.: The Lung. 2nd ed. Chicago, Year Book Medical Publishers, Inc., 1962.)

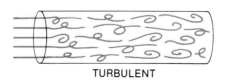

TURBULENT

1. Pressure required is proportional to (flow)^2, i.e., resistance increases as flow is increased.
2. Found in larger airways.
3. Gas density affects flow.

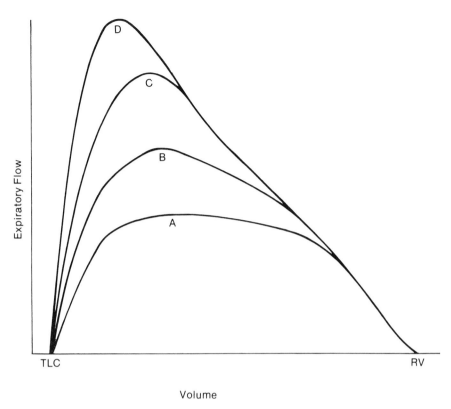

Figure 4–4. Expiratory flow-volume curves with progressively greater effort. Curve A represents the least effort; curve D represents maximal expiratory effort. On the down-sloping part of the curve, beyond the point at which approximately 30 percent of the vital capacity has been exhaled, flow is limited by the mechanical properties of the airways and lungs, not by muscular effort.

Maximal Expiratory Effort

This brief discussion of flow limitation leads us to the next important aspect of the physiology of airflow—the distinction between normal breathing and forced or maximal respiratory efforts. A great deal of information can be obtained by looking at flow during a forced expiration, i.e., breathing out from total lung capacity down to residual volume as hard and as fast as possible. When discussing this concept, it is useful to consider the flow-volume curve, which we mentioned in Chapter 3 and which is shown again in Figure 4–4. In this figure, we have drawn a series of expiratory curves that show the kind of flow rates generated by progressively greater expiratory efforts. Curve A shows expiratory flow with a relatively low effort, while curve D shows flow with a maximal expiratory effort.

As we discussed earlier, during the first part of this curve, perhaps until approximately 30 percent of the vital capacity has been exhaled, the flow rate is quite dependent on the effort expended. That is, with greater expiratory efforts we continue to see increasing expiratory flow rates, resulting from increased pleural pressure and thus the driving force for expiratory airflow. This region of the vital capacity during maximal expiratory flow is often termed the *effort-dependent portion*.

Below 70 percent of vital capacity, there comes a point at which we can no longer increase the flow rate with increasing effort. In other words, something other than our muscular strength (hence, other than the pleural pressure we can generate) limits flow. In fact, the limiting factor is a critical narrowing of the airways. When we try harder, all

During most of a forced expiration, flow is limited by critical narrowing of the airway; further effort does not result in augmented flow.

we do is compress the airway further, without any increase in the flow rate. This part of the flow-volume curve is frequently termed the *effort-independent portion*, where, beyond a certain level of effort, further effort does not result in an augmented flow rate.

There are still two questions we have not answered about maximal expiratory flow. First, why does critical narrowing of the airway occur, so that increasing effort proves fruitless in augmenting flow? Second, at what level in the airways does this critical narrowing occur? These are questions that have been of great interest to pulmonary physiologists, and we will try to distill answers to them from a large amount of theory and research.

During a forced expiration, there are several determinants of airway diameter. First and most obvious is the inherent size of the airway, which depends on its level in the tracheobronchial tree and the tone of the airway smooth muscle. In disease, smooth muscle tone may be increased (as in asthma), or secretions in the airway may narrow the lumen (as in asthma or chronic bronchitis). Second is the amount of radial traction exerted by surrounding lung tissue on the airway walls. We must remember that airways are not isolated structures, but are surrounded by a supporting framework of alveolar walls that are constantly "pulling" or "tethering" the airways open. As we will discuss in Chapter 6, when lung parenchyma is destroyed, as in emphysema, the airways lose some of their normal support and are more likely to collapse. Third, and perhaps most difficult to understand, is the combination of pressures acting on the airway from without and within. This balance of pressures is crucial in determining whether a particular airway remains open or closed during a forced expiration.

Airway diameter depends on the level of the airway in the tracheobronchial tree, airway smooth muscle tone, traction on the airway from surrounding lung tissue, and internal and external pressures on the airway.

The external pressure acting on an airway is determined to a large extent by pleural pressure (Fig. 4–5). When pleural pressure is strongly positive, as with a forced expiration, the airway becomes compressed. It is only because of a counteracting pressure within the airways that they are able to remain open in the face of a strongly positive external pressure. Two factors contribute to this counteracting internal airway

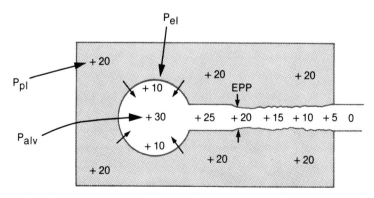

Figure 4–5. Schematic diagram of the equal pressure point (EPP) concept during a forced (maximal) expiration. An alveolus and its airway are shown inside a box, which represents the pleural space. Alveolar pressure (P_{alv}) has two contributing components—pleural pressure (P_{pl}) and the elastic recoil pressure of the lung (P_{el}). In this diagram, P_{pl} = 20 cm H_2O and P_{el} = 10 cm H_2O. P_{alv}, the sum of P_{pl} and P_{el}, is therefore 30 cm H_2O.

pressure: (1) the elastic recoil of the lungs and (2) pleural pressure transmitted to the alveoli and airways. If we look at Figure 4–5, we see that the alveolar wall is like a stretched balloon trying to expel its air. In the same way that the balloon, in trying to collapse, exerts pressure on the air inside, the alveolar wall has its elastic recoil that exerts pressure on the gas within. This pressure results in flow through the airways, but as we mentioned earlier, flow through an airway must result in a pressure drop along the airway. At a certain point along the airway, the pressure falls enough so that pressure within the airway becomes equal to the pressure outside of the airway (i.e., pleural pressure). This point has been called the *equal pressure point*. If one increases the amount of effort, i.e., the amount of pleural pressure, this pressure is exerted both on the alveolus and externally on the airway wall. The driving pressure, the difference between alveolar pressure and the pressure at the equal pressure point, remains the elastic recoil pressure of the lung. One can see from Figure 4–5 that, with additional effort, the increased alveolar driving pressure is exactly balanced by the increased external pressure on the airway. This increased external pressure promotes airway collapse. The net result is that the elastic recoil pressure is an important determinant of maximal expiratory flow, whereas pleural pressure produced by expiratory effort does not play a role, at least in the effort-independent or latter part of a forced expiration. We will see in subsequent chapters that in diseases with altered elastic recoil, maximal expiratory flow rates are affected by this change in the effective driving pressure for airflow.

At the equal pressure point, internal and external pressures on the airway are equal. The net driving pressure from the alveolus to the equal pressure point is the elastic recoil pressure of the lung.

The final question we will address is the level at which this critical narrowing, i.e., the equal pressure point, occurs. The answer actually depends on the lung volume; in other words, the equal pressure point does not remain at a constant position as we go further along the flow volume curve toward residual volume. At higher lung volumes, the elastic recoil pressure is greater (the alveoli are stretched more), and a longer distance separates the alveoli from the equal pressure point. At lung volumes above functional residual capacity, this critical point of narrowing is within relatively large airways, segmental bronchi or larger. At lower lung volumes, the elastic recoil pressure is lower, the distance from alveoli to the equal pressure point is smaller, and critical narrowing occurs more peripherally. Since maximal airflow depends on elastic recoil and the resistance of the airways peripheral ("upstream") to the equal pressure point, the resistance of the small airways is a larger component of the upstream resistance at small lung volumes and is therefore a greater determinant of maximal expiratory flow at lower volumes along the flow-volume curve.

In summary, flow through the tracheobronchial tree reflects a combination of factors—airway size, support or radial traction exerted by the surrounding lung parenchyma, and driving pressure provided by the elastic recoil of the lung. Though pleural pressure contributes to the driving pressure for airflow, it also exerts a counterbalancing external pressure on the airway, promoting airway collapse. When we discuss specific disorders, we will see how these different factors are interrelated as determinants of maximal expiratory airflow and how they can be altered in disease states.

The equal pressure point moves peripherally (toward smaller airways) as lung volume decreases during a forced expiration; hence the resistance of small airways limits maximal expiratory flow more at low than at high lung volumes.

REFERENCES

Comroe, J. H.: Physiology of Respiration. 2nd ed. Chicago, Year Book Medical Publishers, 1974.

Ebert, R. V.: Small airways of the lung: the importance of understanding and assessing the function of pulmonary bronchioles. Ann. Intern. Med. 88:98–103, 1978.

Gail, D. B., and Lenfant, C. J. M.: Cells of the lung: biology and clinical implications. Am. Rev. Respir. Dis. 127:366–387, 1983.

Horsfield, K.: The structure of the tracheobronchial tree. *In* Scadding, J. G., and Cumming, G. (eds.): Scientific Foundations of Respiratory Medicine. Philadelphia, W. B. Saunders Co., 1981, pp. 54–70.

Hyatt, R. E., and Black, L. F.: The flow-volume curve: a current perspective. Am. Rev. Respir. Dis. 107:191–199, 1973.

McFadden, E. R., Jr., and Ingram, R. H., Jr.: Clinical application and interpretation of airway physiology. *In* Nadel, J. A. (ed.): Physiology and Pharmacology of the Airways. New York, Marcel Dekker, Inc., 1980, pp. 297–324.

Murray, J. F.: The Normal Lung: The Basis for Diagnosis and Treatment of Pulmonary Disease. Philadelphia, W. B. Saunders Co., 1976.

Richardson, J. B., and Ferguson, C. C.: Morphology of the airways. *In* Nadel, J. A. (ed.): Physiology and Pharmacology of the Airways. New York, Marcel Dekker, Inc., 1980, pp. 1–30.

Robinson, D. R., Chaudhary, B. A., and Speir, W. A., Jr.: Expiratory flow limitation in large and small airways. Arch. Intern. Med. 144:1457–1460, 1984.

West, J. B.: Respiratory Physiology—The Essentials. 2nd ed. Baltimore, Williams & Wilkins, 1979.

5

Asthma

In Chapter 4, we discussed the normal structure of airways and considered several aspects of airway function. The most common disorders disrupting the normal structure and function of the airways, asthma and chronic obstructive pulmonary disease, will be discussed here and in Chapter 6, respectively, and several other miscellaneous diseases affecting airways will be covered in Chapter 7.

Asthma is a condition characterized by episodes of reversible airway narrowing, associated with contraction of smooth muscle within the airway wall. It is a very common disorder, affecting approximately 3 to 5 percent of the population. Though asthma can occur in any age group, it is particularly common in children and young adults and is probably the most common chronic disease found in these age groups.

The single feature that patients with asthma appear to have in common is *hyperreactivity* of the airways, i.e., an exaggerated response of airway smooth muscle to a wide variety of stimuli. What often varies from patient to patient is the particular constellation of stimuli triggering the attacks, but the net effect—bronchoconstriction—is qualitatively similar. Since asthma is by definition a disease with at least some reversibility, the patient experiences exacerbations, or "attacks," interspersed between relatively symptom-free periods. During an attack, the diagnosis is usually straightforward; during a symptom-free period, the diagnosis may be more difficult to make and may require provocation or challenge tests to induce airway constriction.

Asthma is characterized by hyperreactivity of the airways and reversible episodes of bronchoconstriction.

73

ETIOLOGY AND PATHOGENESIS

Despite the prevalence of asthma in the general population and the many advances that have been made in treating the manifestations of the disease, a great deal about its etiology and pathogenesis remains speculative. In this section, we will discuss two major questions. (1) What causes certain people to have airways that hyperreact to various stimuli? (2) What is the sequence of events from the time of exposure to the stimulus until the time of clinical response?

There appears to be at least some association between asthma and allergy, but the overall importance of an allergic background is quite controversial. A substantial proportion of patients with asthma have an underlying history of allergies, and their asthma is frequently exacerbated by exposure to various allergens to which they have been previously sensitized. In patients with an allergic component to their asthma, there is also often a strong family history of asthma or other allergies, suggesting that genetic factors may play a role in the development of asthma.

The particular trait that seems to be inherited is the tendency to form antibodies of the IgE class, called reaginic antibodies, to a variety of antigens in the environment. The ready production of these antibodies is associated not only with asthma but also with other common forms of allergy, such as allergic rhinitis (hayfever) or eczema. A person who has this predisposition for hyperproduction of IgE, often with one or more of the associated clinical problems, is said to be *atopic*, and the condition is termed *atopy*.

Though some asthmatic patients have allergies, many do not, and the overall relationship between allergies and asthma is not clear.

However, not all asthmatics fall into the allergic category; many have no other evidence for atopy and do not experience exacerbations as a result of antigen exposure. In this latter group, asthma is sometimes called "idiosyncratic" and is often exacerbated by upper respiratory tract infections.

Other names that have been used for identifying these types of asthma (but have largely fallen out of favor) are "extrinsic" and "intrinsic." The term *extrinsic asthma*, which has been used for allergic asthma, implies an external factor such as an allergen that precipitates an attack. In contrast, the term *intrinsic asthma*, which refers to the idiosyncratic disorder, connotes an innate problem that results in asthma for undetermined reasons.

Despite the different names, the single feature that these two categories of patients have in common is the hyperreactivity of their airways to a variety of stimuli. As we will soon discuss, we can explain at least part of the mechanism leading from allergen exposure to bronchoconstriction, but we do not yet know the reason for increased airways reactivity in either of the groups.

An intriguing (but as yet unproven) hypothesis to explain why asthmatics have hyperreactive airways relates to the autonomic nervous system. But whether or not autonomic nervous system abnormalities contribute to a predisposition to develop asthma, knowledge about the effects of sympathetic and parasympathetic activity on airway tone (and on release of chemical mediators that affect airway tone) has allowed many advances in the therapy of asthma. Adrenergic receptors, which respond to the catecholamine output from sympathetic nerves and from the adrenal medulla, are found on large as well as small airways. The main adrenergic receptor subtype on airways is the beta-2 receptor, which when stimulated results in bronchodilation. Airways also have alpha-receptors, whose stimulation results in bronchoconstriction. Interestingly, though both of these receptor types are found on airways, airways do not appear to have any significant innervation by sympathetic nerves. The natural question to ask then is why these receptors are present. We are not entirely sure, but we do know that they can be stimulated by circulating catecholamines originating from the adrenal medulla.

Stimulation of beta-2-adrenergic receptors produces bronchodilation; stimulation of cholinergic or alpha-adrenergic receptors results in bronchoconstriction.

Cholinergic receptors are also present on airways, and they have corresponding innervation from the parasympathetic nervous system via the vagus nerve. The vagus primarily innervates the larger airways, stimulating cholinergic receptors and resulting in bronchoconstriction. There is no circulating acetylcholine, so the cholinergic receptors are stimulated only by the local nerve supply from the vagus.

Now that we have briefly outlined the basic aspects of the autonomic nervous system and airway tone, we can consider how abnormalities of this system might predispose someone to develop asthma. In 1968, Szentivanyi proposed that decreased responsiveness or blockade of beta receptors might be the underlying defect in bronchial asthma. Though this hypothesis has generally fallen out of favor, recently the idea that autonomic dysfunction may play an important role in asthma has been revived. Besides an abnormality in beta receptor responsiveness, other alternative possibilities include either increased alpha adrenergic responsiveness or heightened cholinergic activity. For example, Kaliner and co-workers have found decreased beta-receptor and increased alpha- and cholinergic-receptor sensitivity in allergic asthmatics. Since other allergic subjects without asthma also had equivalent beta-adrenergic and cholinergic abnormalities, they postulated that alpha hyperresponsiveness might be a fundamental defect in asthma. At this time, however, the issue remains unresolved.

One theory suggests that autonomic nervous system abnormalities contribute to the pathogenesis of asthma.

For the asthmatic patient, a substantial amount is now known about the sequence of events occurring from time of exposure to a stimulus until the clinical response of bronchoconstriction. We will specifically consider four stimuli that can result in bronchoconstriction: (1) allergen (antigen) exposure, (2) inhaled irritants, (3) respiratory tract infection, and (4) exercise.

Common stimuli precipitating bronchoconstriction in the asthmatic patient are:
1. exposure to an allergen
2. inhaled irritants
3. respiratory tract infection
4. exercise

Allergens

Allergens to which an asthmatic may be sensitized are widespread in nature. Several of the most common airborne antigens precipitating asthmatic attacks are found in house dust, molds, and animal dander. When an asthmatic has IgE antibody against a particular antigen, the antibody binds to receptors on mast cells and basophils (Fig. 5–1). If the antigen is inhaled, it probably binds to a relatively small number of mast cells in the bronchial lumen that have IgE antibody (against the antigen) bound to their surface. Because of mediators released from these luminal mast cells, permeability of the airway epithelium is increased, allowing the antigen access to the much larger population of specific IgE-containing mast cells that are deeper within the epithelium. The binding of antigen to antibody on the mast cell again initiates

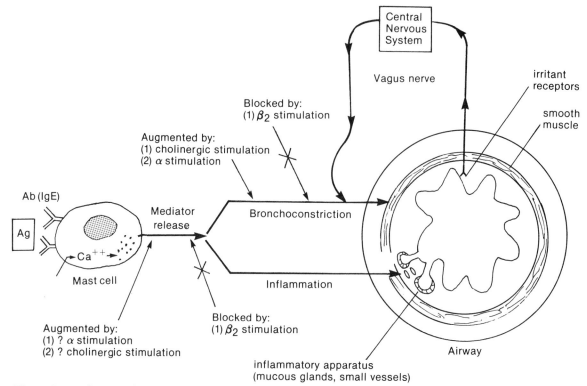

Figure 5–1. Schematic diagram of events in the pathogenesis of asthma, focusing on antigen-induced bronchoconstriction and airway inflammation. Note that the mast cell (shown on the left) is found both in the airway lumen and within the airway wall.

a sequence of events leading to release of chemical mediators capable of inducing bronchoconstriction and inflammation.

Whenever an IgE antibody attached to a mast cell combines with its specific antigen, it is thought that this reaction initiates movement of calcium ion (Ca^{++}) into the intracellular space. Increasing the concentration of free intracellular Ca^{++} results in release of a variety of chemical mediators from the mast cell, as shown in Figure 5–1. A large number of such mediators have now been recognized (Table 5–1), but we will limit discussion to the few that have been primarily implicated in the pathogenesis of allergic asthma. The major mediators and their potential effects include:

Histamine. This relatively small (M.W. 111) compound is found

Table 5–1. POTENTIAL CHEMICAL MEDIATORS IN ASTHMA

Histamine
SRS-A (leukotrienes)
Eosinophil chemotactic factor of anaphylaxis
Neutrophil chemotactic factor of anaphylaxis
Prostaglandins
Bradykinin
Serotonin
Kallikrein
Platelet-activating factor

preformed within the mast cell and is released upon exposure to the appropriate antigen. Histamine has several effects that may be important in asthma, including contraction of bronchial smooth muscle, augmentation of vascular permeability with formation of airway edema, and stimulation of irritant receptors (which can trigger a reflex neurogenic pathway via the vagus, causing secondary bronchoconstriction). Despite these varied effects, the fact that the clinical manifestations of asthma do not respond to antihistamines suggests that histamine is not the most important chemical mediator involved.

SRS-A (Slow-reacting Substance of Anaphylaxis). Unlike histamine, SRS-A is not preformed in the mast cell but is synthesized after antigen exposure and then released. To some extent, its actions are similar to those of histamine; it also has a direct bronchoconstrictor action on smooth muscle and can increase vascular permeability. The structure of SRS-A has only recently been elucidated, and it appears to be composed of members of the class of compounds known as *leukotrienes*. The leukotrienes are synthesized from arachidonic acid (also the precursor for prostaglandins) but along a somewhat different pathway, involving a lipoxygenase enzyme as opposed to the cyclooxygenase enzyme used for prostaglandin synthesis (Fig. 5–2). Some of the leukotrienes are extraordinarily potent bronchoconstrictors, and they may indeed have a crucial role in the pathogenesis of bronchial asthma. An interesting sidelight is provided by knowledge that some asthmatics experience exacerbations of their disease after taking aspirin or other nonsteroidal anti-inflammatory drugs. These drugs are known to be inhibitors of the cyclooxygenase enzyme and may result in preferential shifting of the pathway outlined in Figure 5–2 toward production of the bronchoconstrictor leukotrienes.

The role of the other mediators listed in Table 5–1 in the

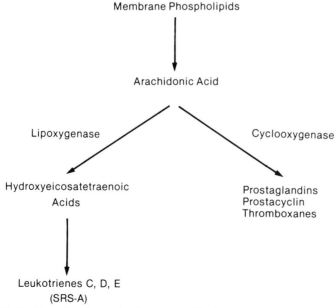

Figure 5–2. Outline of pathway for formation of leukotrienes (SRS-A) and prostaglandins. Aspirin and other nonsteroidal anti-inflammatory drugs are inhibitors of the enzyme cyclooxygenase.

pathogenesis of asthma is less clear. Two of the chemical mediators, eosinophil chemotactic factor of anaphylaxis (ECF-A) and neutrophil chemotactic factor (NCF), may be important in attracting inflammatory cells into the bronchial wall.

Inhaled Irritants

Inhaled irritants such as cigarette smoke and inorganic dusts are also common precipitants of bronchoconstriction in asthmatic patients. These airborne irritants appear to stimulate *irritant receptors* located primarily in the walls of the larynx, trachea, and large bronchi. Stimulation of the receptors initiates a reflex arc which travels to the central nervous system and back to the bronchi via the vagus nerve. This efferent vagal stimulation of the bronchi completes the reflex arc and induces bronchoconstriction. As we also mentioned in the discussion about chemical mediators, histamine is capable of stimulating irritant receptors, and at least part of its bronchoconstrictive effect may be mediated indirectly via stimulation of the irritant receptors.

Respiratory Tract Infection

The third common stimulus for bronchoconstriction, respiratory tract infection, is a factor for patients with nonallergic as well as allergic asthma. Viral infections are the most common ones in this category, but bacterial infections of the tracheobronchial tree can also sometimes be implicated. The mechanism by which respiratory infections precipitate bronchoconstriction in asthmatics is not entirely clear but may be related to airway inflammation. The resultant epithelial damage may then stimulate the irritant receptors or lower their threshold for stimulation by other environmental irritants.

Exercise

Finally, exercise frequently can provoke bronchoconstriction in patients with hyperreactive airways. Recent work has demonstrated that the crucial factor here is airway cooling. During exercise, subjects have a high minute ventilation, and the large amounts of relatively cool and dry inspired air must be warmed and humidified by the tracheobronchial mucosa. When the air is warmed and humidified, water evaporates from the epithelial surface, resulting in cooling of the airway epithelium. The phenomenon of exercise-induced bronchoconstriction can be reproduced by having an asthmatic subject voluntarily breathe cold, dry air at a high minute ventilation. At the same minute ventilation, inhalation of warm, saturated air does not produce a similar effect.

Autonomic nervous system mechanisms and mediators from mast cells interact to produce the bronchoconstriction and airway inflammatory response of asthma.

In discussing the pathogenesis of bronchoconstriction in asthma, we must also reiterate the role of adrenergic and cholinergic influences in modifying airway tone. As we mentioned earlier, airways have beta-2, alpha, and cholinergic receptors. Stimulation of these receptors, either by drugs, circulating hormones, or firing of nerves, eventually changes airway tone via an effect on cyclic nucleotides. Stimulation of beta-2 receptors activates the enzyme adenyl cyclase, resulting in increased amounts of intracellular cyclic AMP (cAMP) in smooth muscle and mast cells. High levels of cAMP block Ca^{++} entry and therefore result in bronchodilation. Cyclic AMP also affects mediator release from mast cells—increases in cAMP inhibit mediator release, while decreases augment release. Some evidence suggests that in contrast to beta-2 receptors, stimulation of alpha-receptors decreases cAMP levels and results in bronchoconstriction and augmentation of mediator release. It has also been proposed that the activity of cholinergic receptors may be modulated not by cAMP but by a related compound, cyclic GMP (cGMP). Cyclic GMP often has different effects than cAMP and could be responsible for bronchoconstriction and increased mediator release from mast cells. By this mechanism, stimulation of cholinergic receptors, e.g., from firing of the vagus nerve, would have effects opposite to those of beta-2 stimulation both on bronchial smooth muscle and on mast cells. These concepts are summarized in Figure 5–1.

PATHOLOGY

Information about the pathologic findings in asthma has generally been obtained at autopsy studies and thus is limited to particularly severe disease. In these cases, there is marked overdistention of the lungs, and the airways are occluded by thick, tenacious mucous plugs. Examination of the airways by microscopy demonstrates the following findings:

1. Hypertrophy of the smooth muscle layer
2. Thickening of the epithelial basement membrane
3. Enlargement of the mucus-secreting apparatus, with hypertrophy of mucous glands and an increased number of goblet cells
4. Infiltrates of eosinophils within the bronchial wall

We presume that milder attacks of asthma have similar but less pronounced morphologic changes. In between attacks, many of these pathologic changes can apparently revert to normal. Therefore, in the same way that we speak about the reversible physiologic changes in asthma, we can also view the pathologic changes as similarly reversible.

PATHOPHYSIOLOGY

The pathophysiologic features of asthma largely follow from the pathologic abnormalities we have just described. Contraction of smooth muscle in the bronchial walls, mucosal edema, and secretions within the airway lumen all contribute to a decrease in airway diameter, which increases airway resistance. The pathologic changes are present at many levels of the tracheobronchial tree, from large airways down to the peripheral airways of less than 2 mm diameter.

As a result of narrowed airways with increased resistance, patients have difficulty with airflow during both inspiration and expiration. However, since intrathoracic airways are subjected to relatively negative external pressure (transmitted from negative pleural pressure) during inspiration, lumen size is larger during the inspiratory phase of the respiratory cycle. During expiration, relatively positive pleural pressure is transmitted to intrathoracic airways, thus decreasing their diameter. Hence greater difficulty with airflow during expiration than inspiration is characteristic of asthma, as it is of any of the diseases causing obstruction or narrowing of airways within the thorax. The greatest difficulty with expiration is seen when the patient is asked to perform a forced expiration, i.e., to breathe out as hard and as fast as possible. With a forced expiration, pleural pressure becomes much more positive, thereby promoting airway closure and air trapping.

In asthma and other diseases associated with obstruction of intrathoracic airways, airflow is most compromised during expiration.

The effects of increased airways resistance are readily seen by measuring pulmonary function in asthmatics. During an attack, pulmonary function studies show decreases in forced expiratory flow rates as well as evidence of air trapping. On the forced expiratory spirogram, patients generally exhibit a decrease in both FVC and FEV_1, with the decrease in FEV_1 usually more pronounced than the decrease in FVC. Hence the ratio FEV_1/FVC, reflecting the proportion of the forced vital capacity that can be exhaled during the first second, is decreased. In addition, the maximal mid-expiratory flow rate (MMFR) is also diminished.

Measurement of lung volumes shows evidence of air trapping, with increases in FRC, RV, and sometimes TLC. Of all these lung volumes, the most impressive increase is in RV, the volume left in the lungs at the end of a maximal exhalation, which may be greater than 200 percent of the predicted value. The increase in RV is thought to be due at least partly to premature airway closure as a result of all the processes we discussed—smooth muscle constriction, mucous plugs, and inflammatory changes of the mucosa.

It is not entirely clear whether TLC truly increases or how this might occur. There are two main factors that determine TLC—inspiratory muscles acting to expand the chest, and elastic recoil of the lung acting to decrease lung volume. For reasons that are not certain, some evidence suggests that elastic recoil is decreased during acute asthma attacks, and it has also been suggested that inspiratory muscle strength (or the efficiency of contraction) may be increased.

Pulmonary function tests with asthma generally demonstrate a decreased FEV_1, FVC, and FEV_1/FVC ratio; air trapping and hyperinflation are demonstrated by increases in RV, FRC, and sometimes TLC.

Functional residual capacity (FRC), the resting point of the lungs after a normal expiration, may also be increased for at least two reasons. First, since more time is required for expiration when airways are obstructed, patients may not have sufficient time before the next breath to exhale fully the volume from the previous breath. This phenomenon is sometimes called *dynamic hyperinflation* and is particularly a problem when the asthmatic patient is breathing at a rapid respiratory rate. Another reason for the increase in FRC is related to a possible change in the lung's elastic recoil. As we mentioned in Chapter 1, two factors normally determine FRC—the inward elastic recoil of the lung acting to decrease lung volume, and the outward recoil of the chest wall acting to increase the volume. If the elastic recoil of the lung is decreased during acute asthma, the restraining force for the outward recoil of the chest wall is less, and FRC is therefore increased.

We have so far described the pulmonary function and physiologic abnormalities with an asthma attack of significant severity. In between attacks, pulmonary function may return to normal. However, it is important to realize that even when a patient is not having an acute attack, subtle abnormalities in pulmonary function may be present, such as a decrease in MMFR and an increase in RV. These abnormalities may reflect some residual disease in the small airways of the lung, which are frequently the last region to become normal after an attack.

The increased resistance to airflow also exerts its toll on gas exchange, which is generally disturbed during acute attacks. The most common pattern of arterial blood gases in asthma consists of a low P_{O_2} accompanied by a low P_{CO_2} (respiratory alkalosis). The mechanism for the hypoxemia is ventilation-perfusion mismatch. The increased airways resistance in asthma is not evenly distributed, i.e., some airways are affected more than others. Therefore, inspired air is not distributed evenly, but tends to go to less diseased areas. However, blood flow remains relatively preserved in the regions that are ventilating poorly. The regions of low ventilation-perfusion ($\dot{V}/\dot{Q}$) ratio result in a decreased P_{O_2} of arterial blood that cannot be made up for by increases in the $\dot{V}/\dot{Q}$ ratio from other regions of lung (see Chapter 1).

Despite the abnormality in P_{O_2}, the patients are able to hyperventilate, and P_{CO_2} is usually low. When P_{CO_2} increases to normal or to a frankly elevated level, it often means worsening airflow obstruction or a tiring patient who is no longer able to maintain normal or high minute ventilation in the face of significant airflow obstruction. The stimulus or mechanism for the hyperventilation is not clear. During an acute asthma attack, it is possible that activation of irritant receptors stimulates ventilation or that other reflexes originating in the airways, lung, or chest wall may serve to stimulate ventilation.

The most common pattern of arterial blood gases in asthma is a low P_{O_2} (due primarily to $\dot{V}/\dot{Q}$ mismatch) and a low P_{CO_2}.

following hyperventilation

CLINICAL FEATURES

The onset of asthma occurs most frequently during childhood and young adulthood, though it is also common to see older patients develop asthma for the first time. In the majority of patients, particularly those in whom asthma started before age 16, the disease eventually regresses, and they are no longer subject to repeated episodes of reversible airway obstruction.

The symptoms most commonly noted by patients during an exacerbation of asthma are cough, dyspnea, wheezing, and chest tightness. It is important to realize that patients do not necessarily present classically with several or all of these complaints, but may merely have an unexplained cough or breathlessness on exertion. In some cases, patients can clearly identify a precipitating factor for an attack, such as exposure to an allergen, respiratory tract infection, exercise, exposure to cold air, emotional stress, or exposure to irritating dusts, fumes, or odors. In other cases, there is no identifiable precipitant. As we discussed earlier, some asthmatics are particularly sensitive to ingestion of aspirin, which perhaps favors production of leukotrienes from arachidonic acid. These patients often have nasal polyps associated with their asthma and aspirin sensitivity. Other nonsteroidal anti-inflammatory drugs (which also inhibit the cyclooxygenase enzyme) may also produce bronchoconstriction in these patients.

On examination, patients experiencing an asthma attack are usually tachypneic, and on auscultation of the chest are found to have prolonged expiration and evidence of wheezing. The wheezing is generally more

Major symptoms during an acute asthma attack are:
1. cough
2. dyspnea
3. wheezing
4. chest tightness

Despite its prominence, the presence of wheezing is not synonymous with asthma and merely reflects airflow through narrowed airways.

prominent during expiration than inspiration, and it may be brought out by having the patient exhale forcefully. Though we often equate wheezing and asthma, the presence of wheezing does not at all necessarily indicate a diagnosis of asthma. Wheezing only reflects airflow through narrowed airways; it can also be seen in such diverse disorders as congestive heart failure and chronic obstructive pulmonary disease, or in the case of a foreign body in the airway. On the other hand, not all asthmatics wheeze. Of particular importance is the common observation that very severe asthma may be associated with no wheeze if airflow is too impaired to generate an audible wheeze.

When asthmatics have a particularly severe attack that is refractory to treatment with bronchodilators, they are said to be in *status asthmaticus*. These patients provide difficult therapeutic challenges, may require assisted ventilation, and unfortunately may even die as a result of the acute attack.

DIAGNOSTIC APPROACH

A clinical history of reversible episodes of bronchoconstriction is often crucial to the diagnosis of asthma. Helpful additional features in the history include other evidence for atopy (such as hayfever or eczema) or a positive family history of allergies or asthma. Physical examination during an attack provides confirmatory evidence for airway obstruction.

The chest roentgenogram, though important for ruling out other causes of wheezing or complications of asthma, is generally not particularly helpful in the diagnosis. It is usually normal, but it may demonstrate hyperinflation with relatively large lung volumes.

If the patient is producing sputum, microscopic examination frequently shows many eosinophils on the sputum smear. An increased percentage of eosinophils in peripheral blood is also common, even when the asthma has no clear relationship to allergies.

There is much debate about the usefulness of skin testing and inhalation testing with allergens in an attempt to identify antigens to which the patient is sensitized. Unfortunately, these tests do not necessarily correlate with each other and do not establish that antigens causing positive tests have been responsible for exacerbations of asthma.

Other types of provocation tests used to make a diagnosis of asthma rely on the principle that asthmatics have hyperreactive airways. Therefore, when tested with inhalation of either methacholine (a cholinergic agent) or histamine, asthmatics respond with bronchoconstriction to comparatively small doses of either agent. Recently, inhalation of cold air at high minute ventilations with P_{CO_2} kept constant (termed *isocapneic hyperpnea*) has been used as a challenge test to induce transient bronchoconstriction in patients in whom the diagnosis of asthma is uncertain.

Testing of pulmonary function is particularly useful in the patient with suspected or known asthma. The abnormalities that appear were mentioned earlier in the discussion of pathophysiology, and even measurement of just the FEV_1 and FVC can provide invaluable information. Documentation of reversible airflow obstruction, either during attacks or with the challenge tests mentioned above, is frequently sufficient to make the diagnosis of asthma. In practice, the diagnosis of asthma is most commonly made by the history of episodic dyspnea, wheezing, or cough, with documentation of reversible airflow obstruction by pulmonary function testing.

A diagnosis of asthma includes a history of episodic dyspnea, wheezing, or cough, along with reversible airflow obstruction documented by pulmonary function testing.

TREATMENT

Several categories of drugs are used to treat asthma, ranging from those that dilate smooth muscle of the bronchial wall to those that inhibit release of chemical mediators from mast cells. These categories are outlined in Table 5–2. Several of the drugs are used for other types of pulmonary disease, particularly chronic obstructive pulmonary disease, and will be mentioned in other chapters in this book.

Probably the most common agents in use for treatment of asthma are those that increase intracellular cAMP levels in both bronchial smooth muscle cells and mast cells. As we mentioned earlier, increased levels of cAMP in bronchial smooth muscle result in bronchodilation, while in mast cells cAMP inhibits release of chemical mediators that secondarily cause bronchoconstriction. Agents in the sympathomimetic category act on beta receptors, thus activating adenyl cyclase and increasing intracellular cAMP. A few examples of these drugs are listed in Table 5–2. Recently, interest has focused on limiting the action of these drugs to stimulation of beta-2 receptors, in order to avoid some of the adverse cardiac effects induced by stimulation of beta-1 receptors. Some of the more beta-2-specific agents are metaproterenol, terbutaline, and albuterol (salbutamol). Sympathomimetic agents can be given

Sympathomimetic agents increase intracellular cyclic AMP by activating adenyl cyclase; newer agents preferentially stimulate beta-2 receptors and decrease potential adverse cardiac effects caused by stimulation of beta-1 receptors.

↑ cAMP = bronchodilat⁰ⁿ

Table 5–2. DRUG THERAPY OF ASTHMA

Drug	Examples	Possible Routes of Administration	Mechanism of Action
Bronchodilators Sympatho- mimetics	Epinephrine Isoproterenol Isoetharine Metaproterenol Terbutaline Albuterol	Inhaled, oral, parenteral (depending on particular drug)	↑ cAMP via stimulation of adenyl cyclase
Xanthines	Theophylline Aminophylline	Oral Oral, parenteral	↑ cAMP via inhibition of phosphodiesterase *wh. normally degrades cAMP*
Anti- cholin- ergics	Atropine Ipratropium	Inhaled	Blockade of cholinergic (bronchoconstrictor) effect on airways
Cromolyn (disodium cromoglycate)		Inhaled	Inhibition of mediator release from mast cells; ? additional mechanisms *prophylaxis*
Corticosteroids		Oral, parenteral, inhaled	Unknown

Methylxanthines (aminophylline, theophylline) increase cyclic AMP by inhibiting the enzyme phosphodiesterase, which degrades cyclic AMP.

by several different routes, including oral or parenteral administration and inhalation.

The second class of agents, the methylxanthines, consists of inhibitors of the enzyme phosphodiesterase, which normally is responsible for the metabolic degradation of cAMP. Since degradation is inhibited, the levels of cAMP in smooth muscle and mast cells increase, resulting again in bronchodilation and decreased mediator release from mast cells. The most commonly used methylxanthines are theophylline and aminophylline. Theophylline is available only for oral administration, while aminophylline (a water-soluble salt of theophylline) can be given either orally or intravenously.

A third type of treatment, used less frequently, includes drugs that have an anticholinergic action. Atropine is the primary example of this class, though other experimental agents have also been used. By decreasing cholinergic stimulation, atropine dilates bronchial smooth muscle and may inhibit mediator release from mast cells. When used for asthma, atropine is usually given via inhalation.

The fourth type of treatment for asthma is quite different from the first three, its major action being inhibition of mediator release from mast cells. The drug in this class, disodium cromoglycate (cromolyn) is believed to inhibit mediator release by stabilizing the membrane of mast cells. This drug is inhaled as a powder, and in itself can be fairly irritating to the airways. Hence it has no role in the treatment of the acute asthmatic attack. Rather, it is generally given during a period of remission, with the goal of preventing future exacerbations.

The final category of drugs used to treat asthma includes the corticosteroids. Though these agents have been used for years in the treatment of asthmatic attacks, their mechanism of action is still unknown. Several hypotheses have been proposed, including suggestions that they decrease the overall inflammatory process in the airways, or that they enhance the cAMP response to adrenergic stimulation. Frequently, steroids such as hydrocortisone or prednisone are started at high doses during an attack and then are tapered relatively rapidly. Because of the potential for significant adverse effects with long-term use of steroids, chronic administration is avoided if the asthma can be managed with other modes of therapy.

REFERENCES

Reviews

Reed, C. E.: Asthma. *In* Simmons, D. H. (ed.): Current Pulmonology. Vol. 2. Boston, Houghton Mifflin, 1980, pp. 69–101.

Reed, C. E.: Asthma. *In* Simmons, D. H. (ed.): Current Pulmonology. Vol. 4. New York, John Wiley & Sons, 1982, pp. 25–42.

Saunders, N. A., and McFadden, E. R., Jr.: Asthma—an update. DM 24(11):1–49, 1978.

Etiology and Pathogenesis

Austen, K. F., and Orange, R. P.: Bronchial asthma: the possible role of the chemical mediators of immediate hypersensitivity in the pathogenesis of subacute chronic disease. Am. Rev. Respir. Dis. 112:423–436, 1975.

Boushey, H. A., Holtzman, M. J., Sheller, J. R., and Nadel, J. A.: Bronchial hyperreactivity. Am. Rev. Respir. Dis. 121:389–413, 1980.

Kaliner, M., Shelhamer, J. H., Davis, P. B., Smith, L. J., and Venter, J. C.: Autonomic nervous system abnormalities and allergy. Ann. Intern. Med. 96:349–357, 1982.

Leff, A.: Pathogenesis of asthma: neurophysiology and pharmacology of bronchospasm. Chest 81:224–229, 1982.

McFadden, E. R., Jr., and Ingram, R. H., Jr.: Exercise-induced asthma: observations on the initiating stimulus. N. Engl. J. Med. 301:763–769, 1979.

Nadel, J. A., and Barnes, P. J.: Autonomic regulation of the airways. Ann. Rev. Med. 35:451–467, 1984.

Clinical Aspects

Corrao, W. M., Braman, S. S., and Irwin, R. S.: Chronic cough as the sole presenting manifestation of bronchial asthma. N. Engl. J. Med. 300:633–637, 1979.

McFadden, E. R., Jr.: Exertional dyspnea and cough as preludes to acute attacks of asthma. N. Engl. J. Med. 292:555–559, 1975.

McFadden, E. R., Jr., Kiser, R., and DeGroot, W. J.: Acute bronchial asthma: relations between clinical and physiologic manifestations. N. Engl. J. Med. 288:221–225, 1973.

McFadden, E. R., Jr., and Lyons, H. A.: Arterial-blood gas tension in asthma. N. Engl. J. Med. 278:1027–1032, 1968.

Diagnostic Approach

Deal, E. C., Jr., McFadden, E. R., Jr., Ingram, R. H., Jr., Breslin, F. J., and Jaeger, J. J.: Airway responsiveness to cold air and hyperpnea in normal subjects and in those with hay fever and asthma. Am. Rev. Respir. Dis. 121:621–628, 1980.

Myers, J. R., Corrao, W. M., and Braman, S. S.: Clinical applicability of a methacholine inhalational challenge. JAMA 246:225–229, 1981.

Pepys, J.: Inhalation challenge tests in asthma. N. Engl. J. Med. 293:758–759, 1975.

Pepys, J., and Hutchcroft, B. J.: Bronchial provocation tests in etiologic diagnosis and analysis of asthma. Am. Rev. Respir. Dis. 112:829–859, 1975.

Pratter, M. R., and Irwin, R. S.: The clinical value of pharmacologic bronchoprovocation challenge. Chest 85:260–265, 1984.

Treatment

Paterson, J. W., Woolcock, A. J., and Shenfield, G. M.: Bronchodilator drugs. Am. Rev. Respir. Dis. 120:1149–1188, 1979.

VanArsdel, P. P., Jr., and Paul, G. H.: Drug therapy in the management of asthma. Ann. Intern. Med. 87:68–74, 1977.

Webb-Johnson, D. C., and Andrews, J. L., Jr.: Bronchodilator therapy. N. Engl. J. Med. 297:476–482; 758–764, 1977.

6

Chronic Obstructive Pulmonary Disease

The term chronic obstructive pulmonary disease (COPD) generally refers to chronic disorders that disturb airflow, whether the most prominent process is within the airways or within the lung parenchyma. The two most common disorders that fall into this category are chronic bronchitis and emphysema. Although the pathophysiology of airflow limitation is different in these two disorders, in practice patients frequently have features of both, making it most appropriate to discuss them together. Though asthma could also logically fall within this category, it is considered in a separate chapter (Chapter 5), since common usage of the term COPD usually does not include bronchial asthma.

There are several other terms that are basically synonymous with COPD, e.g., chronic airflow limitation, chronic airflow obstruction (CAO), and chronic obstructive lung disease (COLD). We will be using the expression COPD, since it is the one in most common usage, realizing it is not necessarily the most suitable one for describing these processes. We are also taking the liberty of including emphysema within the section of this book dealing with airways disease, even though the most obvious pathology affects the lung parenchyma.

Chronic bronchitis is a clinical diagnosis given to patients with chronic cough and sputum production. It has certain pathologic features, but the diagnosis refers to the specific clinical presentation. For epidemiologic purposes, a more formal definition has been used, requiring that a chronic productive cough be present on most days during at least three consecutive months for not less than two successive years. However, for clinical purposes, the physician does not necessarily adhere to this formal time requirement. Patients with chronic bronchitis frequently have periods of worsening or exacerbation, often precipitated by respiratory tract infection. Unlike patients with asthma, though, the patient with pure chronic bronchitis usually has residual clinical disease even between exacerbations, and his disease is not primarily one of airways hyperreactivity. In those patients who have chronic bronchitis along with a prominent component of airways hyperreactivity, the diagnosis of *asthmatic bronchitis* is often given, since features of both disorders are present.

Chronic bronchitis is a diagnosis based on chronic cough and sputum production.

In contrast to the clinical diagnosis of chronic bronchitis, *emphysema* is formally a pathologic diagnosis, though certain clinical and laboratory features are also highly suggestive of the disease. Pathologically, emphysema is characterized by dilatation and destruction of air spaces distal to the terminal bronchiole. The region of the lung from the respiratory bronchioles down to the alveoli is involved, and determination of the particular type of emphysema depends on the pattern of destruction within the acinus. An ante-mortem diagnosis of emphysema obviously does not have the kind of confirmation offered by post-mortem examination of the lung, but indirect support for the diagnosis is still useful and reasonably reliable.

Emphysema is a diagnosis based on dilatation and destruction of air spaces distal to the terminal bronchiole.

Since chronic bronchitis and emphysema coexist to a variable extent in different patients, the broader term chronic obstructive pulmonary disease is frequently more accurate. That these two diagnoses are tied so closely together is not at all surprising, since a single etiologic factor—cigarette smoking—is primarily responsible for both processes. In our subsequent discussions, we will often refer specifically to chronic bronchitis or to emphysema, because some of the clinical and pathophysiologic features are distinct enough to warrant separate consideration. However, one must remember that patients do not necessarily fit neatly into these separate diagnostic categories.

The public health problems posed by chronic obstructive pulmonary disease are enormous. It has been estimated that between 10 and 25 percent of adult Americans have some degree of chronic bronchitis, and approximately 50,000 deaths per year in the United States can be attributed to COPD. The morbidity, in terms of chronic symptoms, days lost from work, or permanent disability, is even more staggering. Unlike many diseases that the physician encounters, COPD is preventable in the large majority of cases, since the main etiologic factor has been well established and is totally avoidable. Despite this fact, the popularity of smoking continues, and women, who are smoking more and more, are now part of an epidemic that was once largely limited to men.

ETIOLOGY AND PATHOGENESIS

Chronic Bronchitis

Several factors have been implicated in the etiology of chronic bronchitis, including smoking, air pollution, infection, and genetics. Of these four, smoking is clearly the most important and will receive most of our attention. From epidemiologic studies, it is apparent that there is a significant correlation between cigarette smoking and the symptoms of cough and sputum production. Pipe and cigar smoking also predisposes to the development of chronic bronchitis, but the risk is significantly less than that from cigarette smoking, probably because pipe and cigar smoke is generally not inhaled. Experimental information about the induction of chronic bronchitis in animals is limited, but the evidence suggests that smoke and other airway irritants can induce some of the pathologic changes observed in patients with chronic bronchitis. In particular, animals exposed to inhaled irritants develop changes of submucosal gland enlargement and an increased number of mucus-secreting goblet cells within the airways, similar to the changes seen in affected patients.

Smoking is the key etiologic factor for chronic bronchitis; air pollutants and respiratory tract infection cause exacerbations but have little role in etiology.

The other factors implicated in the pathogenesis of chronic bronchitis—air pollution, infection, and genetics—are quantitatively much less important than smoking. Air pollutants and respiratory tract infection are important because of their potential for causing exacerbations of pre-existing chronic bronchitis, not for initiating the disorder. Of the different types of respiratory tract infection, viral infection appears to be responsible for a large number of clinical exacerbations of symptoms. Bacterial infections probably play a less important role but can cause superinfection of patients already harboring an acute viral infection. The importance of genetic factors in determining susceptibility to chronic bronchitis is, to a large extent, unknown. As we will discuss, a well-identified hereditary factor can predispose to the development of emphysema. In contrast, no specific genetic factors have been associated with an increased risk of chronic bronchitis. One possibility under active investigation is that a subject's degree of airway reactivity, which perhaps has some genetic determinants, may be related to the potential for developing chronic bronchitis from cigarette smoke inhalation. However, to date, no constitutional risk factor for chronic bronchitis has good supportive evidence.

Emphysema

Cigarette smoking is responsible for most cases of emphysema; deficiency of serum alpha-1-protease inhibitor predisposes to emphysema in a small proportion of cases.

Currently, two main etiologic factors have been identified for emphysema—cigarette smoking and a hereditary predisposition. The best defined hereditary factor predisposing to the development of emphysema is deficiency of a serum protein called *alpha-1-protease inhibitor* (A1PI). This protein, formerly called alpha-1-antitrypsin, is a glycoprotein with a molecular weight of 54,000 that is made in the liver and normally circulates in blood. The fact that patients with low serum levels of this protein (as a result of a genetic defect) are strongly predisposed to the premature development of emphysema has been important in furthering our understanding of the pathogenesis of emphysema in general, even when a genetic defect is not involved. We will first discuss the relationship between A1PI deficiency and emphysema and then proceed to a more general consideration of cigarette smoking and emphysema.

Over a number of years, studies on the biochemistry of A1PI have demonstrated more than 20 phenotypes of this particular protein. In other words, minor changes in the gene coding for A1PI produce alterations in the structure of the protein that can be detected by biochemical methods. Each of these phenotypes has been given a name, preceded by the letters Pi, for "protease inhibitor." Everyone has two genes coding for A1PI, one of maternal and one of paternal origin. The normal (and most common) phenotype is termed Pi M, and the normal complement of two M genes is called Pi MM. When a person has the Pi MM genotype, he or she has approximately 200 mg per dl of the M type of protease inhibitor circulating in the blood. With one of the variant Pi types, termed Pi Z, the amino acid sequence of the protein is slightly altered, affecting transport of the protein from its site of production in the liver. Hence the abnormal protein remains in globules in the liver, where it may result in liver disease, and only small amounts enter the blood. Individuals who are homozygous for the Z gene (Pi ZZ) have circulating levels of A1PI that are approximately 10 percent of normal, or 20 mg per dl. Heterozygotes, with one M and one Z gene (Pi MZ), have intermediate levels of circulating A1PI, in the range of 50 to 60 percent of normal levels.

It is now well recognized that having the Pi ZZ genotype is a strong risk factor for the premature development of emphysema, particularly if the individual is also a smoker. Patients with the Pi ZZ genotype (who are commonly said to have A1PI or alpha-1-antitrypsin deficiency because of the low serum levels) frequently develop emphysema as early as the third or fourth decade of life. Therefore, an adequate amount of A1PI may be important in hindering or protecting against the development of emphysema.

In A1PI deficiency, A1PI transport from its site of production in the liver is impaired, with accumulation of A1PI in the liver and low serum levels.

In order to arrive at the current hypothesis about the role of A1PI deficiency in emphysema, we must also mention information obtained from studies on experimental emphysema in animals. Injection of several proteolytic (i.e., capable of breaking down protein) enzymes into the airways of animals results in pathologic and physiologic changes similar to those of clinical emphysema. However, the only enzymes that can induce these changes are ones capable of breaking down elastin, a complex structural protein found in the walls of alveoli. Additionally, the greater the elastolytic activity of the enzyme, the more pronounced the pathologic changes of emphysema. Other evidence also suggests that changes in elastin are important in the pathogenesis of emphysema. For example, animals with defective ability to form normal crosslinks between elastin molecules develop characteristic changes of emphysema.

Two types of cells are important in certain inflammatory processes in the lung, namely alveolar macrophages and polymorphonuclear leukocytes (PMN's). Both of these cells produce an enzyme called elastase, which is capable of breaking down the structural protein elastin. Of these two cell types, the PMN is thought to be the major source of elastase in the lung. If this enzyme were allowed to exert its proteolytic effect on elastin whenever it was released from a PMN,

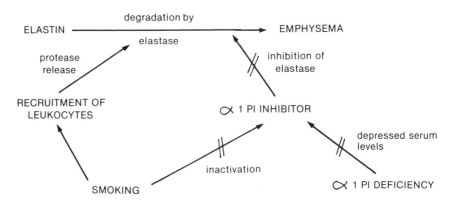

Figure 6–1. Schematic diagram of the hypothesized relationship between elastase and the alpha-1-protease inhibitor (A1PI), indicating how smoking and A1PI deficiency alter the balance, leading to degradation of elastin.

Current theories claim that proteolytic enzymes (especially elastase) are balanced by A1PI; disturbance of this balance in favor of proteolytic enzymes, either due to smoking or a deficiency of A1PI, may result in emphysema.

destruction of this important structural protein of the alveolar wall would ensue. Fortunately, there is normally an inhibitor of elastase present in the lung, and this inhibitor happens to be the alpha-1-protease inhibitor just discussed. According to current thinking, there is a balance between elastase and its inhibitor, so that wanton destruction of the alveolar wall does not occur. When this balance is disturbed, either by an increase in elastase activity or a decrease in anti-elastase (A1PI) activity, damage to elastin and to the alveolar wall can result, with the eventual production of emphysema. In the case of patients with A1PI deficiency, lack of the elastase inhibitor is believed to permit elastase action to proceed in an unchecked fashion, and the early development of emphysema may be the consequence.

Although this theory is an attractive one to explain why patients with A1PI deficiency are predisposed to develop emphysema, we must remember that the homozygous ZZ state is quite uncommon and is probably responsible for less than 1 percent of patients with emphysema. However, there are reasons to believe that the principles just discussed are also important in the pathogenesis of emphysema due to cigarette smoking. The balance between elastase and anti-elastase is thought to be disturbed in more than one way by cigarette smoke. First of all, an increased number of PMN's and alveolar macrophages can be found in the lungs of smokers, thus providing a source for increased amounts of elastase. Additionally, there is now evidence that cigarette smoke can oxidize a critical amino acid residue of A1PI at or near the site where the protease inhibitor binds to elastase. Oxidation of this amino acid interferes with the inhibitory activity of A1PI, again tipping the balance in favor of increased elastase activity. Hence, cigarette smoking may be a double-edged sword, increasing the amount of elastase in the lung and decreasing the normal inhibitory mechanism that serves to limit uncontrolled elastin breakdown by the enzyme. This pathogenetic sequence hypothesized for the development of emphysema is summarized in Figure 6–1.

PATHOLOGY

A great deal of the pathology in chronic bronchitis relates to mucus and to the mucus-secreting apparatus in the airways. As we mentioned in Chapter 4, both mucus-secreting glands and goblet cells are responsible for the production of bronchial secretions, but the mucous glands are quantitatively the more important source. In chronic bronchitis, we find enlargement (hypertrophy and hyperplasia) of the mucus-secreting glands, which has been objectively assessed by comparing the relative thickness of the mucous glands with the total thickness of the airway wall. This ratio, known as the Reid index, is increased in patients with chronic bronchitis. In general, the number of goblet cells in the airways is increased as well, and these particular cells are also abundant in airways more peripheral than usual. As we will discuss in the section on pathophysiology, changes in the small airways may be particularly important in the genesis of symptoms and may be seen quite early in the disease process. As a result of these alterations in the mucus-secreting apparatus, the quantity of airway mucus is increased, and it is likely that the composition may be altered as well. In practice, the secretions found in these patients are often thick and apparently more viscous than usual. The bronchial walls also demonstrate evidence of an inflammatory process, with cellular infiltration and variable degrees of fibrosis.

Chronic bronchitis is characterized by enlargement of the mucus-secreting glands and an increased number of goblet cells.

In the smaller airways, any changes in the lumen or in the airway walls may have particularly important clinical sequelae. Since the resistance of airways varies inversely with the fourth power of the radius, even small changes in bronchiolar size as a result of secretions, inflammation, fibrosis, or an increase in goblet cells may result in major impairment to airflow at the level of the small airways. Young cigarette smokers show abnormalities of the small airways, such as pigmented macrophages around the respiratory bronchioles, which may be the precursors of some of the more advanced lesions of chronic bronchitis and emphysema.

Pathologic changes from smoking often start in small airways, predating the advanced findings associated with chronic bronchitis and emphysema.

The pathology of emphysema is characterized by destruction of alveolar walls and enlargement of terminal airspaces (Fig. 6–2). Several types of emphysema have distinct pathologic features, primarily dependent on the distribution of the lesions. The most important types are panacinar (or panlobular) emphysema and centriacinar (or centri-

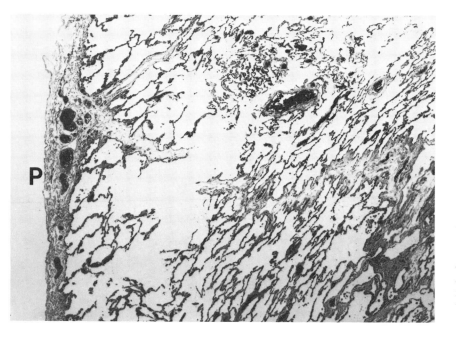

Figure 6–2. Low-power photomicrograph demonstrating a localized region of emphysema in the left half of the figure, adjacent to the pleural surface (P). Since the emphysema here is localized, the destruction of alveolar walls and enlargement of terminal airspaces can be contrasted with the appearance of normal lung in the right half of the figure. (Courtesy of Dr. Earl Kasdon.)

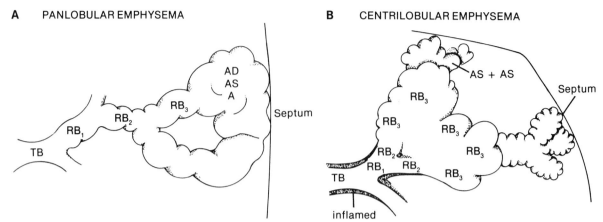

A   PANLOBULAR EMPHYSEMA   **B**   CENTRILOBULAR EMPHYSEMA

Figure 6–3. Diagram of panlobular (A) and centrilobular (B) emphysema. In panlobular (panacinar) emphysema, the enlargement of airspaces is relatively uniform throughout the acinus. In centrilobular (centriacinar) emphysema, enlargement of airspaces is primarily at the level of respiratory bronchioles. TB = terminal bronchiole; RB_1 through RB_3 = three generations of respiratory bronchioles; AD = alveolar duct; AS = alveolar sac; A = alveolus. (From Thurlbeck, W.M.: Chronic obstructive lung disease. *In:* Sommers, S.C., ed. Pathology Annual. Vol. 3. New York, Appleton-Century-Crofts, 1968. Reproduced with permission.)

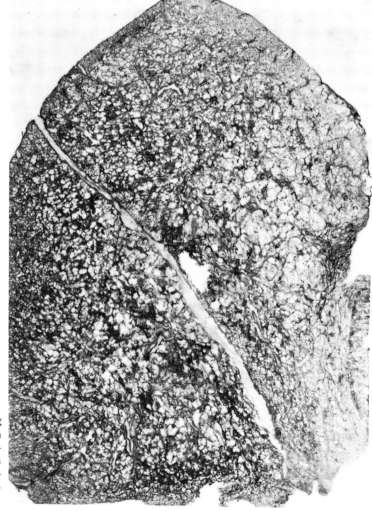

Figure 6–4. Mounted section of whole lung demonstrating diffuse involvement seen with panacinar emphysema. (From Thurlbeck, W.M.: Chronic Airflow Obstruction in Lung Disease. Philadelphia, W.B. Saunders Co., 1976. Reproduced with permission.)

lobular) emphysema (Fig. 6–3). Panacinar emphysema is characterized by a more or less uniform involvement of the acinus, i.e., the region beyond the terminal bronchiole, including respiratory bronchioles, alveolar ducts, and alveolar sacs. Examination of a section of lung with panacinar emphysema shows that the damage in an involved area is relatively diffuse (Fig. 6–4). Panacinar emphysema is the usual type of emphysema described in patients who have A1PI deficiency, though it is by no means limited to this particular clinical setting.

In centriacinar (centrilobular) emphysema, the predominant involvement and dilatation are found in the proximal part of the acinus, namely the respiratory bronchiole. The appearance of a lung section with centriacinar emphysema is different from that of panacinar emphysema. In centriacinar emphysema, the involvement in an affected area seems to be more irregular, with apparently spared alveolar tissue

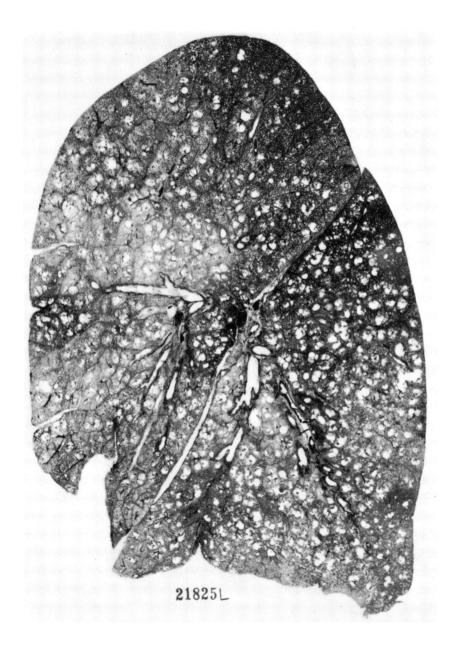

21825L

Figure 6–5. Mounted section of whole lung demonstrating centrilobular emphysema. Adjacent to the emphysematous spaces (which represent dilated respiratory bronchioles) are spared areas of lung parenchyma (representing alveolar ducts and alveolar spaces). (From Thurlbeck, W.M.: Chronic Airflow Obstruction in Lung Disease. Philadelphia, W.B. Saunders Co., 1976. Reproduced with permission.)

between the dilated respiratory bronchioles at the center of the acinus (Fig. 6–5). This type of emphysema is especially common in smokers and is frequently accompanied by the airway changes of chronic bronchitis.

PATHOPHYSIOLOGY

For purposes of discussion here, we will consider chronic bronchitis and emphysema as relatively pure and separate entities, even though most patients with chronic obstructive pulmonary disease have features of both. In both situations, expiratory airflow (particularly during a forced expiration) is reduced. However, the mechanisms of flow reduction are quite different in the two conditions.

Functional Abnormalities in Chronic Bronchitis

In chronic bronchitis, the decrease in airway size as a result of secretions, increase in the mucus-secreting apparatus, and inflammation frequently leads to an increase in airway resistance, commonly abbreviated R_{aw}. Other measurements of airflow, such as the FEV_1/FVC ratio and the MMFR, are also depressed in many patients with chronic bronchitis and associated obstruction. It is of interest that some patients with apparent chronic bronchitis (i.e., chronic cough and sputum production) do not exhibit abnormally high resistance or changes in other measurements of airflow. In these patients, the major pathology is probably located within the small airways. Since these peripheral airways contribute only about 10 to 20 percent of the overall airways resistance, total resistance is preserved unless there are considerable changes in the small airways or additional pathology in the larger airways.

A decrease in airway size from secretions, increase in the mucus-secreting apparatus, and inflammation is responsible for the decreased expiratory flow rates in chronic bronchitis.

Measurement of lung volumes in patients with chronic bronchitis demonstrates several abnormalities. Before discussing these changes, it will be useful to review the factors determining the major lung volumes, namely TLC, FRC, and RV. Total lung capacity (TLC) is the point at which the force of the inspiratory muscles acting to expand the lungs is equaled by the elastic recoil of the respiratory system (primarily lung recoil) resisting expansion. At functional residual capacity (FRC), the resting point of the respiratory system, there is a balance between the elastic recoil of the lungs and the chest wall, which act in opposite directions—the lungs inward and the chest wall outward. The determinants of residual volume (RV) depend to some extent upon age. In a normal young person, RV is the point at which the relatively stiff chest wall can be compressed no further by the expiratory muscles. With increasing age, a sufficient number of airways close at low lung volumes to limit further expiration, and airway closure is an important determinant of RV. In disease states in which airways are likely to close at low lung volumes, airway closure is associated with an elevated RV, even if the patient is young.

In chronic bronchitis, TLC theoretically remains relatively close to normal, since neither the elastic recoil of the lung nor inspiratory muscle strength is altered. Similarly, FRC should remain normal, since the recoil of both the lung and the chest wall is unchanged. However, if expiration is prolonged and the respiratory rate is quite high, then the patient may not have sufficient time during expiration to reach his or her normal resting end-expiratory point. In this case, FRC is increased. Residual volume is generally increased in chronic bronchitis, since the narrowing and occlusion of small airways by secretions and inflammation result in air trapping during expiration.

Functional Abnormalities in Emphysema

The pathophysiology of low expiratory flow rates in pure emphysema is somewhat different from that in chronic bronchitis. The primary problem in emphysema is the loss of elastic recoil, i.e., loss of the lung's natural tendency to resist expansion. One of the consequences of decreased elastic recoil is a decreased driving pressure expelling air from the alveoli during expiration. A simple analogy would be a balloon filled with air, where the elastic recoil is the "stiffness" of the balloon. With a given volume of air inside an unsealed balloon, a stiffer balloon will expel air more rapidly than a less stiff balloon. An emphysematous lung is like a less stiff balloon—a smaller than normal force drives air out of the lungs during expiration.

However, loss of driving pressure is not the only consequence of emphysema. There is also an indirect effect on the collapsibility of airways. Normally, traction is exerted on the walls of airways by a supporting structure of tissue from the lung parenchyma. When the alveolar tissue is disrupted, as in emphysema, the supporting structure for the airways is diminished, and less radial traction is exerted to prevent airway collapse (Fig. 6–6). During a forced expiration, the strongly positive pleural pressure promotes collapse; airways lacking an adequate supporting structure are more likely to collapse (and have diminished flow rates and air trapping) than normally supported ones.

The decrease in elastic recoil in emphysema also alters the compliance curve of the lung and the measured lung volumes. The compliance curve, as discussed in Chapter 1, relates transpulmonary pressure and the associated volume of gas within the lung. Since a

In emphysema, decreased expiratory flow rates are largely due to loss of elastic recoil of the lung, resulting in:
1. a lower driving pressure for expiratory airflow
2. loss of radial traction on the airways provided by supporting alveolar walls, thus promoting airway collapse during expiration

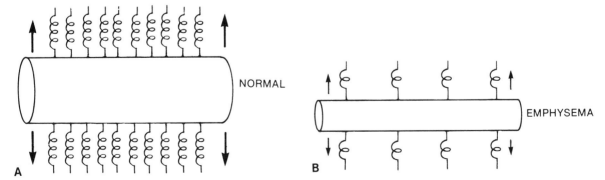

Figure 6–6. Schematic diagram of radial traction exerted by alveolar walls (represented as springs), acting to keep airways open. The normal situation is shown in *(A)*, whereas loss of radial traction, as seen in emphysema, is shown in *(B)*.

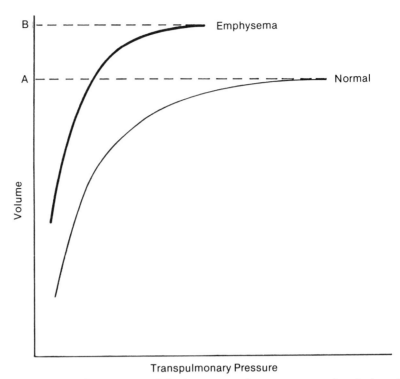

Figure 6–7. Compliance curve of the lung in emphysema compared with that of the normal lung. In addition to the shift of the curve upward and to the left, it can be seen that TLC in emphysema (point B on the volume axis) is greater than the normal TLC (point A). In pure chronic bronchitis without emphysema, the compliance curve is normal.

lung with emphysema has less elastic recoil, i.e., is less stiff, it resists expansion less than its normal counterpart. Hence, the compliance curve is shifted upward and to the left, and the lung has more volume at any particular transpulmonary pressure (Fig. 6–7). Total lung capacity is increased, since loss of elastic recoil results in a smaller force opposing the action of the inspiratory musculature. Functional residual capacity is also increased, since the balance between the outward recoil of the chest wall and the inward recoil of the lung is shifted in favor of the chest wall. As in bronchitis, RV is also substantially increased in emphysema, since poorly supported airways are more susceptible to closure during a maximal expiration.

Mechanisms of Abnormal Gas Exchange

In obstructive lung disease, many of the observed pathologic changes affecting airflow are not uniformly distributed. For example, in chronic bronchitis some airways are extensively affected by secretions and plugging, while others remain relatively uninvolved. Therefore, ventilation is not uniformly distributed throughout the lung—regions of the lung supplied by more diseased airways receive diminished ventilation in comparison with regions supplied by less diseased airways. Though there may be a compensatory decrease in blood flow to underventilated alveoli, the compensation is not totally effective, and inequalities and mismatching of ventilation and perfusion result. As we discussed earlier, this type of ventilation-perfusion disturbance, with some areas of lung having low $\dot{V}/\dot{Q}$ ratios and contributing desaturated blood, leads to arterial hypoxemia.

In obstructive lung disease, non-uniformity of the disease process results in $\dot{V}/\dot{Q}$ mismatch and hypoxemia.

Carbon dioxide elimination is also impaired in some patients with obstructive lung disease. The mechanism of alveolar hypoventilation and CO_2 retention, however, is less clear than the mechanism of hypoxemia. Several factors probably contribute, including increased work of breathing (resulting from impaired airflow), abnormalities of central ventilatory drive, and ventilation-perfusion mismatch creating some areas with high $\dot{V}/\dot{Q}$ ratios, which effectively act as dead space.

Mechanisms contributing to alveolar hypoventilation and CO_2 retention in obstructive lung disease:
1. increased work of breathing
2. abnormalities of ventilatory drive
3. $\dot{V}/\dot{Q}$ mismatch

An additional problem, fatigue of inspiratory muscles, has received attention recently as a factor contributing to acute CO_2 retention when these patients are in respiratory failure (see Chapter 19). The importance of diaphragmatic fatigue in the stable patient with chronic hypercapnia is less certain. However, it is clear that contraction of the diaphragm, the major muscle of inspiration, is less efficient and less effective in patients with obstructive lung disease. When FRC is increased, the diaphragm is lower and flatter, and its fibers are shortened even before the initiation of inspiration. A shortened, flattened diaphragm is at a mechanical disadvantage compared with a longer, curved diaphragm, and it is less effective as an inspiratory muscle.

Pulmonary Hypertension

A potential complication of COPD is the development of pulmonary hypertension, or high pressures within the pulmonary arterial system. Long-standing pulmonary hypertension puts an added workload onto the right ventricle, which hypertrophies and eventually may fail. The term used to describe disease of the right ventricle secondary to lung disease (either COPD or other forms of lung disease) is *cor pulmonale*, a topic that will be discussed further in Chapter 14. The primary feature of COPD that leads to pulmonary hypertension and eventually to cor pulmonale is hypoxia. A decrease in Po_2 is a strong stimulus to constriction of pulmonary arterioles. With correction of the hypoxia, the pulmonary vasoconstriction may be reversible.

Several additional but less important factors may contribute to elevated pulmonary artery pressure—hypercapnia, polycythemia, and reduction in area of the pulmonary vascular bed. Hypercapnia, like hypoxia, is also capable of causing pulmonary vasoconstriction; to a large extent, this effect may be mediated by the change in pH resulting from an increase in Pco_2. An elevation in hematocrit, i.e., polycythemia, is often found in the chronically hypoxemic patient, producing an increased blood viscosity and contributing to an elevated pulmonary artery pressure. Finally, in emphysema, the destruction of alveoli is accompanied by a loss of pulmonary capillaries. Therefore, in extensive disease, the limited pulmonary vascular bed may result in a high resistance to blood flow and consequently an increase in pulmonary artery pressure.

The major cause of pulmonary hypertension in COPD is hypoxia; additional factors include hypercapnia, polycythemia, and destruction of the pulmonary vascular bed.

Two Types of Presentation

In practice, it is often useful to distinguish two pathophysiologic types of chronic obstructive pulmonary disease, termed Types A and B, or more colloquially, *pink puffer* and *blue bloater*, respectively. Originally, Type A (pink puffer) physiology was associated with underlying emphysema, whereas Type B (blue bloater) physiology was equated with chronic bronchitis. Though the association with a particular pathologic process appears to be an oversimplification, the pathophysiologic types of presentation are useful clinically, as different clinical problems result from the two types. In many cases, a patient does not fall clearly into one category or the other, but has some features suggestive of both.

The Type A patient is referred to as a "pink puffer" because (1) arterial Po_2 tends to be reasonably well preserved, so the patient is "pink", i.e., not cyanotic; and (2) dyspnea and high minute ventilation are prominent features, with the patient appearing to be working hard to get air, i.e., "puffing." Not only is the Po_2 not markedly decreased, but the Pco_2 also is not abnormally high. If we use the general (though oversimplified) concept that emphysema is the primary process in these patients, relative preservation of the Po_2 may be related to a simultaneous and matched loss of ventilation and perfusion when alveolar walls are destroyed. Because gas exchange abnormalities are not a striking feature of Type A patients, no prominent stimulus of hypoxia leads to pulmonary hypertension. In addition, an elevation of the hematocrit, often a result of hypoxemia, is not seen.

Type B patients, on the other hand, are characterized by major problems with gas exchange, namely hypoxemia and hypercapnia. They are termed "blue bloaters" because (1) cyanosis can result from significant hypoxemia; and because (2) they are frequently obese and can have peripheral edema resulting from right ventricular failure. Again, if we use the oversimplified concept that Type B patients have primarily chronic bronchitis, it is reasonable to attribute hypoxemia to ventilation-perfusion mismatch. Presumably, regions of lung supplied by diseased airways are underventilated, while perfusion is relatively preserved. Ventilation-perfusion mismatch results in arterial hypoxemia because of desaturated blood coming from areas with a low ventilation-perfusion ratio. As we discussed earlier, several mechanisms may contribute to the development of CO_2 retention, though the primary differences explaining why Type A patients do not retain CO_2 while Type B patients often do are not entirely clear. As a consequence of the gas exchange abnormalities (particularly hypoxemia) in Type B patients, pulmonary hypertension, cor pulmonale, and elevations in the hematocrit ("secondary polycythemia") commonly accompany the clinical picture.

Two presentations of obstructive lung disease are the "pink puffer" (Type A) and the "blue bloater" (Type B), but a clear distinction between their underlying processes is an oversimplification.

Despite the common association of Type B pathophysiology with chronic bronchitis, these patients frequently also have pathologic evidence of emphysema, particularly of the centrilobular variety. How much of the clinical picture is secondary to bronchitis and how much is secondary to coexisting centrilobular emphysema is difficult to determine.

CLINICAL FEATURES

Symptoms most commonly experienced by patients with chronic obstructive lung disease include dyspnea and cough, frequently with sputum production. Dyspnea is the most prominent symptom in those patients with Type A pathophysiology, whereas Type B patients generally complain of chronic cough and sputum production. Many patients have features of both, while some patients with COPD actually are asymptomatic and may have their disease diagnosed by pulmonary function tests.

Frequently, patients have a certain level of chronic symptoms, but their disease course is then punctuated by periods of exacerbation. The precipitating factor producing an exacerbation is often a respiratory tract infection, particularly of viral origin. Patients may also have bacteria chronically in their tracheobronchial tree, which should normally be sterile, and an acute bacterial infection can sometimes be implicated in acute exacerbations. Other factors that cause acute deterioration of these patients include exposure to air pollutants, bronchospasm (particularly if patients have a superimposed asthmatic component to their disease), and congestive heart failure, just to name a few. When exacerbations are severe, patients may go into frank respiratory failure, a complication that will be discussed further in Chapter 26.

The precipitating factor for an exacerbation of COPD is often a viral infection.

In addition to chronic symptoms of dyspnea and/or cough, which may worsen during periods of acute exacerbation, patients also may experience secondary cardiovascular complications of their lung disease, i.e., cor pulmonale. As we mentioned, the patient with Type B physiology is more susceptible to this complication than the Type A patient.

On physical examination, patients with Type A physiology often appear thin (if not cachectic), and they frequently may be leaning forward and resting on their extended arms. They are not cyanotic and do not demonstrate peripheral edema characteristic of right ventricular failure. In contrast, the Type B patient is often obese and may be cyanotic, but generally appears to be in less respiratory distress than his Type A counterpart.

Examination of the chest often discloses an increase in the anteroposterior diameter, indicating hyperinflation of the lungs. Patients may be using accessory muscles of respiration, such as the sternocleidomastoid and trapezius muscles, and the intercostal muscles may retract with each inspiration. When diaphragmatic excursion is assessed by percussion of the lung bases during inspiration and expiration, diminished movement is noted. Breath sounds are generally decreased in intensity, and expiration is prolonged. Wheezing may also be heard, but unfortunately does not necessarily reflect reversible bronchospasm. Some patients do not have wheezing on their normal tidal breathing, but they will have this finding when asked to give a forced exhalation. In those patients with chronic bronchitis and profuse airway secretions, rhonchi are frequently heard. When cor pulmonale is present, with or without frank right ventricular failure, patients have the cardiac findings that will be described in Chapter 14.

Continuation of smoking is a major risk factor affecting the prognosis in COPD.

Smoking is not only the primary factor initiating chronic obstructive pulmonary disease, it is also a major risk factor determining the prognosis of a patient's illness. Those patients who continue to smoke appear to have the greatest further deterioration of pulmonary function over time, whereas respiratory tract infections, though they may cause acute deterioration, do not appear to affect the rate at which pulmonary function is lost.

A wide spectrum of severity is characteristic of chronic obstructive lung disease, and therefore the morbidity that patients experience from their disease varies tremendously. Patients with mild disease are able to continue their usual work and lifestyle with minimal, if any, changes. Those with severe disease are quite limited in their capacity for any exertion, are subject to frequent hospitalizations, and may have a life expectancy of less than 5 years.

DIAGNOSIS

In most cases, the diagnosis of chronic obstructive pulmonary disease is made by a combination of history and physical examination. As we mentioned earlier, chronic bronchitis is actually a clinical diagnosis, and it is here that the history is particularly crucial. Though emphysema is formally a pathologic diagnosis, lung biopsy is not performed in order to make this diagnosis. Pathologic confirmation is generally obtained only at post-mortem examination, if one is done.

A valuable study for assessing the lungs of patients with COPD on a macroscopic level is the chest roentgenogram. Patients with chronic bronchitis alone frequently have a normal chest roentgenogram. Minor changes of increased markings through the lungs may be present, but it is difficult to know whether these can be attributed to coexisting emphysema, particularly of the centrilobular variety. When these patients develop cor pulmonale, secondary cardiac changes may also be seen, indicative of right ventricular hypertrophy or dilatation.

Characteristic radiographic findings in the more frequently recognized arterial deficiency pattern of COPD:
1. large lung volumes
2. flat diaphragms
3. increased anteroposterior diameter
4. loss of vascular markings

In patients with emphysema, two radiographic patterns are well described. In the first, which is the type most frequently recognized, patients have hyperinflation, with large lung volumes, flat diaphragms, and an increase in the anteroposterior diameter (seen on the lateral view). Additionally, a paucity of vascular markings in the lung results from destruction of alveolar septae and dilatation of alveolar spaces. This pattern is known as the *arterial deficiency* pattern of emphysema because of the changes in vascular markings and is often associated with underlying panacinar emphysema (Fig. 6–8). In patients with A1PI deficiency and early onset of emphysema, the arterial deficiency pattern is quite striking in the lower lobes, where there may be almost a complete loss of vascular markings.

The other radiographic pattern in patients with emphysema is termed the *increased markings* pattern. In this pattern, the radiograph demonstrates prominent lung markings and may also give evidence of pulmonary hypertension and cor pulmonale. Patients with this type of picture are often the ones with coexisting chronic bronchitis and Type B physiology, and their radiographic findings are probably related to coexistent centrilobular emphysema.

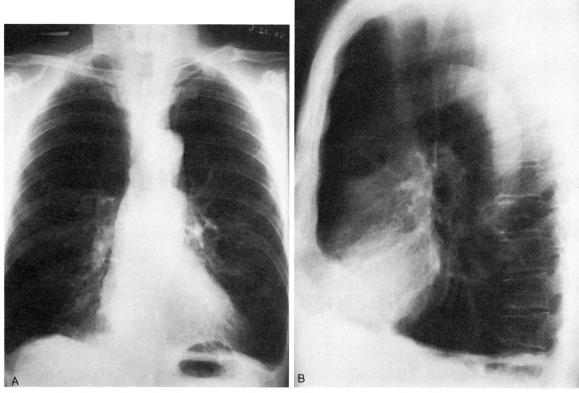

Figure 6–8. Chest radiograph of a patient with severe chronic obstructive lung disease, showing the arterial deficiency pattern of emphysema. The lungs are hyperinflated, the diaphragms are low and flat (in this case they are actually inverted on the lateral film), and there is a paucity of vascular markings. Posteroanterior *(A)* and lateral *(B)* views.

The most useful physiologic adjuncts in evaluating patients with COPD are pulmonary function tests and arterial blood gases. Pulmonary function tests demonstrate airflow obstruction, with a decrease in FVC, FEV$_1$, the FEV$_1$/FVC ratio, and MMFR. The tests generally give evidence of air trapping, with an elevation in RV. In patients whose lung compliance is increased, i.e., those with emphysema, TLC is generally elevated. FRC is elevated either as a result of decreased compliance in emphysema or as a consequence of insufficient expiratory time in the face of significant airflow obstruction. Whether emphysema is present can be indirectly assessed by measuring the diffusing capacity for carbon monoxide. In patients with emphysema, in whom the surface area for gas exchange is lost, the diffusing capacity is decreased. In pure airways disease, e.g., chronic bronchitis without emphysema, the diffusing capacity is generally normal.

The results of arterial blood gases depend to a large extent on the pathophysiologic type of disease, and in fact the blood gases are an important criterion for classifying the patient in one of the two pathophysiologic categories. Patients with Type A pathophysiology have a normal or mildly decreased arterial Po$_2$ with a normal or slightly decreased arterial Pco$_2$. Those with Type B physiology have more strikingly abnormal blood gases—often marked hypoxemia as well as

Pulmonary function tests in COPD show:
1. airflow obstruction (decreased FVC, FEV$_1$, FEV$_1$/FVC, MMFR)
2. air trapping (increased RV, FRC, and often TLC)
3. diffusing capacity generally decreased in emphysema, normal in chronic bronchitis

Type B patients are more hypoxemic than Type A patients and often have hypercapnia.

Table 6–1. CLINICAL DISTINCTIONS BETWEEN TYPE A AND TYPE B
PATHOPHYSIOLOGY

Feature	Type A	Type B
Commonly used name	pink puffer	blue bloater
Disease association	predominant emphysema	predominant bronchitis
Major symptom	dyspnea	cough and sputum
Appearance	thin, wasted, not cyanotic	obese, cyanotic
P_{O_2}	↓	↓ ↓
P_{CO_2}	normal or ↓	normal or ↑
Elastic recoil of lung	↓	normal
Diffusing capacity	↓	normal
Hematocrit	normal	often ↑
Cor pulmonale	infrequent	common

CO_2 retention. With chronic elevation in the P_{CO_2}, the kidneys retain bicarbonate in an attempt to compensate and return the pH toward normal. With acute exacerbations of COPD, the hypoxemia frequently becomes even worse, and the CO_2 retention more pronounced, so that the pH may drop from the stable compensated value.

Many of the clinical features characterizing patients with Type A and Type B pathophysiology are summarized in Table 6–1.

TREATMENT

There are several modalities of treatment available for the patient with chronic obstructive pulmonary disease, the usefulness of each varying greatly from patient to patient. Though bronchoconstriction in COPD patients is considerably less than that in patients with bronchial asthma, bronchodilators remain an important part of the treatment of many patients with COPD. The actual agents used are identical to the ones discussed in Chapter 5, including phosphodiesterase inhibitors (methylxanthines) and the wide variety of sympathomimetic agents.

For those patients in whom airway secretions cause significant symptomatic problems, chest physiotherapy and postural drainage frequently offer a great deal in helping to mobilize and clear the secretions. These techniques utilize percussion of the chest wall to loosen secretions and induce cough, followed by positional changes to allow gravity to aid in drainage of the secretions.

When patients with COPD develop acute respiratory tract infections, or even if they have an exacerbation of their disease without a clear precipitant, they are often treated with antibiotics. The primary usefulness of antibiotics is for bacterial infections, but a bacterial etiology is often difficult to document with certainty. In practice, patients are frequently treated with antibiotics when there is a change in the quantity and/or nature of their chronic sputum production, even though a bacterial infection may or may not be present. Of the potential bacterial pathogens, *Streptococcus pneumoniae* and *Hemophilus influenzae* are often implicated, and the choice of antibiotic allows coverage for these organisms.

The use of corticosteroids for the treatment of these patients is a controversial topic, and a discussion of its pros and cons is clearly beyond the scope of this chapter. When steroids are given, it is frequently at the time of an acute exacerbation, though occasional patients with severe disease are placed on a chronic regimen of corticosteroids.

Finally, an important adjunct to therapy is the administration of supplemental oxygen to those patients who are significantly hypoxemic (e.g., arterial P_{O_2} less than 55 to 60 torr). Fortunately, the P_{O_2} of hypoxemic patients with COPD usually responds quite well to even relatively small amounts of supplemental oxygen (in the range of 24 to 28 percent O_2). A low flow rate of oxygen (1 to 2 liters per minute) given by nasal prongs is an effective and well tolerated method for achieving these concentrations of inspired oxygen. Oxygen is particularly important in those patients with pulmonary hypertension and in those with secondary polycythemia, since each of these complications is largely caused by (and responsive to treatment for) hypoxemia. Evidence also suggests that survival of hypoxemic patients with COPD can be improved by the administration of supplemental oxygen. This is actually the first demonstration of a form of therapy capable of altering the natural history and improving the long-term survival of these patients.

The goal of oxygen therapy is to get the P_{O_2} into the range where hemoglobin is almost fully saturated, i.e., P_{O_2} greater than 60 to 65 torr. Ideally, oxygen saturation should be well maintained on a continuous basis, i.e., throughout the day and night. In some patients with COPD who are not significantly hypoxemic during the day, a substantial drop in their P_{O_2} and oxygen saturation can occur at night; in these patients, nocturnal oxygen may be of benefit.

When respiratory failure supervenes as a part of COPD, all of the above modalities are frequently utilized for therapy. In addition, mechanical ventilation may be necessary for supporting gas exchange and maintaining acceptable arterial blood gases. Other considerations of the treatment of acute respiratory failure superimposed upon chronic disease of the obstructive variety will be covered further in Chapter 26. A discussion of mechanical ventilation can be found in Chapter 28.

Modalities available for treatment of COPD:
1. bronchodilators
2. chest physiotherapy
3. antibiotics
4. corticosteroids
5. supplemental oxygen

REFERENCES

Reviews

Hugh-Jones, P., and Whimster, W.: The etiology and management of disabling emphysema. Am. Rev. Respir. Dis. 117:343–378, 1978.

Petty, T. L. (ed.): Chronic Obstructive Pulmonary Disease. New York, Marcel Dekker, Inc., 1978.

Snider, G. L. (ed.): Emphysema. Clin. Chest Med. 4:329–482, 1983.

Thurlbeck, W. M.: Aspects of chronic airflow obstruction. Chest 72:341–349, 1977.

Thurlbeck, W. M.: Chronic Airflow Obstruction in Lung Disease. Philadelphia, W. B. Saunders Co., 1976.

Etiology and Pathogenesis

Hoidal, J. R., and Niewoehner, D. E.: Pathogenesis of emphysema. Chest 83:679–685, 1983.

Lieberman, J.: Elastase, collagenase, emphysema, and alpha₁–antitrypsin deficiency. Chest 70:62–67, 1976.

Morse, J. O.: Alpha₁–antitrypsin deficiency. N. Engl. J. Med. 299:1045–1048; 1099–1105, 1978.

Snider, G. L.: The pathogenesis of emphysema—twenty years of progress. Am. Rev. Respir. Dis. 124:321–324, 1981.

Clinical Features

Black, L. F.: Early diagnosis of chronic obstructive pulmonary disease. Mayo Clin. Proc. 57:765–772, 1982.

Diener, C. F., and Burrows, B.: Further observations on the course and prognosis of chronic obstructive lung disease. Am. Rev. Respir. Dis. 111:719–724, 1975.

Fletcher, C., and Peto, R.: The natural history of chronic airflow obstruction. Br. Med. J. 1:1645–1648, 1977.

Treatment

Anthonisen, N. R.: Long-term oxygen therapy. Ann. Intern. Med. 99:519–527, 1983.

Make, B.: Medical management of emphysema. Clin. Chest Med. 4:465–482, 1983.

Sahn, S. A.: Corticosteroids in chronic bronchitis and pulmonary emphysema. Chest 73:389–396, 1978.

7

Miscellaneous Airway Diseases

Bronchiectasis
  Etiology and Pathogenesis
  Pathology
  Pathophysiology
  Clinical Features
  Diagnostic Approach
  Treatment
Cystic Fibrosis
  Etiology and Pathogenesis
  Pathology
  Pathophysiology
  Clinical Features
  Diagnostic Approach
  Treatment
Upper Airway Disease
  Etiology
  Pathophysiology
  Clinical Features
  Diagnostic Approach
  Treatment

In this chapter, we consider a few additional selected disorders that affect airways, chosen because of their clinical or physiologic importance. The first of these, bronchiectasis, is a disease that used to be much more common. The use of effective antibiotics for the control of respiratory tract infections has made this problem less prevalent and has also diminished its clinical consequences. The second disorder, cystic fibrosis, is a genetic disease that generally becomes clinically manifest in childhood, and is notable for the often devastating clinical consequences that ensue. Finally, we will briefly consider abnormalities of the upper airway (which for our purposes here includes the airway at or above the level of the trachea) to acquaint the reader with the physiologic principles allowing detection of these disorders.

BRONCHIECTASIS

Bronchiectasis is defined as an irreversible dilatation of airways due to inflammatory destruction of airway walls. Since the most common etiologic factor is a prior localized infection that has damaged the airway wall, the term bronchiectasis usually refers to a localized area of involvement. However, patients may certainly have more than one area of bronchiectasis, and they often have coexisting chronic bronchitis as a generalized process involving other airways.

Etiology and Pathogenesis

Prior infection and/or obstruction are the most common problems leading to bronchiectasis.

Infection and obstruction are the two underlying problems that contribute to the development of dilated or bronchiectatic airways. The old infection(s) may have been viral or bacterial; some years ago, measles or pertussis (whooping cough) pneumonia were common problems eventuating in bronchiectasis. Currently, a variety of other viral and bacterial infections are often responsible, with tuberculosis being one important example. At times, fungal infections may be responsible, as with an entity called bronchopulmonary aspergillosis. This latter problem, found almost exclusively in patients with underlying asthma, is characterized by colonization of airways with *Aspergillus* organisms and by thick mucous plugs and bronchiectasis in relatively proximal airways.

When obstruction of an airway is associated with bronchiectasis behind the obstruction, a superimposed infection may also contribute to destruction of the airway wall. Tumors, foreign bodies, or thick mucus is commonly the cause of bronchial obstruction resulting in bronchiectasis.

An additional factor that plays a role in some patients is a defect in the ability of the airway to clear itself of, or protect itself against, bacterial pathogens (see Chapter 22). Such a defect predisposes to recurrent infections and eventually to airway dilatation and bronchiectasis. The abnormality may involve inadequate humoral immunity and insufficient antibody production (hypogammaglobulinemia), defective leukocyte function, or impaired cellular immunity. Another problem that has received significant attention recently is that of ciliary dysfunction, which affects the ability of the ciliary blanket lining the airway to clear bacteria and to protect the airway against infection. The ciliary dysfunction is not limited to the lower airways; it also affects the nasal mucosa and, in males, may affect sperm motility and hence fertility. Pathologically, the dynein arms that are a characteristic feature of the ultrastructure of cilia are frequently absent in this disorder. One specific

Abnormalities of ciliary structure and function can result in recurrent infections and bronchiectasis.

syndrome associated with bronchiectasis and ciliary dysfunction is called *Kartagener's syndrome*, which includes a triad of sinusitis, bronchiectasis, and situs inversus (discovered by the presence of dextrocardia).

Pathology

The primary pathologic feature of bronchiectasis is evident on gross inspection of the airways, which are markedly dilated in the

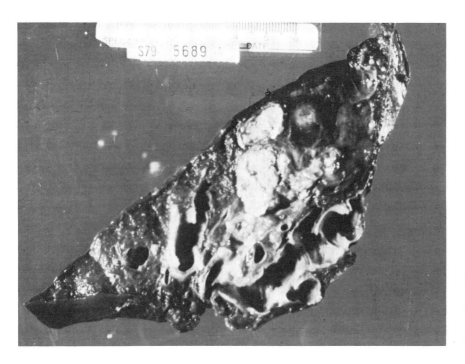

Figure 7–1. Surgically removed specimen of lung demonstrating extensive bronchiectasis. Some of the grossly dilated airways are filled with large amounts of mucoid and purulent material.

involved region (Fig. 7–1). Three specific patterns of dilatation have been described; these have been termed cylindrical, varicose, and saccular bronchiectasis. The dilated airways are generally filled with a considerable amount of secretions, which may be grossly purulent. Microscopic changes of the bronchial wall epithelium, consisting of ulceration and squamous metaplasia, are also seen.

As a result of the exuberant inflammatory changes in the bronchial wall, the blood supply, provided by the bronchial arteries, is increased. The arteries enlarge and increase in number as well, and new anastomoses may form between the bronchial and pulmonary artery circulations. Inflammatory erosion or mechanical trauma at the site of these vascular changes is often responsible for the hemoptysis seen so frequently in patients with bronchiectasis.

Vessels from the bronchial arterial circulation supplying a bronchiectatic region are often a source of bleeding and hemoptysis.

Coexisting disease in the remainder of the tracheobronchial tree is not at all uncommon. Either other areas of bronchiectasis may be present, or the generalized changes of chronic bronchitis may occur, as we described earlier in Chapter 6.

Pathophysiology

Once the airways have become irreversibly dilated, their defense mechanisms against infection are disturbed. The normal propulsive action of cilia is lost in the involved area, even if it was intact prior to the development of bronchiectasis. Bacteria colonize the enlarged airways, and secretions pool in the dilated sacs of patients with saccular bronchiectasis. In many cases, the relationship established between the colonizing bacteria and the host is relatively stable over a period of time, but it may also be punctuated by acute exacerbations of the airway infection.

Functionally, patients with a localized area of bronchiectasis are not impaired in the same way that other patients with generalized obstructive lung disease are. Measurement of their pulmonary function may in fact reveal surprisingly few if any abnormalities. When seen, functional abnormalities are either the result of extensive bronchiectasis involving a large area of one or both lungs or the result of coexistent generalized airway disease, primarily chronic bronchitis.

Clinical Features

The most prominent symptom in patients with bronchiectasis is generally cough and copious sputum production. The sputum may be frankly purulent, and it is often the profuse amount of yellow or green sputum production that raises the physician's suspicion of bronchiectasis. However, it is important to realize that not all patients with bronchiectasis have significant sputum production. It has been estimated that approximately 10 to 20 percent of patients are free of copious sputum production, and these patients are said to have "dry" bronchiectasis.

Common clinical features of bronchiectasis:
1. cough
2. copious and purulent sputum
3. hemoptysis
4. localized rales or rhonchi
5. clubbing

The other frequent symptom in patients with bronchiectasis is hemoptysis, which may be impressive in amount. The hypertrophied bronchial artery circulation to the involved area is probably responsible for this symptom in the majority of cases.

Physical examination of the patient with bronchiectasis may reveal few abnormalities, even over the area of involvement. On the other hand, the examiner may hear strikingly abnormal findings in a localized area, such as rales or rhonchi. Clubbing is frequently present. Although the mechanism is not clear, it is thought to be associated with the chronic suppurative process.

Whether arterial blood gases are abnormal in these patients often depends upon the extent of involvement and the presence or absence of underlying chronic bronchitis. With well-localized disease, both P_{O_2} and P_{CO_2} may be normal. At the other extreme, patients may have the blood gas changes seen in the Type B pattern of chronic obstructive lung disease, namely hypoxia and hypercapnia, and they may also develop the complication of cor pulmonale.

Diagnostic Approach

The diagnosis of bronchiectasis is usually suggested by the history of copious sputum production and/or hemoptysis. Evaluation on a macroscopic level generally includes a chest roentgenogram, the findings of which are often nonspecifically abnormal in the involved area. The radiograph may show an area of increased markings, crowded vessels, or "ring" shadows corresponding to dilated or saccular airways. However, none of the findings on the routine radiograph is considered diagnostic of bronchiectasis. The definitive diagnosis depends on bronchography, a radiographic procedure in which an opaque contrast material is used to outline part of the tracheobronchial tree (Fig. 7–2). Usually, bronchography is not done as part of the patient's evaluation

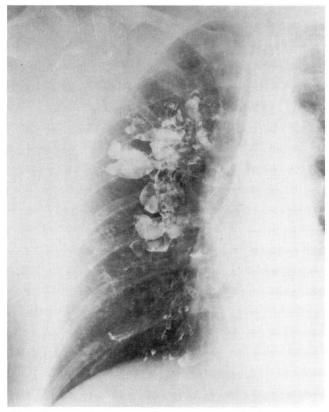

Figure 7–2. Bronchogram of patient with extensive saccular bronchiectasis, primarily in the right upper lobe.

unless a surgical procedure to remove the bronchiectatic area is being considered.

Evaluation on a microscopic level does not offer much for the patient with presumed bronchiectasis, except for examination of the sputum for microorganisms, particularly during an acute exacerbation of the disease. The findings on functional evaluation have already been discussed in the Pathophysiology and Clinical Features sections of this discussion and will not be considered further here.

Treatment

There are currently three major aspects of treatment of the patient with bronchiectasis—bronchopulmonary drainage (clearance of airway secretions), antibiotics, and bronchodilators. Chest physical therapy and positioning to allow better drainage of secretions, i.e., postural drainage, are particularly important for the patient with copious secretions and sputum. Antibiotics are used in various ways in these patients. Sometimes patients are only treated when there is a clear change in the quantity or appearance of the sputum. In other cases, patients are given a regimen of intermittent or even continuous antibiotics in an attempt to keep a chronic infection under control. Bronchodilators may be useful in patients who have coexisting airway obstruction that is at least partially reversible.

*Treatment of bronchiectasis
includes bronchopulmonary
drainage, antibiotics, and
bronchodilators; surgical
therapy with resection of the
diseased area is infrequent.*

In the past, surgery was used for many patients with localized bronchiectasis. Since medical therapy is frequently effective in limiting symptoms and impairment, resection of the diseased area is now done much less frequently. In general, surgery is reserved for selected patients who have significant, poorly controlled symptoms attributable to a single localized area, and who do not have other areas of bronchiectasis or significant evidence of generalized chronic obstructive pulmonary disease.

CYSTIC FIBROSIS

Cystic fibrosis, the most common lethal genetic disease affecting the Caucasian population, is inherited as an autosomal recessive trait and is present in approximately 1 in 2000 live births. Onset of the disease is often in childhood, though cases are being recognized in adults, and children with the disease are living longer into adulthood. The clinical picture is dominated by severe lung disease and by pancreatic insufficiency, resulting from thick and tenacious secretions produced by exocrine glands.

Etiology and Pathogenesis

*Major defects in cystic fibrosis:
(1) production of thick,
tenacious secretions from
exocrine glands
(2) elevated concentrations of
sodium, chloride, and
potassium in sweat*

Two major defects have been recognized in this disease, but the mechanism of each and the possible interrelationship between the two have so far defied elucidation. The first defect is the quality of the secretions produced by various exocrine glands. These secretions are thick and tenacious and block the tubes into which the secretions are normally deposited (especially airways and pancreatic ducts). Second, electrolyte abnormalities have been observed in the sweat produced by affected patients—elevated concentrations of sodium, chloride, and potassium. These abnormalities have proved to be crucial in the diagnosis of the disorder, but the underlying defect causing the electrolyte disturbances is unknown.

Research into the basic abnormality in cystic fibrosis has focused on a variety of areas. Though water and electrolyte transport for exocrine secretions is deranged, it is not clear if this is a primary problem or secondary to defective control of the secretory process by the autonomic nervous system. There has been some speculation that abnormal glycoproteins might alter the physicochemical properties of mucus. Some investigators have also found evidence for a circulating factor in these patients that might be responsible for ciliary dysfunction. Further consideration of the extensive body of research on cystic fibrosis is beyond the scope of this discussion but may be found in several excellent articles listed at the end of this chapter.

Pathology

The pathologic findings in cystic fibrosis appear to result from obstruction of ducts or tubes by tenacious secretions. In the pancreas, this obstruction of the ducts eventually produces fibrosis, atrophy of the acini, and cystic changes. In the airways, thick mucous plugs appear in the bronchi and obstruct airflow as well as the normal drainage of the tracheobronchial tree. Early in the course of the disease, the airway changes are found predominantly in the bronchioles, which are plugged and obliterated by the secretions. Later, the findings are more extensive, superimposed areas of pneumonitis appear, and frank bronchiectasis and areas of abscess formation may be found. As we will discuss, cardiac complications of cor pulmonale frequently occur, and pathologic examination of the heart shows evidence of right ventricular hypertrophy.

Pathophysiology

In the pancreas, the pathologic process leads to pancreatic insufficiency with maldigestion and malabsorption of foodstuffs, particularly fat. In the lung, the major problem is with recurrent episodes of tracheobronchial infection resulting from bronchial obstruction and from defective mucociliary transport. The major organisms that eventually colonize the airways are *Staphylococcus aureus* and *Pseudomonas aeruginosa*. Difficulty with these organisms seems to be entirely a result of the local (airway) host defense mechanisms; the humoral immune system, i.e., the ability to form antibodies, appears to be intact.

Major clinical problems from cystic fibrosis:
(1) pancreatic insufficiency
(2) recurrent episodes of tracheobronchial infection

As a result of the airways obstruction, patients develop functional changes characteristic of obstructive airways disease, along with the finding of air trapping. These patients also exhibit the pathophysiologic changes seen in Type B patients with COPD, i.e., ventilation-perfusion mismatch, hypoxemia (sometimes with CO_2 retention), pulmonary hypertension, and cor pulmonale.

Clinical Features

Approximately 10 to 20 percent of patients with cystic fibrosis develop their first clinical problem in the neonatal period, with intestinal obstruction from thick meconium. This obstruction is called "meconium ileus." The remainder of patients usually present in childhood, with pancreatic insufficiency and/or recurrent bronchial infections. Occasionally, patients are first diagnosed as adults. Almost all males with the disease are sterile, though females are often capable of having children.

The physical examination of patients with cystic fibrosis reveals the findings to be expected with severe airflow obstruction as well as plugging of airways with secretions. Wheezing and coarse rales or rhonchi are frequent and clubbing is common.

Patients may develop several complications as a result of their disease. Pneumothorax and hemoptysis, which may be massive, can be major problems in management. Eventually, patients develop frank respiratory insufficiency and cor pulmonale. Though patients certainly may live into adult life when good care has been provided, their lifespan is significantly reduced.

Serious complications of cystic fibrosis:
1. pneumothorax
2. massive hemoptysis
3. respiratory insufficiency
4. cor pulmonale

Diagnostic Approach

Diagnosis of cystic fibrosis is made by demonstration of an elevated concentration of sweat chloride.

Definitive diagnosis of cystic fibrosis is made by analysis of sweat electrolytes. The concentrations of sodium, chloride, and potassium are elevated in sweat from these patients, and a sweat chloride concentration greater than 60 meq per L is generally considered diagnostic. Only individuals homozygous for the cystic fibrosis gene demonstrate this abnormality, as heterozygous carriers have normal sweat electrolytes. At the present time, there is no accurate way to diagnose carriers or to detect homozygous individuals in utero.

The chest radiograph (Fig. 7–3) often demonstrates an increase in markings along with the findings of bronchiectasis that were described in the previous section. There may also be evidence of focal pneumonitis at times during the course of the disease.

Early in the disease, functional assessment of these patients shows evidence of obstruction of small airways. As the disease progresses, there is evidence of more generalized airway obstruction (decreased FEV_1, FVC, and FEV_1/FVC ratio) and air trapping (increased RV/TLC ratio) is evident. The elastic recoil of the lung is generally preserved, and TLC is most commonly within the normal range. Since emphysematous changes are not generally seen in patients with cystic fibrosis and since the alveolar-capillary interface remains relatively preserved, the diffusing capacity is also most frequently normal. Arterial blood gases often demonstrate hypoxemia, and hypercapnia may also be seen as the disease progresses.

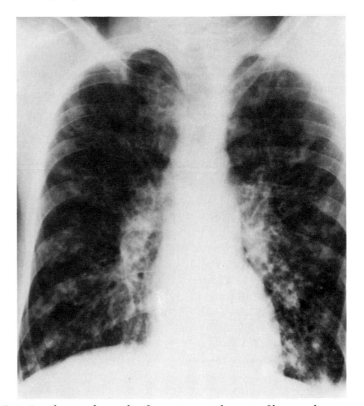

Figure 7–3. PA chest radiograph of a patient with cystic fibrosis, demonstrating a diffuse increase in markings throughout both lungs. These findings represent extensive fibrotic changes and bronchiectasis. (Courtesy of Dr. Mary Ellen Wohl.)

Treatment

Unfortunately, there is no treatment for the primary defect in cystic fibrosis, and therapy is based upon an attempt to diminish the clinical consequences and manage complications when they occur. The principles of therapy are similar to those used for bronchiec-tasis—bronchopulmonary drainage (chest physical therapy and postural drainage), antibiotics, and bronchodilators. Agents used to decrease the viscosity of the sputum appear to offer benefit in some patients. Though therapy has significantly improved prognosis in this disease, the natural history is still one of progressive pulmonary dysfunction and eventual death as a result of the disease or its complications.

UPPER AIRWAY DISEASE

So far, the obstructive diseases that we have considered primarily affect the airways below the level of the main carina, i.e., bronchi and bronchioles. In contrast to disease of these lower airways, a variety of other disorders affect the pharynx, larynx, or trachea and produce what is termed upper airway obstruction. Our discussion of these disorders will be limited and will include a brief consideration of representative etiologies, as well as a discussion of some of the tests used to make the diagnosis. In particular, we will discuss the use of the flow-volume loop to define the location of upper airway obstruction.

Etiology

The upper airway may be affected by either acute problems or ones that have followed a more subacute or chronic course. Acutely the larynx is probably the major area subject to obstruction. Potential causes include infection (epiglottitis, which is most often due to *Hemophilus influenzae*), thermal injury and the resulting laryngeal edema from smoke inhalation, aspiration of a foreign body, and laryngeal edema from an allergic (anaphylactic) reaction.

On a chronic basis, the upper airway may be partially obstructed by hypertrophy of the tonsils, by tumors (particularly of the trachea), by strictures of the trachea (often resulting from previous instrumentation of the trachea), or by vocal cord paralysis. Some patients are also subject to recurrent episodes of upper airway obstruction during sleep; this entity is one variety of what is termed *sleep apnea syndrome*, which will be considered further in Chapter 18.

Pathophysiology

The resistance of a tube to airflow varies inversely as the fourth power of the radius, and hence even small changes in airway size may produce dramatic changes in resistance and in the work of breathing. If the airways under consideration were always stiff, or if a disorder did not allow any flexibility in the size of the airway, then inspiration and expiration would be impaired by the same amount, and the flow rate generated during inspiration would be essentially identical to the flow rate during expiration. This type of obstruction is termed a *fixed* obstruction.

If, on the other hand, airway diameter changes during the respiratory cycle, then the greatest impairment to airflow occurs during the time that airway diameter is smallest. This type of obstruction is termed a *variable* obstruction. If the obstruction is within the thorax, then changes in pleural pressure during the respiratory cycle affect the size of the airway and therefore the magnitude of the obstruction. During a forced expiration, the positive pleural pressure causes airway narrowing, making the obstructing lesion more critical. In contrast, during inspiration, the airways increase their diameter, and the effects of a partial obstruction are less pronounced (Fig. 3–19).

The location and respiratory variability of an upper airway obstruction affect the appearance of the flow-volume curve and the findings on physical examination.

If the obstruction is above the level of the thorax (i.e., outside), then changes in pleural pressure are not directly transmitted to the airway in question. Rather, the negative airway pressure during inspiration tends to create a vacuum-like effect on extrathoracic upper airways, narrowing them and therefore augmenting the effect of any partial obstruction. During expiration, the pressure generated by the flow of air from the intrathoracic airways tends to widen the extrathoracic airways and to decrease the net effect of a partially obstructing lesion (Fig. 3–19).

Clinical Features

Symptomatically, patients with upper airway obstruction may have dyspnea or cough and on physical examination may have evidence of flow through narrowed airways. If the lesion is variable and intrathoracic, the primary difficulty with airflow takes place during expiration and the patients demonstrate expiratory wheezing. If it is variable and extrathoracic, obstruction is more marked during inspiration, and the patient frequently manifests inspiratory stridor, a high-pitched continuous inspiratory sound often best heard over the trachea.

Diagnostic Approach

In the evaluation of suspected disorders of the upper airway, radiography and direct visualization provide the most information about the macroscopic appearance of the airway. Tomography of the upper airway may reveal the localization, extent, and character of a partially obstructing lesion. Though routine tomography has been most frequently used in the past, computed tomography may offer additional information, since it provides a cross-sectional view of the airways from the larynx down to the carina. Direct visualization of the upper airway may be done by laryngoscopy or bronchoscopy, during which the physician may observe whether edema, vocal cord paralysis, or an obstructing lesion such as a tumor is present. However, direct visualization of the airways by these techniques is not entirely without risk, since the instrument used occupies part of the already compromised airway and may induce airway spasm that further obstructs the airway.

The functional assessment of the patient with presumed upper airway obstruction is useful in localizing the obstruction, since the functional consequences of a fixed versus a variable obstruction and an extrathoracic versus an intrathoracic obstruction are quite different. In order to understand these differences, we must consider the flow-volume loop and the principles just discussed under Pathophysiology.

With a fixed lesion causing a relatively critical obstruction, the maximum flow rates generated during inspiration and expiration are approximately equal, and a "plateau" marks both the inspiratory and expiratory parts of the flow-volume curve. When the lesion is variable, the effect of the obstruction depends on whether it is intrathoracic or extrathoracic. With an intrathoracic obstruction, the critical narrowing is during expiration, and the expiratory part of the flow-volume curve displays a plateau. With an extrathoracic obstruction, the expiratory part of the loop is preserved, and the inspiratory portion now displays the plateau. A schematic diagram of the flow-volume loops observed in these various types of upper airway obstruction is presented in Figure 3–20.

Treatment

Since many different types of disorders result in upper airway obstruction, treatment varies greatly depending upon the particular underlying problem. Discussion of each disorder is beyond the scope of this chapter but may be found in more detailed textbooks and in some of the articles mentioned at the end of this chapter.

REFERENCES

Bronchiectasis

Crofton, J.: Diagnosis and treatment of bronchiectasis—I. Diagnosis and II. Treatment and prevention. Br. Med. J. 1:721–723; 783–785, 1966.
Eliasson, R., Mossberg, B., Camner, P., and Afzelius, P. A.: The immotile-cilia syndrome: a congenital ciliary abnormality as an etiologic factor in chronic airway infections and male sterility. N. Engl. J. Med. 297:1–6, 1977.
Ellis, D. A., Thornley, P. E., Wightman, A. J., Walker, M., Chalmers, J., and Crofton, J. W.: Present outlook in bronchiectasis: clinical and social study and review of factors influencing prognosis. Thorax 36:659–664, 1981.
Sanderson, J. M., Kennedy, M. C. S., Johnson, M. F., and Manley, D. C. E.: Bronchiectasis: results of surgical and conservative management. Thorax 29:407–416, 1974.

Cystic Fibrosis

Bowman, B. H., and Mangos, J. A.: Cystic fibrosis. N. Engl. J. Med. 294:937–938, 1976.
Davis, P. B., and di Sant'Agnese, P. A.: Diagnosis and treatment of cystic fibrosis. Chest 85:802–809, 1984.
di Sant'Agnese, P. A., and Davis, P. B.: Research in cystic fibrosis. N. Engl. J. Med. 295:481–485; 534–541; 597–602, 1976.
di Sant'Agnese, P. A., and Davis, P. B.: Cystic fibrosis in adults: 75 cases and a review of 232 cases in the literature. Am. J. Med. 66:121–132, 1979.
Holsclaw, D. S.: Cystic fibrosis: overview and pulmonary aspects in young adults. Clin. Chest Med. 1:407–421, 1980.
Shwachman, H., Kowalski, M., and Khaw, K–T.: Cystic fibrosis: a new outlook. Medicine 56:129–149, 1977.

Upper Airway Disease

Acres, J. C., and Kryger, M. H.: Upper airway obstruction. Chest 80:207–211, 1981.
Kryger, M., Bode, F., Antic, R., and Anthonisen, N.: Diagnosis of obstruction of the upper and central airways. Am. J. Med. 61:85–93, 1976.
Miller, R. D., and Hyatt, R. E.: Obstructing lesions of the larynx and trachea: clinical and physiologic characteristics. Mayo Clin. Proc. 44:145–161, 1969.
Proctor, D. F.: The upper airways. II. The larynx and trachea. Am. Rev. Respir. Dis. 115:315–342, 1977.

8

Anatomic and Physiologic Aspects of the Pulmonary Parenchyma

Anatomy
Physiology

In the next section, encompassing Chapters 8 through 11, we will focus on the region of the lung directly involved in gas exchange. Specifically, this region includes the alveolar walls and spaces (with the alveolar-capillary interface), whether at the level of the alveolar sacs, ducts, or respiratory bronchioles. Some authors use the term pulmonary interstitium when referring to the alveolar walls and describe diseases of this region as *interstitial lung disease,* a convention we will also use.

As a prelude to our consideration of specific diseases, we will describe the normal anatomy of the gas-exchanging region of the lung and then discuss some aspects of its normal physiology. In Chapters 9 through 11, we will primarily discuss those disorders, generally subacute or chronic, whose main pathology appears to reside within the alveolar wall. We are deliberately excluding pneumonia, acute pulmonary injury (adult respiratory distress syndrome), and diseases of the pulmonary vasculature, since they are different pathologic processes and are considered separately in other parts of this book.

In Chapter 9, we will provide an overview of the interstitial lung diseases, emphasizing how disturbances in the structure of this region are closely linked with aberrations in function. Though a wide variety of disorders affect the alveolar wall, many of the pathophysiologic features are common to a large number of individual diseases. Knowledge of these general pathophysiologic features and their effect on the normal function of the lung is useful for understanding the consequences of the individual disease entities. Where specific diseases have special characteristics, we will also consider these individual features.

ANATOMY

For the lung to function efficiently as a gas-exchanging organ, it makes sense that a large surface area should be available where oxygen can be taken up and carbon dioxide released. At the alveolar wall, where this gas exchange occurs, an extensive network of capillaries coursing through and coming into close contact with alveolar gas facilitates this exchange. In the normal lung, the capillaries are closely apposed to the alveolar lumen, and there is little tissue extraneous to the gas-exchanging process (Fig. 8–1).

The surface of the alveolar walls, i.e., the region bordering the alveolar lumen, is lined by a continuous layer of epithelial cells. Two different types of these lining epithelial cells, called Type I and Type II cells, can be identified. *Type I cells* are less numerous than Type II cells, but they have impressively long cytoplasmic extensions that line more than 95 percent of the alveolar surface (Fig. 8–2). The Type I

Type I alveolar epithelial cells have long cytoplasmic processes that line almost the entire alveolar surface.

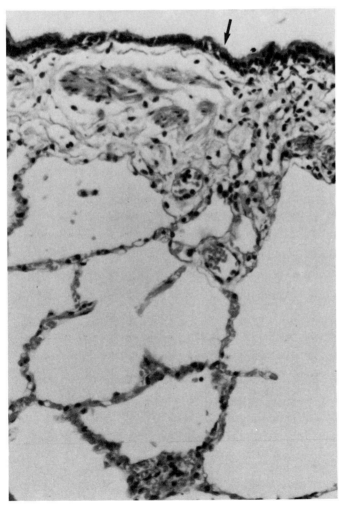

Figure 8–1. Photomicrograph of alveolar walls, demonstrating the normal thin, lacy appearance. At the top of the photo is a bronchial lumen, lined by bronchial epithelial cells (arrow). Peribronchial tissue lies between the bronchial epithelium and the alveolar walls. (Courtesy of Dr. Earl Kasdon.)

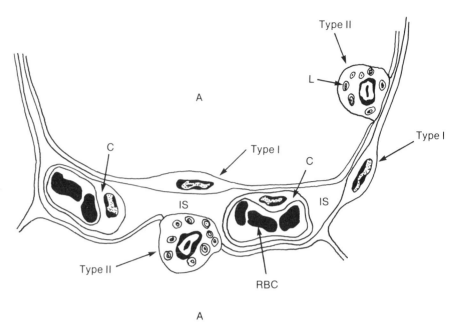

Figure 8–2. Schematic diagram of normal alveolar structure. Type I and Type II epithelial cells are shown lining the alveolar wall. Type I cells are relatively flat and are characterized by long cytoplasmic processes. Type II cells are cuboidal and have cytoplasmic lamellar bodies (L), the source of surfactant. Two capillaries, with capillary endothelial cells (C) and erythrocytes (RBC) in the capillary lumen, are shown. The interstitial space (IS) is the relatively acellular region of the alveolar wall. A = alveolar space.

cells have very few cytoplasmic organelles, and they appear to function primarily as a barrier preventing the free movement of material such as fluid from the alveolar wall into the alveolar lumen.

In contrast, the more numerous *Type II cells* do not have long cytoplasmic extensions, but they do have many cytoplasmic organelles (mitochondria, rough endoplasmic reticulum, Golgi apparatus), suggesting an important synthetic role for these cells. The product of the Type II cells is a material of high lipid content called *surfactant*. Specific inclusion bodies within the Type II cells, termed lamellar inclusions, appear to be the packaged form of surfactant that is eventually released into the alveolar lumen. Surfactant acts like a detergent to reduce the surface tension of the alveoli. It "stabilizes" the alveolus in the same way that a bubble is prevented from collapsing by a detergent material, and it therefore prevents microatelectasis (collapse on a microscopic level). The Type II epithelial cells have a cuboidal shape and are often seen to bulge into the alveolar lumen. However, since they do not have long cytoplasmic extensions, they cover less than 5 percent of the alveolar surface.

Type II cells have an additional function relating to maintenance and repair of the injured alveolar epithelium. The Type I epithelial cells are quite susceptible to a variety of injurious agents, whether the agents reach the alveolar wall via the airways or via the bloodstream. When Type I cells are damaged, the reparative process involves hyperplasia of the Type II cells and eventual differentiation into cells with the characteristics of Type I cells.

Pulmonary capillaries course through the alveolar walls as part of an extensive network of intercommunicating vessels. Unlike the alveolar epithelial cells, which are quite impermeable under normal circumstances, junctions between capillary endothelial cells permit passage of small molecular weight proteins. The permeability features of the alveolar epithelial and capillary endothelial cells will become important when we discuss the adult respiratory distress syndrome in Chapter

Type II cells produce surfactant and are important in the reparative process when Type I cells are damaged.

27, since this disorder is characterized by increased permeability and leakage of fluid and protein into alveolar spaces.

Both the alveolar epithelial and capillary endothelial cells rest upon a basement membrane. At some regions of the alveolar wall, nothing stands between the epithelial and endothelial cells other than their basement membranes, which are fused to form a single basement membrane. At other regions, a space called the interstitial space intervenes, consisting of relatively acellular material (Fig. 8–2). The major components of the interstitial space are collagen and elastin, some nerve endings, and some fibroblast-like cells. There are also small numbers of lymphocytes as well as cells that appear to be in a transition state between blood monocytes and alveolar macrophages (which are derived from circulating monocytes).

Within the alveolar lumen a thin layer of liquid covers the alveolar epithelial cells. This extracellular alveolar lining layer is composed of an aqueous phase immediately adjacent to the epithelial cells, covered by a surface layer of lipid-rich surfactant produced by the Type II epithelial cells. Within the alveolar lining layer are also alveolar macrophages, a type of phagocytic cell important in protecting the distal lung against bacteria and in clearing inhaled dust particles.

PHYSIOLOGY

Though we briefly covered some of the physiologic principles relating to the pulmonary parenchyma in Chapter 1, we will now expand on two topics that will be important when we discuss pathophysiologic abnormalities of interstitial lung disease. We will start with a review of gas exchange at the alveolar-capillary level, and then proceed to a discussion of how disturbances within the pulmonary parenchyma affect the mechanical properties of the lung.

Gas exchange between the alveolus and the capillary depends on the passive diffusion of gas from a region of higher to one of lower partial pressure. The partial pressure of oxygen in the alveolus is normally in the range of 100 torr, while the blood entering the pulmonary capillary has a Po_2 of approximately 40 torr. This difference gives rise to a driving pressure for oxygen to diffuse from the alveolus to the pulmonary capillary, where it binds with hemoglobin in the erythrocyte. The barrier to diffusion—which includes the thin cytoplasmic extension of the Type I cell, the basement membrane of the Type I and capillary endothelial cells, and the capillary endothelial cell itself—is extremely thin, measuring approximately 0.5 micron. In some areas of the alveolar wall, there is also a thin layer of interstitium, but presumably diffusion and gas exchange preferentially occur at the thinnest region where the interstitium is sparse or absent.

Though the rate of gas transfer across the alveolar-capillary interface depends upon the thickness of the barrier, oxygen uptake by the blood is usually complete early during the transit through the capillaries. The total period of time spent by a red blood cell traveling through the pulmonary capillaries is approximately 0.75 second, and equilibration with oxygen occurs within the first third of this time period. Therefore, extra time is available for diffusion should there be disease

Oxygen uptake and CO_2 elimination at the alveolar-capillary interface are completed early during an erythrocyte's transit through the pulmonary vascular bed.

affecting the alveolar-capillary interface and impairing the normal process of diffusion. Carbon dioxide diffuses even more readily than oxygen, so that there is also reserve time available for its diffusion.

Rarely, abnormalities of the alveolar-capillary interface in the setting of interstitial lung disease impair gas exchange by virtue of hindering diffusion of gases. We will consider this issue in more detail in Chapter 9, when we discuss abnormalities in gas exchange in patients with diseases affecting the alveolar wall.

Another important aspect of physiology relating to the lung parenchyma is that of compliance, or more simply, the stiffness of the lung. As we discussed earlier in Chapter 1, the lung is elastic and behaves like a balloon or a rubber band in terms of resisting expansion. Therefore, pressure must be exerted through the airway to inflate a lung; or conversely, negative pressure can also be applied around the lung to cause it to expand. For any given volume of air in the lungs, a certain pressure is required to achieve this degree of inflation, and a curve can be drawn relating volume on the Y axis to pressure on the X axis (Fig. 1–3A). Since the net pressure producing expansion is the difference between the pressure exerted on the alveoli (via the airway) and the absolute pressure outside the lung, the term transpulmonary pressure is used to describe this distending pressure. In vivo, when the lung is sitting within the chest, pressure outside the lung is the

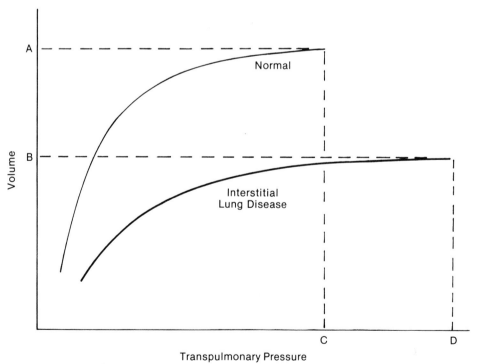

Figure 8–3. Compliance curve of the lung in interstitial lung disease compared with that of the normal lung. In addition to the shift of the curve downward and to the right, it can be seen that the TLC in interstitial lung disease (point B on the volume axis) is characteristically less than the normal TLC (point A). The maximal pressure at TLC is called the maximal static recoil pressure (Pst_{max}), represented for the normal lung and the lung with interstitial disease by points C and D, respectively. Compare with Figure 6–7.

pleural pressure. If a lung is removed and dealt with in isolation, the pressure outside the lung would be atmospheric pressure.

The normal compliance relationship between volume and pressure in the lung is a curve that flattens out at high distending pressures, when the lung reaches its upper limit of expansion. At this point, the elastic tissues of the lung can be stretched no further, and additional pressure does not add extra volume to the lung.

Diseases affecting the alveolar walls commonly disturb this pressure-volume relationship, either making the lung stiffer (more resistant to expansion) or less stiff (easier to expand). For the stiffer, less compliant lung, the compliance curve is shifted to the right, i.e., a lower volume is achieved for any given transpulmonary pressure. Most of the diseases covered in this section, which are included in the category of interstitial lung disease, affect the compliance of the lung in this way (Fig. 8–3). In contrast, as we discussed in Chapter 6 and illustrated in Figure 6–7, patients with emphysema, whose lungs are less resistant to expansion (i.e., more compliant), have compliance curves that are shifted to the left. This principle of compliance is an important one in pulmonary physiology. We have already alluded in Chapters 1 and 6 to the role compliance plays in determining lung volumes measured in pulmonary function testing, particularly TLC and FRC. We will touch upon this principle again in the next chapter, when we discuss the pathophysiology of diseases affecting the alveolar walls.

The compliance curve of the lung in interstitial lung disease is shifted downward and to the right.

REFERENCES

Anatomy

Corrin, B.: The cellular constituents of the lung. *In* Scadding, J. G., and Cumming, G. (eds.): Scientific Foundations of Respiratory Medicine. Philadelphia, W. B. Saunders Co., 1981, pp. 78–91.

Gail, D. B., and Lenfant, C. J. M.: Cells of the lung: biology and clinical implications. Am. Rev. Respir. Dis. 127:366–387, 1983.

Kuhn, C., III.: The cells of the lung and their organelles. *In* Crystal, R. G. (ed.): The Biochemical Basis of Pulmonary Function. New York, Marcel Dekker, Inc., 1976, pp. 3–48.

Morgan, T. E.: Pulmonary surfactant. N. Engl. J. Med. 284:1185–1193, 1971.

Physiology

Murray, J. F.: The Normal Lung: The Basis for Diagnosis and Treatment of Pulmonary Disease. Philadelphia, W. B. Saunders Co., 1976.

West, J. B.: Respiratory Physiology—The Essentials. 2nd ed. Baltimore, Williams and Wilkins, 1979.

9

Overview of the Interstitial Lung Diseases

A large group of disorders affects the alveolar wall, generally in a fashion that may ultimately lead to diffuse scarring or fibrosis. As we mentioned in Chapter 8, these disorders are commonly referred to as the interstitial lung diseases, though the term is something of a misnomer. The interstitium formally refers just to the region of the alveolar wall exclusive of and separating the alveolar epithelial and the capillary endothelial cells. These diseases, on the other hand, affect all components of the alveolar wall—epithelial cells, endothelial cells, and the cellular and noncellular components of the interstitium. Since the convention has been established, however, we will also refer to these diseases as interstitial lung diseases, but the reader must remember that the pathologic processes are certainly not limited to the interstitium.

There have now been more than 130 disorders so described. Since it is difficult even for the pulmonary specialist to know about all of these diseases, it is obviously not appropriate for the novice in pulmonary medicine to worry about amassing knowledge about each individual entity. Rather, we hope that the reader will first develop an understanding of the pathologic, pathogenetic, pathophysiologic, and clinical features that these disorders have in common. We will attempt to cover these areas in this chapter and will refer to individual diseases only when necessary. In the subsequent two chapters, we will then focus on the major types of interstitial lung disease. Chapter 10 will include those disorders associated with an identifiable etiologic agent. Overall, perhaps 35 percent of patients with interstitial lung disease fall into this category. In Chapter 11, we will cover interstitial lung diseases for which a specific etiologic agent has not been identified. The majority of patients with interstitial disease fall into this second category. In these chapters, we will discuss only a small number of the described etiologies. Throughout, the goal is to include the ones that the reader is most likely to encounter.

The diseases covered in this section of the book are basically chronic diseases affecting the alveolar wall. An additional group of diseases is associated with acute injury to various components of the alveolar wall. These latter disorders are of clinical importance as causes of acute respiratory failure, and they will be discussed in Chapter 27 of this book, entitled Adult Respiratory Distress Syndrome.

PATHOLOGY

By and large, the interstitial diseases, regardless of etiology, have two major pathologic components—an inflammatory process in the alveolar wall (sometimes called an *alveolitis*), and a scarring or fibrotic process (Fig. 9–1). Both features generally occur simultaneously, though the relative proportions of inflammation and fibrosis vary with the particular etiology and the duration of the disease. The presumption has generally been that active inflammation is the primary process and that fibrosis follows as a secondary feature.

Interstitial lung diseases are characterized pathologically by alveolitis and fibrosis.

As part of the alveolitis, a variety of inflammatory cells infiltrate the alveolar wall—macrophages, lymphocytes, neutrophils, eosinophils, and plasma cells. Individual etiologies of interstitial disease are

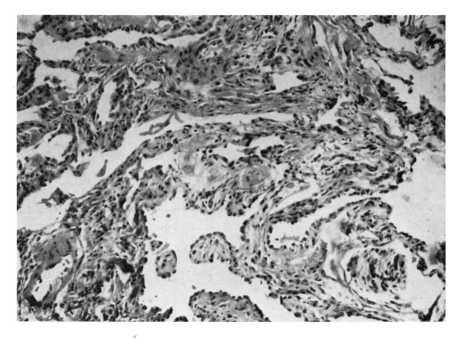

Figure 9–1. Photomicrograph of interstitial lung disease, demonstrating markedly thickened alveolar walls. A cellular inflammatory process and fibrosis are both present. Compare with the appearance of normal alveolar walls in Figure 8–1.

often associated with a particular prominence of one or another of these cell types. In addition to the presence of inflammatory cells, certain disorders have other characteristic pathologic features associated with the alveolitis. These individual patterns are useful and in many cases critical to the diagnosis of a specific pathologic entity.

One of the most important of the pathologic features associated with certain interstitial lung diseases is the *granuloma*. A granuloma is a localized collection of cells called epithelioid histiocytes, which are essentially tissue cells of the phagocytic or macrophage series (Fig. 9–2). Within or around granulomas there may also be multinucleated giant cells, which result from a fusion of several phagocytic cells into a single large cell with abundant cytoplasm and many nuclei (Fig. 9–2). Examples of interstitial lung diseases that have granulomas as part of the pathologic process include sarcoidosis and hypersensitivity pneumonitis. Granulomas are often considered to reflect some underlying immune process, specifically an immune reaction to an exogenous agent. In the case of hypersensitivity pneumonitis, many such agents have been identified. However, in the case of sarcoidosis, no specific exogenous agent has ever been identified. Granulomas in the lung have many other causes (e.g., tuberculosis, certain fungal infections, and foreign bodies), but these will not be covered here, since the granulomas are generally not associated with diffuse interstitial lung disease.

For many of the interstitial lung diseases not associated with granulomas, surprisingly few if any distinguishing features of the alveolitis appear on pathologic examination. For example, in idiopathic pulmonary fibrosis, there is a mixed inflammatory cell infiltrate in the alveolar wall, consisting of macrophages, lymphocytes, neutrophils, eosinophils, and plasma cells in variable numbers. A similar pathologic picture is seen with the interstitial lung diseases secondary to under-

Interstitial diseases with granulomas include sarcoidosis and hypersensitivity pneumonitis.

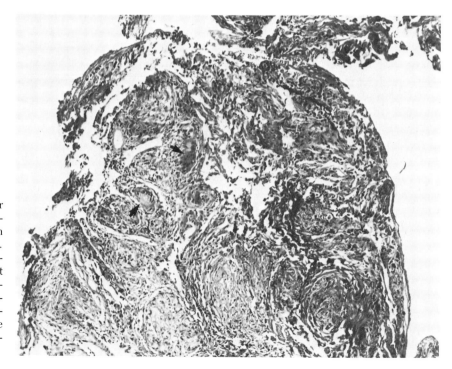

Figure 9–2. Low-power photomicrograph of a transbronchial lung biopsy from a patient with sarcoidosis. Numerous confluent granulomas appear throughout the entire specimen, obliterating the normal pulmonary architecture. Two multinucleated giant cells are marked by arrows. (Courtesy of Dr. Earl Kasdon.)

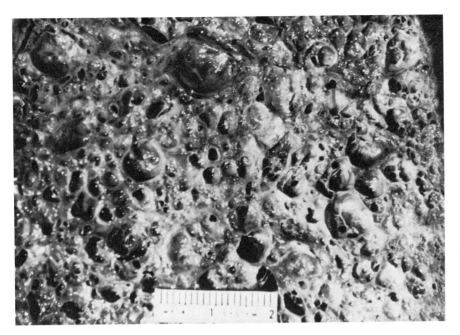

Figure 9–3. Appearance of "honeycomb lung" from a patient with severe interstitial lung disease. There are many cystic areas between the bands of extensively scarred and retracted pulmonary parenchyma.

lying rheumatologic disease, so that a background history of a specific connective tissue disease may be the only way to make this diagnostic distinction.

The other important aspect of the interstitial lung diseases that is obvious on pathologic examination is the presence of fibrosis. When tissue sections are stained by a special technique for identifying collagen, such as a Masson trichrome stain, increased staining indicates collagen deposition and hence fibrosis. The amount of fibrosis is quite variable, depending on the nature and duration of the particular disorder.

When interstitial lung diseases have been present for a fairly long period and are associated with significant fibrosis, often any distinctive features of a prior alveolitis are lost. For example, any of the granulomatous lung diseases may no longer demonstrate the characteristic granulomas after a sufficient time period and a substantial degree of fibrosis. Therefore, at a certain point all of the interstitial lung diseases, if sufficiently severe and chronic, follow a final common pathway toward what is called "end-stage" interstitial lung disease. Along with severe fibrosis, the end-stage lung has a great deal of distortion that can be seen both grossly and microscopically, with areas of contraction and other areas showing formation of cystic spaces. In many cases, the picture is described as one of *honeycomb lung*, since the dense scarring and intervening cystic regions may make areas of the lung resemble a honeycomb (Fig. 9–3).

PATHOGENESIS

For most of the individual interstitial diseases that we will discuss, some etiologic or pathogenetic points are specific to the particular disease and will be considered accordingly. However, a few general concepts are worth discussing separately in this chapter, since their applicability is not limited to a specific disease.

Recent work has suggested that it may be worthwhile to separate the interstitial diseases into two categories, each with a somewhat different pathogenesis. In the first of these, which corresponds to diseases that exhibit a granulomatous component to the alveolitis (e.g., sarcoidosis, hypersensitivity pneumonitis), the lymphocyte is thought to play a crucial role. Therefore, these disorders are said to have a *lymphocytic alveolitis*. In the second category, granulomas are generally not part of the pathology, and the neutrophil is believed by some investigators to play a crucial role in the pathogenesis. These disorders are described as having a *neutrophilic alveolitis*.

According to a current theory about the diseases associated with lymphocytic alveolitis, the initiating event is exposure to an antigen (see Fig. 11–2). In the case of hypersensitivity pneumonitis, many such antigens have been identified, as will be discussed in Chapter 10. In the case of sarcoidosis, no antigen has been identified, but the presumption is that at least one unknown antigen plays an important role. Upon exposure to the offending antigen, T-lymphocytes are recruited to and activated in the lung. Alveolar macrophages may have an accessory role in this process, perhaps being necessary for optimal activation of the T-lymphocytes. Once the T-lymphocytes are activated, they release a chemotactic factor directed at circulating monocytes (the precursors of macrophages), attracting them to the lung parenchyma and perhaps initiating their accumulation into granulomas. Evidence for this theory includes the finding of many activated T-lymphocytes in the lung in these disorders, as well as demonstration of a monocyte chemotactic factor produced by the activated T-lymphocytes.

The corresponding theory to explain diseases with a neutrophilic alveolitis suggests that antigen-antibody complexes are crucial in initiating the chain of events (see Fig. 11–1). These complexes activate macrophages, which as a result release a chemotactic factor for neutrophils. The neutrophils are responsible for producing a variety of chemical mediators potentially toxic to components of the alveolar wall. One such mediator is the enzyme collagenase, which has been identified in the lower respiratory tract of patients with idiopathic pulmonary fibrosis. Evidence for this theory includes the finding of antigen-antibody complexes in serum and in lung tissue of these patients, and the demonstration of release of a chemotactic factor for neutrophils in response to activation of macrophages by antigen-antibody complexes. Whatever the validity of this theory, no definite antigens comprising the antigen-antibody complexes have yet been identified.

These theories about the pathogenesis of the two main types of interstitial lung disease are intriguing, and it seems likely that evidence either supporting or disputing the theories will be forthcoming in the near future. However, even if the theories are correct, a great deal of research must yet be done to elucidate the nature of the antigen(s) initiating the entire process.

PATHOPHYSIOLOGY

With minor exceptions and variations, the pathophysiologic features of all the interstitial lung diseases are quite similar and will

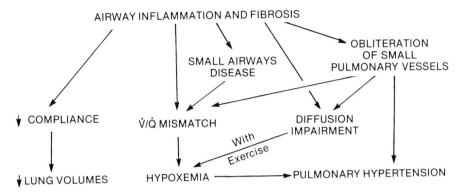

Figure 9–4. Schematic diagram illustrating interrelationships between the various pathologic and physiologic features of interstitial lung disease.

therefore be discussed here as a single group. As a result of the inflammation and fibrosis affecting the alveolar walls, the following abnormalities are generally seen (Fig. 9–4): (1) decreased compliance (increased stiffness) of the lung; (2) a generalized decrease in lung volumes; (3) impairment of diffusion; (4) abnormalities in small airway function without generalized airflow obstruction; (5) disturbances in gas exchange, usually consisting of hypoxemia without CO_2 retention; and (6) in some cases pulmonary hypertension. We will briefly consider each of these features in turn.

Decreased Compliance

The distensibility of the lungs is altered significantly by processes involving inflammation and fibrosis of the alveolar walls. The lungs become much stiffer, have a greatly increased elastic recoil, and therefore require greater distending (transpulmonary) pressures to achieve any given lung volume. The pressure-volume or compliance curve is shifted to the right, as shown in Figure 8–3, and at TLC a much higher elastic recoil pressure is found than in normal lungs. This maximal pressure at TLC is termed the maximum static recoil pressure of the lung or Pst_{max}. Since wider swings in transpulmonary pressure are required to achieve a normal tidal volume during inspiration, the patient's work of breathing is increased. As a result, patients with interstitial lung disease tend to breathe with smaller tidal volumes in order to expend less work, while increasing respiratory frequency to maintain adequate alveolar ventilation.

Compliance curves in interstitial lung disease are shifted downward and to the right, reflecting increased stiffness of the lung.

Decrease in Lung Volumes

Early in the course of interstitial lung disease, the lung volumes may be normal. However, in most cases some reduction in lung volumes will be seen shortly, including a reduction in TLC, VC, FRC, and to a lesser extent RV. The decreases in TLC and FRC are a direct consequence of the change in compliance of the lung. At TLC, the force generated by the inspiratory muscles is balanced by the inward elastic recoil of the lung. Since the recoil pressure is increased, this balance is achieved at a lower lung volume or lower TLC. At FRC, the outward recoil of the chest wall is balanced by the inward elastic

Lung volumes are characteristically decreased in interstitial lung disease.

recoil of the lung. Again, the balance will be achieved at a lower lung volume or lower FRC because of the greater elastic recoil of the lung.

Impairment of Diffusion

Diffusing capacity is reduced with destruction of a portion of the alveolar-capillary interface and reduced surface area for gas exchange.

Measurement of diffusion by the usual techniques involving carbon monoxide shows a decrease in the diffusing capacity. Though thickening of the alveolar-capillary interface (because of interstitial inflammation and fibrosis) might be expected to be responsible for this decrease, it is not the major factor. Rather, the processes of inflammation and fibrosis actually destroy a portion of the alveolar-capillary interface and reduce the surface area available for gas exchange. This decrease in surface area appears to be mainly responsible for the observed diffusion abnormality.

Abnormalities in Small Airway Function

Small airways function is often disturbed in interstitial lung disease; large airways function is generally preserved.

Large airways generally function normally in these patients, and the FEV_1/FVC ratio is usually normal. However, frequently the pathologic process occurring in the alveolar walls also affects small airways within the lung. Light microscopy commonly demonstrates inflammation and fibrosis in the peribronchiolar regions, with narrowing of the lumen of the small airways or bronchioles. Tests of small airways function often show the physiologic effects of this narrowing. The clinical importance of small airways dysfunction in the absence of larger airways abnormalities is uncertain, but it is certainly possible that ventilation-perfusion mismatching and hypoxemia may be a consequence. In a few of the disorders causing interstitial lung disease, evidence of more significant airflow obstruction may be seen. This relatively infrequent problem sometimes results from severe fibrosis and airway distortion.

Disturbances in Gas Exchange

Arterial blood gases in interstitial lung disease generally show hypoxemia (resulting from V̇/Q̇ mismatch) and a normal or decreased P_{CO_2}; with exercise, the P_{O_2} falls even further.

The gas exchange consequences of interstitial lung disease most frequently consist of hypoxemia without CO_2 retention, or in fact with hypocapnia. Though a diffusion block was at one time proposed as the cause of the hypoxemia, most evidence supports ventilation-perfusion mismatch as the major contributor to hypoxemia. The pathologic process in the alveolar walls is an uneven one, and the normal matching of ventilation and perfusion is disrupted. In patients with small airways disease, dysfunction at this level probably also contributes to the ventilation-perfusion mismatch and to hypoxemia. Characteristically, patients with interstitial lung disease become even more hypoxemic with exercise. Though the entire mechanism is not entirely clear, under conditions of exercise diffusion limitation may actually contribute to the hypoxemia. The combination of impaired diffusion plus a decreased transit time of the red blood cell during exercise may prevent complete equilibration of the P_{O_2} in pulmonary capillary blood with alveolar P_{O_2}.

Despite the often profound hypoxemia in patients with severe interstitial fibrosis, P_{CO_2} is generally normal or low, as patients are able to increase their minute ventilation sufficiently to compensate for a decrease in tidal volume and for any additional dead space.

Pulmonary Hypertension

Eventually, patients with severe interstitial lung disease often develop pulmonary hypertension and cor pulmonale. Rarely, the cause of the pulmonary hypertension is a primary process affecting pulmonary vessels as well as alveolar walls. More frequently, the process in the alveolar walls is the cause of the pulmonary hypertension. There are two main contributing factors: (1) hypoxemia and (2) obliteration of small pulmonary vessels by the fibrotic process in the alveolar walls. During exercise, the pulmonary hypertension becomes even more marked. This is due partly to worsening hypoxemia and partly to limited ability of the pulmonary capillary bed to distend and recruit new vessels to handle the exercise-induced increase in cardiac output.

Pulmonary hypertension is common in severe interstitial lung disease, a result of hypoxemia and obliteration of small pulmonary vessels.

CLINICAL FEATURES

Patients with interstitial lung disease most commonly have dyspnea as their presenting symptom. The dyspnea is initially noticed on exertion, but with severe disease may even be experienced at rest. Cough, usually nonproductive, may also be present. On physical examination, auscultation of the chest characteristically reveals dry crackles or rales, which are often most prominent at the bases of the lungs. Clubbing is frequently present, and patients with cor pulmonale may have the cardiac physical findings associated with pulmonary hypertension and right ventricular hypertrophy.

Chest examination is often notable for crackles, particularly at the lung bases.

DIAGNOSTIC APPROACH

The chest radiograph is certainly the most important means for making a macroscopic assessment of interstitial lung disease. The characteristic roentgenographic picture is one of increased linear and small nodular markings, usually referred to as a reticulonodular or interstitial pattern (see Fig. 3–6). This pattern is felt to be indicative of a process involving the alveolar walls, as opposed to the alveolar spaces. However, absence of this abnormality does not exclude the presence of interstitial disease, since up to 10 percent of such patients have been reported to have entirely normal chest radiographs. The roentgenographic pattern is not particularly useful for gauging the relative amounts of inflammation versus fibrosis, each of which may result in a similar pattern. The reticulonodular changes are frequently diffuse throughout both lung fields, though individual causes of interstitial lung disease may be more likely to result in either an upper or a lower lung field predominance of the abnormal markings. Besides the interstitial pattern, certain diseases may have other associated

A reticulonodular pattern on chest x-ray is characteristic of interstitial lung disease; however, up to 10 percent of patients may have a normal x-ray.

findings on chest roentgenogram, such as hilar adenopathy or pleural disease. These additional features will be discussed with each disease in Chapters 10 and 11.

As we mentioned earlier, with long-standing and severe disease, the lungs may become grossly distorted; and there may be regions of cyst formation between scarred and retracted areas of lung (Fig. 9–3). A corresponding pattern of honeycombing on chest radiograph may also be apparent. Cor pulmonale may be suspected on chest roentgenogram by the presence of right ventricular enlargement, best seen on the lateral view.

Another means of making a macroscopic assessment of the pathologic process in the lungs has recently been suggested. This technique involves injecting a radioisotope, gallium-67, into a peripheral vein and scanning the lung with a detector to form a pictorial representation of uptake by the lung. The isotope is taken up by a variety of inflammatory cells and therefore appears to accumulate in regions of active inflammation or alveolitis. It has been suggested that the gallium scan is useful for assessing the activity of the disease, and that serial studies over time may be an objective way to follow the course of the disease or of treatment.

Despite the importance of the macroscopic evaluation, making a diagnostic distinction between the different types of interstitial lung disease usually requires investigation at the microscopic or histologic level. A variety of biopsy procedures have been used to obtain tissue specimens from the lung, which are then subjected to several routine staining techniques. The most frequently used biopsy procedures for this purpose are the open lung biopsy and the transbronchial biopsy (via fiberoptic bronchoscopy). Open biopsy often is the more appropriate of the two procedures in order to obtain a sufficient piece of tissue for examination. However, as we will discuss, when sarcoidosis (or certain other forms of interstitial disease) is suspected, transbronchial biopsy is a particularly suitable initial procedure.

Recently another way of sampling the cell population of the alveolitis has been suggested, a procedure called *bronchoalveolar lavage*. In this procedure, a fiberoptic bronchoscope is placed as distally as possible into an airway, and an irrigation or lavage of fluid through the bronchoscope allows cells from the alveolar spaces to be collected. These cells are thought to be representative of those that are actually within the alveolar wall and responsible for the alveolitis. With this technique, some investigators suggest that a lymphocytic and neutrophilic alveolitis can be distinguished, and also that serial determinations over time reflect the activity of the disease or the response to treatment.

The findings on functional assessment of the patient with interstitial lung disease have basically been reviewed in the Pathophysiology section of this chapter. Briefly, patients have a restrictive pattern on pulmonary function testing, with decreased lung volumes and preserved airflow. Diffusing capacity is usually reduced, indicative of loss of the surface area for gas exchange. Hypoxemia is usually (though not necessarily) present, and the P_{O_2} falls even further with exercise. Hypercapnia is rarely a feature of the disease. When it occurs, hypercapnia usually reflects preterminal disease or an additional, unrelated process.

TREATMENT

Treatment considerations vary greatly from disease to disease. In general, patients with interstitial disease either do not respond to any form of treatment or respond to corticosteroids to a variable extent. The rationale for corticosteroid therapy is to reduce the alveolitis component of the disease, since the fibrosis is generally considered to be irreversible. Specific aspects of treatment will be discussed with the individual diseases in Chapters 10 and 11.

Corticosteroids are used for treating interstitial lung disease to decrease the inflammatory component of the disease.

REFERENCES

Reviews

Crystal, R. G., Bitterman, P. B., Rennard, S. I., Hance, A. J., and Keogh, B. A.: Interstitial lung diseases of unknown cause: disorders characterized by chronic inflammation of the lower respiratory tract. N. Engl. J. Med. 310:154–166; 235–244, 1984.

Crystal, R. G., Gadek, J. E., Ferrans, V. J., Fulmer, J. D., Line, B. R., and Hunninghake, G. W.: Interstitial lung disease: current concepts of pathogenesis, staging and therapy. Am. J. Med. 70:542–568, 1981.

Davis, W. B., and Crystal, R. G.: Chronic interstitial lung disease. *In* Simmons, D. H. (ed.): Current Pulmonology. Vol. 5. New York, John Wiley & Sons, 1984, pp. 347–473.

Fulmer, J. D.: The interstitial lung diseases. Chest 82:172–178, 1982.

Fulmer, J. D.: An introduction to the interstitial lung diseases. Clin. Chest Med. 3:457–473, 1982.

Fulmer, J. D., and Crystal, R. G.: Interstitial lung disease. *In* Simmons, D. H. (ed.): Current Pulmonology. Vol. 1. Boston, Houghton Mifflin, 1979, pp. 1–65.

Keogh, B. A., and Crystal, R. G.: Chronic interstitial lung disease. *In* Simmons, D. H. (ed.): Current Pulmonology. Vol. 3. New York, John Wiley & Sons, 1981, pp. 237–340.

Specific Articles

Epler, G. R., McLoud, T. C., Gaensler, E. A., Mikus, J. P., and Carrington, C. B.: Normal chest roentgenograms in chronic diffuse infiltrative lung disease. N. Engl. J. Med. 298:934–939, 1978.

Wall, C. P., Gaensler, E. A., Carrington, C. B., and Hayes, J. A.: Comparison of transbronchial and open biopsies in chronic infiltrative lung diseases. Am. Rev. Respir. Dis. 123:280–285, 1981.

10

Interstitial Diseases Associated with Known Etiologic Agents

> **Diseases Due to Inhaled Inorganic Dusts**
>   Silicosis
>   Coal Worker's Pneumoconiosis
>   Asbestosis
> **Hypersensitivity Pneumonitis**
> **Drug-Induced Interstitial Lung Disease**
> **Radiation-Induced Lung Disease**

In this chapter, we will consider a few of the major categories of interstitial lung disease for which an etiologic agent has been identified. The general principles discussed in Chapter 9 apply to most of these conditions, and the features we will emphasize here are ones peculiar to or characteristic of each etiology. Considering the vast number of interstitial lung diseases, we will only be scratching the surface of information available. The reader will find that when confronted with a patient having a particular type of interstitial lung disease, it is best to learn or relearn the details of the disease at that time.

DISEASES DUE TO INHALED INORGANIC DUSTS

Many types of interstitial lung disease due to inhalation of inorganic dusts have now been identified, for which the term *pneumoconiosis* has been used. Examples of responsible agents include silica, asbestos, coal, talc, mica, aluminum, and beryllium, just to name a few. In most cases, contact has occurred over a prolonged period of time as a result of occupational exposure. In some of these diseases, the interstitial process is well-known to progress even in the absence of continued exposure.

For an inhaled inorganic dust to initiate an alveolitis, it must be deposited at an appropriate area of the lower respiratory tract. If particle size is too large or too small, deposition tends to be in the upper airway or in the larger airways of the tracheobronchial tree. Particles with a diameter of approximately 0.5 to 5 microns are the ones for which deposition in the respiratory bronchioles or the alveoli is most likely.

Particles between 0.5 and 5 microns are the ones most likely to be deposited in respiratory bronchioles or alveoli.

Unfortunately, no effective treatment is available for interstitial lung disease due to inhaled inorganic dusts. Therefore, at this time, the important issues facing physicians are recognition and prevention of these disorders. Total avoidance of exposure is obviously the optimal form of prevention, but when exposure is necessary, appropriate precautions with effective masks are essential.

We will briefly consider three types of pneumoconiosis that are clinically most important—silicosis, coal-worker's pneumoconiosis, and asbestosis. For information about the numerous other agents, the reader should consult the more detailed references listed at the end of this chapter.

Silicosis

Silicosis is the interstitial lung disease resulting from exposure to silica (silicon dioxide). Of several crystalline forms of silica, quartz is the one most frequently encountered, usually as a component of rock or sand. Persons at risk include sandblasters, rock miners, quarry workers, and stone cutters. In most cases, development of disease requires at least 20 years of exposure, but with particularly heavy doses of inhaled silica, as are found with sandblasters, much shorter periods are sufficient.

Though the pathogenesis of silicosis is not known with certainty, theories have centered around the potential toxicity of silica for macrophages. Silica particles in the lower respiratory tract are engulfed and ingested by alveolar macrophages. In this process, the macrophages are thought to be activated and eventually destroyed by the silica particles. With their destruction, the macrophages release chemical mediators which may initiate or perpetuate an alveolitis. They also release the toxic silica particles, which are now capable of repeating the process after being re-ingested by other macrophages. Some evidence suggests that one of the materials released by the killed macrophages stimulates collagen production by fibroblasts, but this finding has not been universally accepted.

The pulmonary effects of silica may be related to a toxic effect on alveolar macrophages.

Pathologically, the inflammatory process is initially localized around the respiratory bronchioles but eventually becomes more diffuse throughout the parenchyma. Generally, a characteristic acellular nodule composed of connective tissue also appears and is called a silicotic nodule (Fig. 10–1). At first, the nodules are small and discrete; with progression of the disease they become larger and may coalesce.

Initially, the radiographic appearance of silicosis is notable for small, rounded opacities or nodules. At this point, the patient is said to have *simple pneumoconiosis*; when the nodules become larger and coalescent, the pneumoconiosis is *complicated* (Fig. 10–2). As a general rule, in patients with silicosis the upper lung zones are more heavily affected than the lower zones. There may also be enlargement of the hilar lymph nodes, which frequently calcify.

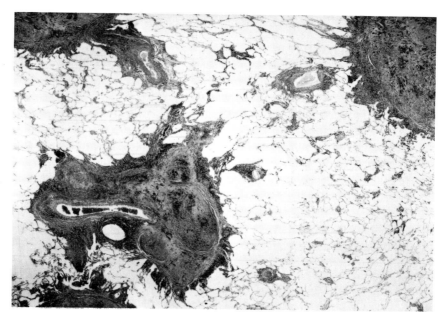

Figure 10–1. Low power view of silicotic lung, demonstrating the characteristic appearance of silicotic nodules. (From Morgan, W. K. C. and Seaton, A.: Occupational Lung Diseases. Philadelphia, W. B. Saunders Co., 1975. Reproduced with permission.)

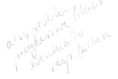

Silicosis predisposes to secondary infections by mycobacteria.

In addition to the potential problem of progressive pulmonary involvement and eventual respiratory failure, patients with silicosis are particularly susceptible to infections with mycobacteria. The specific organisms may be either *Mycobacterium tuberculosis*, the etiologic agent for tuberculosis, or other species of mycobacteria, often called atypical mycobacteria.

Coal Worker's Pneumoconiosis

Tissue reaction to inhaled coal dust is much less than that to silica.

Individuals who have worked as part of the coal mining process and have been exposed to large amounts of coal dust are at risk for the development of *coal worker's pneumoconiosis* (CWP). In comparison with silica, coal dust is a less fibrogenic material, and the tissue reaction is much less marked for equivalent amounts of dust deposited in the lungs.

The pathologic hallmark of CWP is the coal macule, which is a focal collection of coal dust surrounded by relatively little tissue reaction, either in terms of cellular infiltration or fibrosis (Fig. 10–3). The initial lesions tend to be distributed primarily around respiratory bronchioles. Small associated regions of emphysema, termed focal emphysema, may also appear.

Symptoms and pulmonary function changes in CWP occur primarily in patients with extensive radiographic changes.

As with silicosis, the disease is often separated into "simple" and "complicated" forms. In simple CWP, the chest roentgenogram consists of relatively small and discrete densities that are usually more nodular than linear. In this phase of the disease, patients have little in the way of symptoms, and pulmonary function is often relatively preserved. In later stages of the disease, to which fortunately only a small minority of individuals progress, both chest roentgenographic findings and clinical symptoms become more pronounced. With extensive disease and coalescent opacities on chest radiograph, the patients are said to

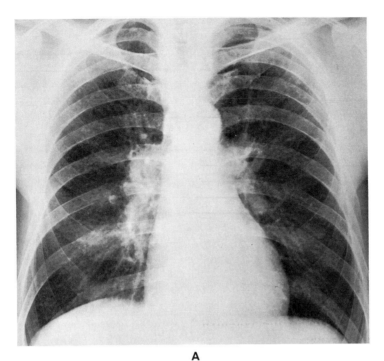

A

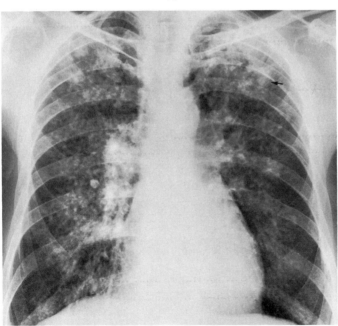

B

Figure 10–2. Radiographic appearance of "simple" *(A)* and "complicated" *(B)* silicosis in the same patient. In *A*, there are small nodules throughout both lungs, particularly in the upper zones, with a reticular component as well. In *B*, the nodules have become larger, and are now coalescent in the upper zones. One of the confluent shadows on the left shows cavitation (arrow). The interval between radiographs *A* and *B* is 11 years. (From Fraser, R. G. and Paré, J. A. P.: Diagnosis of Diseases of the Chest. Vol. III. 2nd ed. Philadelphia, W. B. Saunders Co., 1979. Reproduced with permission.)

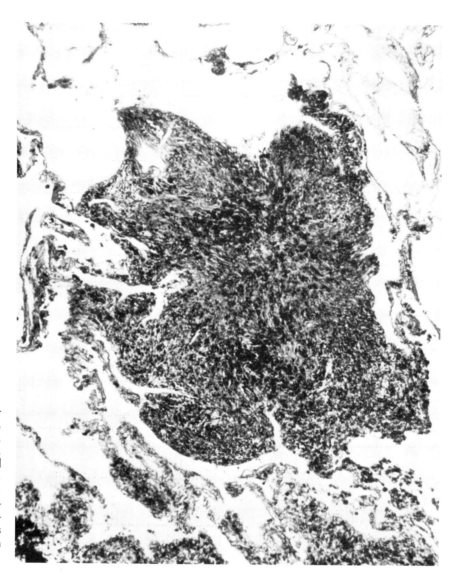

Figure 10–3. Histologic appearance of coal macule, demonstrating coal dust, dust-laden macrophages, and relatively small amounts of fibrous reaction. (From Morgan, W. K. C. and Seaton, A.: Occupational Lung Diseases. Philadelphia, W. B. Saunders Co., 1975. Reproduced with permission.)

have complicated disease, which is also called *progressive massive fibrosis*.

Why some patients with CWP develop complicated disease is not entirely clear. At one time, it was speculated that patients with progressive massive fibrosis had also been exposed to toxic amounts of silica, and that the simultaneous silica exposure was responsible for most of the fibrotic process. However, though some patients do have a mixed form of pneumoconiosis from both coal dust and silica exposure, it appears that progressive massive fibrosis can result from coal dust in the absence of concomitant exposure to silica.

Asbestosis

Asbestos, which has received wide usage in the past because of its thermal and fire resistance, is actually a fibrous derivative of silica, termed a fibrous silicate. Its health hazards include not only the development of diffuse interstitial fibrosis but also the potential for inducing several types of neoplasm, particularly bronchogenic carcinoma and mesothelioma. These latter problems will be discussed in Chapters 20 and 15, respectively. The term *asbestosis* should be reserved for the interstitial lung disease that occurs as a result of asbestos exposure.

Individuals at risk for development of asbestosis include insulation, shipyard, and construction workers, as well as persons who have been exposed by working with brake linings. Even though the health hazards of asbestos have been well recognized and its use consequently curtailed, workers may still be exposed in the course of remodeling or reinsulating pipes or buildings where asbestos has been used. The duration of exposure necessary for development of asbestosis is usually greater than 10 to 20 years, though it may vary depending on the intensity of the exposure.

One theory of the pathogenesis of asbestosis suggests that asbestos fibers activate macrophages and induce the release of mediators, including a chemotactic factor that attracts neutrophils. Unlike silica, asbestos is not cytotoxic to macrophages. It does not destroy or "kill" macrophages in the way that silica does. The mechanism of the often significant fibrotic reaction that occurs with asbestos is not at all clear but presumably follows in some way from an active alveolitis.

The earliest microscopic lesions appear around respiratory bronchioles, with an alveolitis that progresses to peribronchiolar fibrosis. The fibrosis subsequently becomes more generalized throughout the alveolar walls and can become quite marked. Areas of the lung that are heavily involved by the fibrotic process include the lung bases and the subpleural regions.

A characteristic finding of asbestos exposure is the *ferruginous body*, which is a rod-shaped body with clubbed ends (Fig. 10–4) that appears yellow-brown in stained tissue. These ferruginous bodies seem to be asbestos fibers that have been coated by macrophages with an

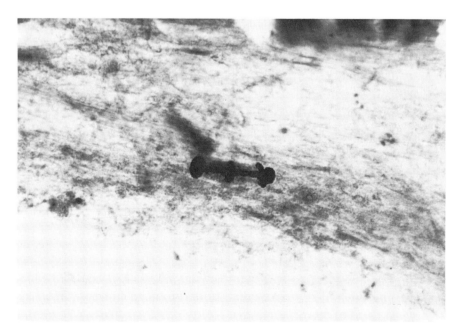

Figure 10–4. High-power photomicrograph of a ferruginous body. This rod–shaped body (with clubbed ends) represents a "coated" asbestos fiber. (Courtesy of Dr. Earl Kasdon.)

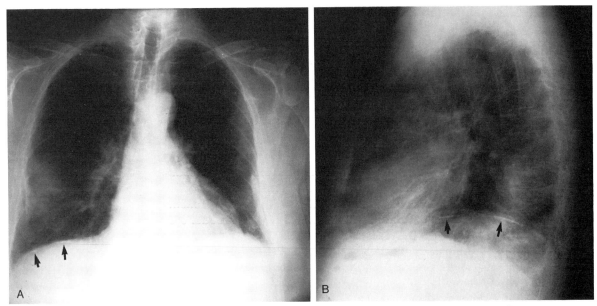

Figure 10–5. Chest radiograph of a patient with parenchymal and pleural disease secondary to asbestos exposure. Interstitial markings are increased at the lung bases, and there is extensive pleural thickening. Diaphragmatic calcification, which strongly suggests prior asbestos exposure, is highlighted by arrows. Posteroanterior (A) and lateral (B) views.

In asbestosis, microscopic examination of lung tissue often shows large numbers of ferruginous bodies.

iron-protein complex. Though it is common to see large numbers of these structures by light microscopy in patients with asbestosis, it is important to note that not all such coated fibers are asbestos, and that ferruginous bodies may be seen even in the absence of parenchymal lung disease. Uncoated asbestos fibers, which are long and narrow, cannot be seen by light microscopy and require electron microscopy for their detection.

The chest radiograph in asbestosis shows a pattern of linear streaking that is generally most prominent at the lung bases (Fig. 10–5). In advanced cases, the findings may be quite extensive and associated with cyst formation and honeycombing. Commonly, there is evidence of associated pleural disease, either in the form of pleural thickening or plaques (which may be calcified) or, much less frequently, in the form of pleural effusions. Since asbestos also predisposes to the development of malignancies of the lung and pleura, either of these complications may also be seen on the chest radiograph.

Pulmonary complications of asbestos exposure:
1. interstitial lung disease (asbestosis)
2. pleural thickening
3. pleural effusions
4. lung cancer
5. pleural malignancy (mesothelioma)

The clinical, pathophysiologic, and diagnostic features of asbestosis usually follow the general description of interstitial lung disease given in Chapter 9. However, it is worth noting that of the pneumoconioses we have discussed, asbestosis is much more likely on physical examination to be associated with clubbing than either silicosis or CWP.

HYPERSENSITIVITY PNEUMONITIS

In the entity called *hypersensitivity pneumonitis*, immunologic phenomena directed against an antigen are responsible for the production of interstitial lung disease. This disorder is also sometimes referred to as *extrinsic allergic alveolitis*, but we will adhere to the more commonly used term.

The antigens that induce the series of immunologic events are inhaled particulate antigens from a variety of sources. Almost all the antigens are derived from microorganisms, plant proteins, or animal proteins, and exposure is generally related either to the patient's occupation or to some avocation. The first of the hypersensitivity pneumonitides to be described was *farmer's lung*, which is due to antigens from microorganisms (thermophilic actinomycetes) that may be present on moldy hay. The list of antigens and types of exposure has now become quite extensive and includes such entities as air conditioner or humidifier lung, in which antigens from microorganisms contaminating a forced air system are involved, and bird breeder's or fancier's lung, in which bird proteins are involved.

Hypersensitivity pneumonitis represents an immunologic response to an inhaled organic antigen.

Interestingly, even when a large number of individuals are exposed to a given antigen by virtue of their occupation or avocation, only a small percentage actually develop the disease. Clearly, additional factors, perhaps genetic, determine who will contract the disease, but these factors have not been identified to date.

Pathogenetically, the hypersensitivity pneumonitides fall into the category of diseases with a lymphocytic alveolitis. It is currently believed that a Type IV immune reaction (cell-mediated or delayed hypersensitivity, mediated by T-lymphocytes) is of prime importance in producing the disease, though a Type III (immune complex disease) mechanism may also have a contributory role. Evidence suggests that T-lymphocytes in the lower respiratory tract become sensitized to the particular organic antigen. They may then release soluble mediators called lymphokines that attract macrophages and possibly induce them to form granulomas in the lung. Antigen-antibody immune complexes may also be involved, with binding of complement and the resulting production of chemotactic factors and activation of macrophages.

IgAb to Ag

both lymphocytic & neutrophilic alveolitis

Pathology of the lung in hypersensitivity pneumonitis reveals the alveolitis as well as the presence of granulomas. The granulomas are often poorly formed, unlike the well-defined granulomas characteristic of sarcoidosis (see Chapter 11). Often, the pathologic changes have a peribronchiolar prominence, thus accounting for the frequent physiologic evidence for obstruction of small airways.

Clinically, hypersensitivity pneumonitis manifests itself in different ways—either in acute episodes of dyspnea, cough, fever, and infiltrates on chest radiograph, occurring approximately 4 to 6 hours after exposure to the offending antigen, or in a chronic form. This latter presentation is a more insidious one, with the patient often complaining of gradual onset of shortness of breath and cough, along with systemic symptoms of fatigue, loss of appetite, and weight loss. Antigen exposure is a more long-term problem in these circumstances, and unfortunately, since acute episodes are not necessarily an important feature, the patient does not associate the symptoms with any particular exposure.

Hypersensitivity pneumonitis presents with either acute episodes 4 to 6 hours after exposure to the offending antigen or with the more insidious course of chronic interstitial lung disease.

Unlike its acute form, the chronic form of hypersensitivity pneumonitis behaves like other forms of interstitial lung disease. Unless the physician is attuned to the possibility that hypersensitivity to an antigen in the environment might be responsible for the patient's lung disease,

after certain no of acute attacks permanent fibrosis results

this entity may easily be missed, and exposure to the antigen may continue.

With an acute episode of hypersensitivity pneumonitis, the chest radiograph has diffuse infiltrates. As the disease becomes chronic, the abnormality may take on a more nodular quality, eventually appearing as the reticulonodular pattern characteristic of the other chronic interstitial lung diseases. In the chronic form of the disease, there is often an upper lobe predominance to the roentgenographic changes.

The diagnosis is certainly more likely to be considered if the patient is able to give a history of acute episodes only or of acute episodes punctuating a more chronic illness. Historical features concerning the patient's occupation and hobbies may provide valuable clues for detecting the responsible exposure. One of the standard diagnostic tests is a search for precipitating antibodies to the common organic antigens known to cause hypersensitivity pneumonitis. Unfortunately, false positive and false negative results for precipitins may cause diagnostic confusion. For instance, the finding of precipitins to thermophilic actinomycetes, the agent responsible for farmer's lung, is relatively common in healthy farmers without any evidence for the disease. In addition, making a diagnosis of hypersensitivity pneumonitis by the finding of precipitins obviously requires that the responsible antigen be included in the panel of antigens tested. If the patient has a lung biopsy performed for diagnosis of interstitial lung disease, findings on microscopic examination may also suggest this entity.

The best treatment again is avoidance of exposure. Unfortunately, the chronic form of the disease often leads to irreversible changes in the lung that persist even after exposure is terminated. Corticosteroids are sometimes administered in patients with persistent disease, but the results are variable.

DRUG-INDUCED INTERSTITIAL LUNG DISEASE

As the list of available pharmacologic agents expands every year, so does the list of potential complications. The lung is certainly one of the target organs for these side effects, and interstitial lung disease is a particularly important (though not the only) manifestation of such drug toxicity. We will not be able to consider each drug in detail, or even give a complete list of the growing number of drugs that have been implicated. We will, however, attempt to discuss briefly the general principles of drug-induced interstitial lung disease and mention the major agents that have been responsible.

Chemotherapeutic and cytotoxic agents are the largest category of drugs associated with interstitial lung disease.

The largest single category of drugs associated with disease of the alveolar wall clearly includes the chemotherapeutic or cytotoxic agents, i.e., those drugs designed primarily as antitumor agents. The most common individual drugs that have been implicated in the development of lung disease are bleomycin, busulfan, cyclophosphamide, methotrexate, and the nitrosoureas, though several others have also been described in smaller numbers of cases. In general, the risk of developing interstitial lung disease increases with higher cumulative doses of a particular agent. However, occasional cases are described with even a relatively low cumulative dose that would not normally be expected to cause problems. In most cases, the development of interstitial lung disease occurs in the time period ranging from one month to several years after use of the agent. Busulfan is particularly notable for the late development of complications, often several years after the onset of therapy.

The pathogenesis of chemotherapy-induced interstitial lung disease is not known with certainty, but in many instances direct toxicity to normal lung parenchymal cells appears to be the crucial factor. One exception is methotrexate, for which hypersensitivity mechanisms may also be involved.

The pathology of interstitial lung disease due to cytotoxic agents is frequently notable for the presence of atypical, bizarre-appearing type II alveolar epithelial cells, with large nuclei. When this feature is associated with the other usual findings of interstitial lung disease, the pathologist should suspect that a chemotherapeutic agent may be responsible. In conjunction with its presumed difference in pathogenesis, methotrexate also does not produce the same degree of epithelial cell atypia as do the other cytotoxic agents.

Drug-induced interstitial lung disease shows atypical, bizarre-appearing alveolar type II epithelial cells.

Clinically, fever is a common accompaniment to the respiratory symptoms associated with drug-induced interstitial lung disease. An increase in eosinophils in peripheral blood is also often noted in patients with methotrexate-induced lung disease.

There are several diagnostic considerations that arise routinely in patients receiving these drugs who develop pulmonary infiltrates, often associated with fever. In addition to the possibility of drug toxicity, concern is directed toward infection (since host defenses are generally impaired by the drug or by the underlying malignancy), dissemination of the malignancy through the lung, bleeding into the lung, or, in patients who have received radiation therapy, toxic effects from the irradiation. When the diagnosis is not clear, patients often undergo a lung biopsy, primarily to rule out an infectious process. If atypical epithelial cells but no infectious agents are found, a drug-induced process is suspected.

For patients who are felt to have a cytotoxic drug-related interstitial lung disease, the particular chemotherapeutic agent is generally discontinued. Steroids may be administered, but as with their use in other interstitial diseases, the results are variable.

Several drugs that are not chemotherapeutic agents have also been implicated in the development of interstitial lung disease. Nitrofurantoin, an antibiotic, has been associated with both acute and chronic reactions. The acute problem, which is presumably a hypersensitivity phenomenon, is often characterized by pulmonary infiltrates, pleural effusions, fever, and eosinophilia in peripheral blood. The chronic problem, which does not appear to be related to prior acute episodes, is characterized by a nonspecific interstitial pneumonitis and fibrosis akin to that of the other interstitial pneumonitides.

Therapy with injections of gold, which is used in rheumatoid arthritis, has also been associated with development of interstitial lung disease. The diagnosis here may be confusing, since the underlying disease (rheumatoid arthritis) can be associated with alveolitis and pulmonary fibrosis. Other individual drugs associated with interstitial lung disease are discussed in recent references listed at the end of this chapter.

other drug
amiodarone
(anti-arrhythmic)

For the sake of completeness, the reader should note that a large number of drugs have been linked with the development of an illness that resembles systemic lupus erythematosus, and patients with this "drug-induced lupus" may have interstitial lung disease as one manifestation of the drug-induced problem. In addition, a variety of drugs have been associated with pulmonary infiltrates and peripheral blood eosinophilia. This constellation of pulmonary infiltrates with eosinophilia, of which drugs are just one of several possible causes, is often abbreviated as the PIE syndrome.

RADIATION-INDUCED LUNG DISEASE

Interstitial lung disease is a potential complication of radiation therapy for tumors within or in close proximity to the thorax, particularly lymphoma (Hodgkin's disease) and carcinoma of the breast or lung. It has been estimated that 5 to 15 percent of patients receiving radiation therapy that includes portions of normal lung will develop signs and symptoms of clinically apparent injury. However, radiographic changes in the absence of symptoms are even more frequent, occurring in 20 to 70 percent of such patients.

Radiation-induced pulmonary disease is generally divided into two phases, early pneumonitis and late fibrosis. The acute phase of radiation pneumonitis develops approximately 1 to 3 months after completion of a course of therapy, depending to a large extent on the total dose and the volume of lung irradiated. The later stage of radiation fibrosis may directly follow earlier radiation pneumonitis, may occur after an asymptomatic latent interval, or may develop without any prior clinical evidence of acute pneumonitis. When fibrosis occurs, it is generally in the period of 6 to 12 months after radiation has been completed.

Radiation-induced lung disease includes an early period of pneumonitis and a later period of radiation fibrosis.

The pathogenesis of radiation-induced lung disease is uncertain at present. Toxicity to capillary endothelial cells and, to a lesser extent, to type I alveolar epithelial cells is believed to be the primary mode of injury, perhaps mediated by oxygen-derived free radicals. In the period preceding chronic fibrosis, an alveolitis probably contributes directly to the development of the fibrotic changes.

Early pathologic changes include swelling of endothelial cells, interstitial edema, mononuclear cell infiltrates, and atypical, hyperplastic epithelial cells. Subsequent changes during the fibrotic stage consist of progressive fibrosis (indistinguishable from pulmonary fibrosis of other etiologies) and sclerosis of small vessels, with obliteration of a major portion of the capillary bed in the involved area.

Clinically, patients may have fever with the acute pneumonitis in conjunction with their respiratory symptoms. On chest radiograph, a reticulonodular pattern characteristically conforms in shape and location to the region of lung irradiated. However, for reasons that are still unclear, some patients may develop additional changes outside the field of radiation. The acute changes of the pneumonitis are potentially reversible, whereas the chronic fibrotic changes are generally permanent.

The interstitial pattern in radiation-induced lung disease conforms in distribution to the region of lung irradiated.

Diagnostic considerations are usually similar to the ones mentioned for drug-induced interstitial lung disease. A history of recent irradiation occurring at the appropriate time is obviously crucial to the diagnosis. Additionally, the finding of roentgenographic changes that conform to the radiation port, often with a relatively sharp cutoff, is strongly suggestive of the diagnosis.

Corticosteroids are frequently used to treat radiation pneumonitis, often with reasonably good results. When the chronic changes of fibrosis have supervened, steroids are much less effective.

REFERENCES

Diseases Due to Inhaled Inorganic Dusts

Becklake, M. R.: Asbestos-related diseases of the lung and other organs: their epidemiology and implications for clinical practice. Am. Rev. Respir. Dis. 114:187–227, 1976.

Becklake, M. R.: Asbestos-related diseases of the lungs and pleura: current clinical issues. Am. Rev. Respir. Dis. 126:187–194, 1982.

Craighead, J. E., and Mossman, B. T.: The pathogenesis of asbestos-related diseases. N. Engl. J. Med. 306:1446–1455, 1982.

Lapp, N. L.: Lung disease secondary to inhalation of nonfibrous minerals. Clin. Chest Med. 2:219–233, 1981.

Morgan, W. K. C., and Lapp, N. L.: Respiratory disease in coal miners. Am. Rev. Respir. Dis. 113:531–559, 1976.

Morgan, W. K. C., and Seaton, A.: Occupational Lung Diseases. 2nd ed. Philadelphia, W. B. Saunders Co., 1984.

Ziskind, M., Jones, R. N., and Weill, H.: Silicosis. Am. Rev. Respir. Dis. 113:643–665, 1976.

Hypersensitivity Pneumonitis

Fink, J. N., et al.: Interstitial lung disease due to contamination of forced air systems. Ann. Intern. Med. 84:406–413, 1976.

Pepys, J.: Clinical and therapeutic significance of patterns of allergic reactions of the lungs to extrinsic agents. Am. Rev. Respir. Dis. 116:573–588, 1977.

Reynolds, H. Y.: Hypersensitivity pneumonitis. Clin. Chest Med. 3:503–519, 1982.

Roberts, R. C., and Moore, V. L.: Immunopathogenesis of hypersensitivity pneumonitis. Am. Rev. Respir. Dis. 116:1075–1090, 1977.

Drug-Induced Interstitial Lung Disease

Batist, G., and Andrews, J. L., Jr.: Pulmonary toxicity of antineoplastic drugs. JAMA 246:1449–1453, 1981.

Ginsberg, S. J., and Comis, R. L.: The pulmonary toxicity of antineoplastic agents. Semin. Oncol. 9:34–51, 1982.

Rosenow, E. C., III.: The spectrum of drug-induced pulmonary disease. Ann. Intern. Med. 77:977–991, 1972.

Sostman, H. D., Matthay, R. A., and Putnam, C. E.: Cytotoxic drug-induced lung disease. Am. J. Med. 62:608–615, 1977.

Weiss, R. B., and Muggia, F. M.: Cytotoxic drug-induced pulmonary disease: update 1980. Am. J. Med. 68:259–266, 1980.

Radiation-Induced Lung Disease

Gross, N. J.: Pulmonary effects of radiation therapy. Ann. Intern. Med. 86:81–92, 1977.

Roswit, B., and White, D. C.: Severe radiation injuries of the lung. Am. J. Roentgenol. 129:127–136, 1977.

11

Interstitial Lung Diseases of Unknown Etiology

> **Idiopathic Pulmonary Fibrosis**
> **Pulmonary Fibrosis Associated with Connective Tissue Disease**
> **Sarcoidosis**
> **Miscellaneous Disorders Involving the Pulmonary Parenchyma**
>   Eosinophilic Granuloma
>   Goodpasture's Syndrome
>   Idiopathic Pulmonary Hemosiderosis
>   Wegener's Granulomatosis

Approximately 65 percent of patients with interstitial lung disease are victims of a process for which no etiologic agent has been identified, even though a specific name may be attached to their disease entity. Included in this category of disease are idiopathic pulmonary fibrosis, pulmonary fibrosis associated with connective tissue disease, sarcoidosis, and eosinophilic granuloma, as well as a variety of other disorders. Since many general aspects of these problems were discussed in Chapter 9, we will now focus on the specific diseases and their particular characteristics.

IDIOPATHIC PULMONARY FIBROSIS

Though the name *idiopathic pulmonary fibrosis* (IPF) has often been used nonspecifically to describe fibrotic interstitial lung disease without an identifiable diagnosis, some have suggested that IPF represents a specific disease entity. We will proceed under this latter assumption and consider pulmonary fibrosis associated with an underlying connective tissue disease as a separate entity. Other names that have been used interchangeably with IPF include cryptogenic fibrosing alveolitis and usual interstitial pneumonitis (UIP).

As implied by the name, idiopathic pulmonary fibrosis does not yet have a recognizable inciting agent. Whether the primary agent, if one exists, reaches the lung via the airways or the bloodstream has also

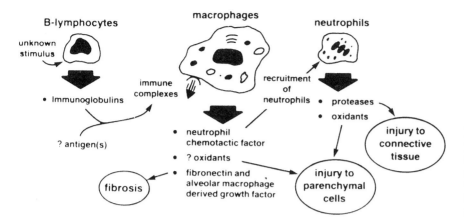

Figure 11–1. Proposed pathogenetic sequence in idiopathic pulmonary fibrosis (IPF). (From Crystal, R. G., et al.: N. Engl. J. Med. 310:154–166, 1984. Reproduced with permission.)

not been settled. A recent theory suggests that IPF is the prototype of diseases associated with a neutrophilic alveolitis (Fig. 11–1). It has been proposed that exposure to an unknown antigen initiates the disease, with local production of specific antibody in the lung resulting in the formation of antigen-antibody complexes. These complexes may stimulate macrophages in the lung to release a chemotactic factor for neutrophils as well as a growth factor for fibroblasts. Neutrophils attracted to the lung are also activated by the chemotactic factor to release a variety of proteolytic enzymes and other mediators that damage lung parenchymal cells and noncellular components of the interstitium.

The pathology of IPF is relatively nonspecific, with components of an alveolitis (consisting of mononuclear cells and neutrophils) and fibrosis (see Fig. 9–1). Though the neutrophilic infiltration of the alveolar walls is often not obvious on microscopic examination, these cells are readily found on bronchoalveolar lavage or by quantitation of cell types obtained from biopsy specimens. As discussed in Chapter 9, extensive fibrosis eventually results in the morphologic picture of honeycombing and end-stage lung.

Some clinicians feel that this form of idiopathic interstitial lung disease is best separated into two entities, termed *usual interstitial pneumonitis* (UIP) and *desquamative interstitial pneumonitis* (DIP). In UIP, the most prominent feature of the pathology is interstitial fibrosis, whereas in DIP numerous cells are found in the alveolar spaces. These cells are actually alveolar macrophages and not desquamated epithelial cells, as the name DIP would imply. Other investigators feel strongly that UIP and DIP are merely different stages of the same disease, IPF, and that any such distinction is artificial.

It is not clear if usual interstitial pneumonitis (UIP) and desquamative interstitial pneumonitis (DIP) are separate diseases or different stages of idiopathic pulmonary fibrosis (IPF).

Clinically, patients with IPF may present at any age from childhood on, though the most common age at presentation is between 40 and 70 years. The symptoms are similar to those of other interstitial lung diseases, with dyspnea being the most prominent complaint. In addition to the classic finding of dry crackles or rales on physical examination, patients frequently have evidence of clubbing of the digits.

clubbing assoc w/ a d/s that involves PMN's

The chest roentgenogram demonstrates an interstitial or reticulonodular pattern that is generally bilateral and relatively diffuse (see Fig. 3–6, which is from a patient with IPF). Neither pleural effusions

The chest x-ray in IPF demonstrates a diffuse interstitial pattern without pleural disease or hilar enlargement.

nor hilar enlargement is found on the roentgenogram. Many patients have serologic abnormalities, such as a positive test for antinuclear antibodies, that are generally found in patients with autoimmune or connective tissue disease. However, in the absence of other suggestive clinical features, these abnormalities are thought to be nonspecific and not indicative of an underlying rheumatologic disease.

The diagnosis is often made on lung biopsy, but only in the appropriate clinical setting when other etiologic factors for interstitial lung disease cannot be identified. Granulomas are not seen on biopsy. If found, they indicate the presence of another disorder.

Prognosis and response to corticosteroid therapy in IPF depend upon relative amounts of inflammation and fibrosis.

From the time of clinical presentation, patients have a very variable prognosis, with survival ranging from months to many years. Depending on the series of reported patients, the mean survival is approximately 4 to 10 years. In general, patients with evidence of a more cellular, active alveolitis (often corresponding to a DIP-like picture) have a better prognosis, while patients with prominent fibrosis (corresponding to a UIP-like picture) have a poorer prognosis. Corticosteroids are frequently used to treat patients with IPF. Patients with greater cellularity generally have a better response to therapy than those with significant fibrosis.

PULMONARY FIBROSIS ASSOCIATED WITH CONNECTIVE TISSUE DISEASE

The connective tissue or collagen vascular diseases, as they are commonly called, include rheumatoid arthritis (RA), systemic lupus erythematosus (SLE), progressive systemic sclerosis (scleroderma), polymyositis-dermatomyositis, Sjögren's syndrome, and an overlap syndrome often called mixed connective tissue disease. Though they form a diverse group of diseases, all are multisystem inflammatory diseases that are immunologically mediated. The particular organ systems that are likely to be involved vary with each disease and will be mentioned briefly as we discuss each entity.

Each of the diseases is complicated and has been the focus of an extensive amount of research into etiology and pathogenesis. Since none of them are disorders primarily affecting the lung, we will not consider them in detail. Rather, we will briefly mention how they affect the respiratory system, particularly with regard to development of pulmonary fibrosis. Some clinicians include additional disorders under the category of connective tissue diseases, but we will limit our discussion to the ones mentioned above, each of which has the potential for pulmonary involvement.

Histologic and physiologic changes suggest that pulmonary involvement in most connective tissue diseases is common.

Four points are worth mentioning that appear to be true of each of these disorders. First, though the patients generally have evidence of the underlying connective tissue disease prior to the development of pulmonary manifestations, some patients have lung disease as the presenting problem, occasionally predating other manifestations of their illness by several years. Second, detailed histologic or physiologic evaluation of patients with these diseases shows that pulmonary involvement is much more common than is clinically suspected. Third, the histopathology of interstitial lung disease associated with connective tissue disorders is, with few exceptions, indistinguishable from that of IPF. Finally, the interstitial lung disease that may develop with each of these entities preferentially affects the lower rather than the upper lung zones. This fact is usually apparent on examination of the chest roentgenogram.

Rheumatoid arthritis is a disorder whose primary manifestations consist of inflammatory joint disease. The most common site of involvement within the thorax is the pleura, in the form of pleurisy and/or pleural effusions. The lung itself may become involved with one or multiple nodules, or with development of interstitial lung disease. The latter is usually relatively mild, though severe cases are occasionally seen.

Systemic lupus erythematosus is a multisystem disease that primarily affects joints and skin but often has more serious involvement of several organ systems, including kidneys, lungs, nervous system, and heart. Its most frequent presentation within the chest is in the form of pleural disease, i.e., pleuritic chest pain and/or pleural effusion. The lung parenchyma may be involved by an acute pneumonitis, in which infiltrates often involve the alveolar spaces as well as the alveolar walls, or by chronic interstitial lung disease. In the latter, extensive fibrosis is usually not a prominent feature of the histology.

In rheumatoid arthritis and lupus erythematosus, pleural disease is more common than clinically evident interstitial lung disease.

Progressive systemic sclerosis or *scleroderma* is a disease whose most obvious manifestations are in the skin and the small blood vessels. Other organ systems, including gastrointestinal tract, lungs, kidneys, and heart, are involved relatively frequently. The interstitial lung disease with scleroderma is notable for the relative predominance of fibrosis and lack of a significant active alveolitis. Of all the connective tissue diseases, scleroderma is the one in which pulmonary involvement is most severe and most likely to be associated with significant scarring of the pulmonary parenchyma. Another potential pulmonary manifestation of scleroderma is disease of the small pulmonary blood vessels, which we will discuss in Chapter 14. This involvement appears to be independent of the fibrotic process affecting the alveolar walls.

Scleroderma lung disease is notable for interstitial fibrosis; disease of the small pulmonary vessels may be independent of the interstitial process.

In *polymyositis-dermatomyositis*, muscles and skin are the primary sites of the inflammatory process. The interstitial lung disease of polymyositis-dermatomyositis is relatively infrequent and has no particular distinguishing features. Patients may also have respiratory problems as a result of their muscle disease, with weakness of the diaphragm or other inspiratory muscles. In addition, difficulty in swallowing may lead to recurrent episodes of aspiration pneumonia.

In *Sjögren's syndrome*, a lymphocytic infiltration affects salivary and lacrimal glands and is associated with dry mouth and dry eyes (keratoconjunctivitis sicca). There are two major types of involvement of the alveolar wall—either a picture indistinguishable from IPF, or a lymphocytic infiltration of the alveolar walls. As a consequence of the latter, patients may occasionally have malignant transformation with development of a lymphoma.

Finally, an overlap syndrome, frequently called *mixed* or *undifferentiated connective tissue disease*, has features of several of these disorders, particularly scleroderma, lupus, and polymyositis. These patients may also develop evidence of interstitial lung disease indistinguishable from that of idiopathic pulmonary fibrosis.

SARCOIDOSIS

Sarcoidosis is a disorder in which multiple organ systems usually have granulomas that are described as noncaseating. The lung is the most frequently involved organ, with manifestations generally including interstitial lung disease and/or enlargement of hilar lymph nodes. Sarcoidosis is a common disorder, which particularly affects young black women, though a substantial number of Caucasians and males are also affected by the disease. Of all the disorders of unknown etiology affecting the alveolar wall, it is clearly the most prevalent.

Sarcoidosis is particularly common in young black women.

In addition to the apparent clinical manifestations, patients with sarcoidosis have a variety of immunologic abnormalities, including depression of the cellular immune (delayed hypersensitivity) system and hyperactivity of the humoral immune system. A great deal of recent research has tried to explain how these immunologic changes relate to the clinical and histopathologic manifestations of sarcoidosis. Research has shown that though the cellular immune system in peripheral blood is depressed, the local cellular immune system in the lung is activated, probably by a specific antigen. The T-lymphocyte, which is the major cell type of the cellular immune system, is crucial in this process, and one theory assigns it primary responsibility for the lymphocytic alveolitis that is so characteristic of the disease.

Presumably, an antigen, as yet unknown, initiates the disease by activating T-lymphocytes in the lung (Fig. 11–2). The specific subtype of T-lymphocyte is the "helper" lymphocyte, which then has two major actions. First, activated helper lymphocytes attract and stimulate macrophages, promoting their migration into the lung and their accu-

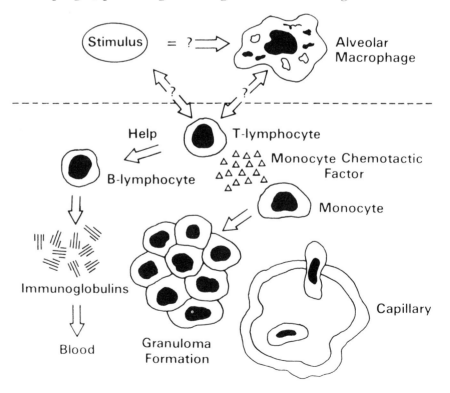

Figure 11–2. Proposed pathogenetic sequence in sarcoidosis. (From Keogh, B. A., and Crystal, R. G.: Chronic interstitial lung disease. *In* Current Pulmonology, Vol. 3. New York, John Wiley & Sons, 1981. Reproduced with permission.)

mulation into discrete collections of cells called granulomas. Second, helper T-lymphocytes stimulate B-cells of the humoral immune system to produce immunoglobulins, accounting for the hyperactivity of the humoral immune system commonly found in sarcoidosis. Accumulation of activated helper T-lymphocytes in the lung possibly depletes the peripheral blood of this population of cells, leaving "suppressor" T-cells in the peripheral circulation to inhibit normal manifestations of delayed hypersensitivity.

Undoubtedly, there is a great deal more to be understood about the etiology and pathogenesis of sarcoidosis, including the nature of any initiating antigen(s). Nevertheless, the recent theories of pathogenesis are intriguing and may offer new insights into this perplexing disease.

The characteristic feature of the pathology of sarcoidosis is the noncaseating granuloma (see Fig. 9–2). This discrete collection of tissue macrophages composing the granuloma does not show evidence of frank necrosis or caseation, as would appear in such disorders as tuberculosis or histoplasmosis. In addition to granulomas, in which multinucleated giant cells are frequently seen (see Fig. 9–2), there is often an alveolitis. The alveolitis is composed of mononuclear cells, including macrophages and lymphocytes, with the latter presumed to be of particular importance in the pathogenesis of the disease.

The characteristic pathology of sarcoidosis is the noncaseating granuloma; an alveolitis composed primarily of mononuclear cells may also occur.

Patients with sarcoidosis present most frequently either as a result of abnormalities detected on an incidental chest radiograph or because of respiratory symptoms, mainly dyspnea or a nonproductive cough. Since many other organ systems may be involved with noncaseating granulomas, other manifestations occur but are less common. Eye involvement (e.g., anterior uveitis or inflammation occupying the anterior chamber) and skin involvement (e.g., skin papules, erythema nodosum) are particularly common extrathoracic manifestations of sarcoidosis, but there may also be cardiac, neuromuscular, hematologic, hepatic, endocrine, and peripheral lymph node findings.

As we mentioned earlier, patients often display abnormalities in the immune system. Clinically, these patients may have anergy, i.e., failure to respond to skin tests requiring intact delayed hypersensitivity, as well as hyperglobulinemia—evidence of a hyperactive humoral immune system.

The chest radiograph in sarcoidosis generally demonstrates one of the following patterns: (1) enlargement of lymph nodes, most commonly bilateral hilar lymphadenopathy, with or without paratracheal node enlargement (Fig. 11–3); (2) interstitial lung disease; or (3) both adenopathy and interstitial disease (Fig. 11–4). The course of these radiographic findings is quite variable. Over time, both the adenopathy and the interstitial lung disease may regress spontaneously. However, at the other extreme, the interstitial disease may progress to a picture of extensive scarring and end-stage lung, at which time the patient has severe respiratory compromise.

The chest x-ray in sarcoidosis shows symmetrically enlarged hilar lymph nodes and/or interstitial lung disease.

Diagnosis of sarcoidosis can be made in several ways. When the clinical diagnosis strongly suggests sarcoidosis, tissue confirmation is not necessary. An example of such a presentation would be bilateral hilar lymphadenopathy found on incidental chest radiograph in an

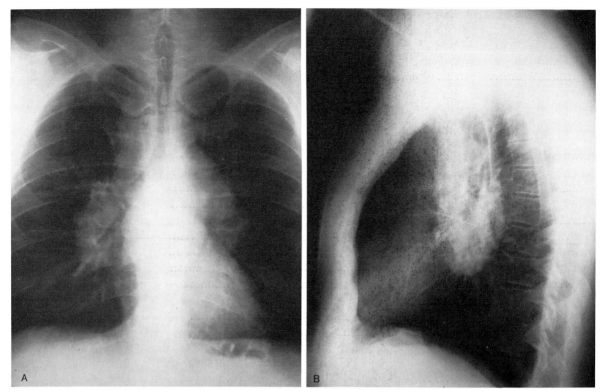

Figure 11–3. Radiographic appearance of stage I sarcoidosis, demonstrating bilateral hilar and paratracheal adenopathy; the enlarged nodes can be seen on both posteroanterior (*A*) and lateral (*B*) views.

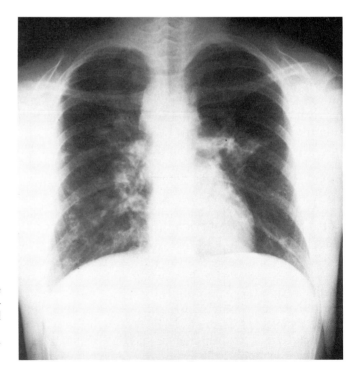

Figure 11–4. Chest radiograph demonstrating the characteristic features of stage II sarcoidosis—bilateral hilar adenopathy and diffuse interstitial lung disease. In stage III sarcoidosis (not shown), patients have diffuse interstitial lung disease without hilar adenopathy.

asymptomatic young black female. On the other hand, when the patient is symptomatic or when there is a question about the diagnosis, tissue sampling is usually undertaken to look for noncaseating granulomas and to rule out other etiologies. The lung is generally the most appropriate source of tissue, samples of which are frequently obtained with a transbronchial biopsy through a fiberoptic bronchoscope. Interestingly, even when the chest radiograph shows only hilar adenopathy without obvious interstitial lung disease, the alveolar walls usually are studded with granulomas that may be seen on a transbronchial lung biopsy. Other ways of obtaining tissue include biopsy of a lymph node in the mediastinum (via mediastinoscopy) or open lung biopsy. Additionally, skin or conjunctival lesions as well as minor salivary glands are occasionally biopsied and may show the characteristic noncaseating granulomas.

In sarcoidosis, transbronchial lung biopsy through a fiberoptic bronchoscope usually demonstrates granulomas in the lung parenchyma, even when the chest x-ray does not show interstitial lung disease.

In some medical centers, measurement of the angiotensin converting enzyme level in blood is used to confirm the diagnosis of sarcoidosis. This enzyme, which is normally synthesized by vascular endothelial cells, is also thought to be produced in the granulomas of sarcoidosis and is elevated in a large percentage of patients with active sarcoidosis. However, it is not specific for sarcoidosis and often is normal in the presence of relatively inactive disease.

The natural history of sarcoidosis is quite variable. Some patients resolve all their manifestations, clinical and radiographic, within 1 to 2 years. Other patients have continued progression of their radiographic abnormalities, with or without additional extrathoracic disease, and may have debilitating respiratory symptoms. In addition to pulmonary function tests, which are most useful for quantitating functional impairment, it has been suggested that patients have serial studies to assess the alveolitis of the disease, either by bronchoalveolar lavage (with a fiberoptic bronchoscope) or by gallium scanning. However, the latter techniques are still largely research tools and have not yet received wide clinical usage in this setting.

The treatment of sarcoidosis consists of administration of corticosteroids. However, it is often difficult to know which patients need to be treated, since the course of the disease is so variable and since the disease of many patients resolves spontaneously. As a general rule, patients are treated when there is evidence of progressive functional impairment of one or more organs, particularly the lung. Serial assessment of the alveolitis has been suggested as a guide to therapy, but its usefulness remains to be determined.

The variable natural history of sarcoidosis often makes decisions about use of corticosteroids difficult.

MISCELLANEOUS DISORDERS INVOLVING THE PULMONARY PARENCHYMA

Though we obviously cannot present an exhaustive description of all the remaining diseases of unknown etiology affecting alveolar walls, we will briefly describe four others to acquaint the reader with their major features. These include eosinophilic granuloma of the lung, Goodpasture's syndrome, idiopathic pulmonary hemosiderosis, and Wegener's granulomatosis.

Eosinophilic Granuloma

Eosinophilic granuloma is an entity that is usually included within the larger category of diseases termed *histiocytosis X*. These diseases are characterized by infiltration of organs with a particular type of histiocytic cell that has been named the histiocytosis X (HX) cell. Within the cytoplasm of the HX cell are peculiar rod-like structures called X-bodies that are seen under electron microscopy.

In eosinophilic granuloma of the lung, infiltration by these cells is generally limited to the lung, though occasionally discrete lesions may be found in the bones. On pathology of the lung, in addition to these histiocytes, there is infiltration by eosinophils, lymphocytes, macrophages, and plasma cells.

Patients with the disease are most frequently young to middle-aged adults, who present with a pattern of nodular or reticulonodular disease on chest roentgenogram, often accompanied by respiratory symptoms of dyspnea and/or cough. Occasionally, patients have a spontaneous pneumothorax, which may be the presenting feature of the disease. The radiographic findings tend to be more prominent in the upper lung zones and may in some cases progress to a pattern with extensive cystic disease and honeycombing.

The natural history of the disease is variable. In some patients, the disease is self-limited, and the radiographic and functional changes may stabilize over a period of time. In others, extensive disease and significant functional impairment follow. There is no known effective treatment for the disease. Though eosinophilic granuloma of the lung is not a common disorder, it should always be considered in the young or middle-aged adult with the clinical and radiographic features of interstitial lung disease.

P/E no crackles

Eosinophilic granuloma of the lung (histiocytosis X) enters into the differential diagnosis of unexplained interstitial disease, particularly in the young or middle-aged adult.

Goodpasture's Syndrome

Goodpasture's syndrome is a disease that has become well known not because of its incidence, which is extremely low, but because of its interesting pathogenetic and immunologic features. In this syndrome two organ systems are involved—the lungs and the kidneys. In the lungs, patients have episodes of pulmonary hemorrhage and may develop pulmonary fibrosis, presumably as a consequence of the recurrent episodes of bleeding. In the kidneys, patients have a glomerulonephritis characterized by linear deposits of antibody along the glomerular basement membrane. Studies on peripheral blood have demonstrated that these patients have circulating antibodies against their own glomerular basement membrane, often abbreviated anti-GBM antibodies. It is believed that these antibodies crossreact with the basement membrane of the alveolar wall, and that their deposition in the kidney and lung is responsible for the clinical manifestations of the disease.

Why patients with Goodpasture's syndrome develop these true autoantibodies is not entirely clear. In some patients, onset of the disease appears to follow influenza infection or exposure to a toxic hydrocarbon. Presumably, injury to basement membranes and release

In Goodpasture's syndrome, autoantibodies directed against the glomerular basement membrane may crossreact with the basement membrane of alveolar walls.

of previously unexposed antigenic determinants are involved, or there may be incidental formation of antibodies (against an unrelated antigen) that happen to crossreact with alveolar and glomerular basement membranes.

Idiopathic Pulmonary Hemosiderosis

Idiopathic pulmonary hemosiderosis is a disease with some similarity to Goodpasture's syndrome but with important differences as well. Patients have recurrent episodes of pulmonary hemorrhage and also may develop pulmonary fibrosis. However, no evidence for circulating antibodies against alveolar or glomerular basement membranes is available, and the disorder is not associated with renal disease. The mechanism of this disorder is totally unknown.

Wegener's Granulomatosis

Finally, a group of disorders termed the *granulomatous vasculitides* may affect the alveolar wall as part of a more generalized disease. The most well-known of these disorders is *Wegener's granulomatosis*, a disease characterized primarily but not exclusively by involvement of the upper respiratory tract, the lungs, and the kidneys. The pathologic process in the lungs and the upper respiratory tract consists of a necrotizing, granulomatous vasculitis, while a focal glomerulonephritis is present in the kidney. On chest radiograph, patients commonly have one or several nodules (often large) or infiltrates, commonly with associated cavitation of the lesion(s). Unlike most of the other disorders of the pulmonary parenchyma discussed in Chapters 10 and 11, diffuse interstitial lung disease is not the characteristic radiographic finding in this entity.

Wegener's granulomatosis is characterized pathologically by granulomatous vasculitis of the lung and upper respiratory tract and by glomerulonephritis; the clinical corollary is pulmonary, upper respiratory tract, and renal disease.

Though Wegener's granulomatosis had been considered an aggressive and fatal disease, its prognosis has dramatically improved since cytotoxic agents, specifically cyclophosphamide, have been used in its treatment. Whereas the mean survival time without treatment was 5 months, patients are now achieving complete and long-term remissions with institution of appropriate therapy.

REFERENCES

Idiopathic Pulmonary Fibrosis

Carrington, C. B., Gaensler, E. A., Coutu, R. E., FitzGerald, M. X., and Gupta, R. G.: Natural history and treated course of usual and desquamative interstitial pneumonia. N. Engl. J. Med. 298:801–809, 1978.

Crystal, R. G., Bitterman, P. B., Rennard, S. I., Hance, A. J., and Keogh, B. A.: Interstitial lung diseases of unknown cause: disorders characterized by chronic inflammation of the lower respiratory tract. N. Engl. J. Med. 310:154–166; 235–244, 1984.

Crystal, R. G., Fulmer, J. D., Roberts, W. C., Moss, M. L., Line, B. R., and Reynolds, H. Y.: Idiopathic pulmonary fibrosis: clinical, histologic, radiographic, physiologic, scintigraphic, cytologic, and biochemical aspects. Ann. Intern. Med. 85:769–788, 1976.

Crystal, R. G., Gadek, J. E., Ferrans, V. J., Fulmer, J. D., Line, B. R., and Hunninghake, G. W.: Interstitial lung disease: current concepts of pathogenesis, staging and therapy. Am. J. Med. 70:542–568, 1981.

Jackson, L. K.: Idiopathic pulmonary fibrosis. Clin. Chest Med. 3:579–592, 1982.

Pulmonary Fibrosis Associated with Connective Tissue Disease

Eisenberg, H.: The interstitial lung diseases associated with collagen-vascular disorders. Clin. Chest Med. 3:565–578, 1982.

Hunninghake, G. W., and Fauci, A. S.: Pulmonary involvement in the collagen vascular diseases. Am. Rev. Respir. Dis. 119:471–503, 1979.

Sarcoidosis

Crystal, R. G., Roberts, W. C., Hunninghake, G. W., Gadek, J. E., Fulmer, J. D., and Line, B. R.: Pulmonary sarcoidosis: a disease characterized and perpetuated by activated lung T-lymphocytes. Ann. Intern. Med. 94:73–94, 1981.

Israel, H.: Sarcoidosis. In Simmons, D. H. (ed.): Current Pulmonology. Vol. 1. Boston, Houghton Mifflin, 1979, pp. 163–182.

Mitchell, D. N., and Scadding, J. G.: Sarcoidosis. Am. Rev. Respir. Dis. 10:774–802, 1974.

Thrasher, D. R., and Briggs, D. D., Jr.: Pulmonary sarcoidosis. Clin. Chest Med. 3:537–563, 1982.

Miscellaneous Disorders Involving the Pulmonary Parenchyma

Basset, F., et al.: Pulmonary histiocytosis X. Am. Rev. Respir. Dis. 118:811–820, 1978.

Bradley, J. D.: The pulmonary hemorrhage syndromes. Clin. Chest Med. 3:593–605, 1982.

Fauci, A. S., Haynes, B. F., Katz, P., and Wolff, S. M.: Wegener's granulomatosis: prospective clinical and therapeutic experience with 85 patients for 21 years. Ann. Intern. Med. 98:76–85, 1983.

Friedman, P. J., Liebow, A. A., and Sokoloff, J.: Eosinophilic granuloma of lung: clinical aspects of primary pulmonary histiocytosis in the adult. Medicine 60:385–396, 1981.

Matthay, R. A., Bromberg, S. I., and Putnam, C. E.: Pulmonary renal syndromes—a review. Yale J. Biol. Med. 53:497–523, 1980.

12

Anatomic and Physiologic Aspects of the Pulmonary Vasculature

Anatomy
Physiology
    Distribution of Pulmonary Blood Flow
    Pulmonary Vascular Response to Hypoxia
    Other Aspects of Pulmonary Vascular Physiology

The pulmonary vasculature is responsible for transporting desaturated blood to the lungs and then carrying freshly oxygenated blood back to the left atrium and ventricle for pumping to peripheral tissues. Though the pulmonary circulation is often called the "lesser circulation," in fact the lungs are the only organ system that receives the entire cardiac output. This extensive system of pulmonary vessels is susceptible to a variety of disease processes, ranging from those that primarily affect the vasculature to those that are either secondary to airway or pulmonary parenchymal disease or due to transport of material that is "foreign" to the pulmonary vessels, including blood clots.

Before considering diseases of the pulmonary vasculature in Chapters 13 and 14, we will describe a few of the general anatomic and physiologic aspects of the pulmonary vessels. Included in the discussion on physiology will be several topics relating to hemodynamics of the pulmonary circulation, as well as a brief consideration of some nonrespiratory, metabolic functions of the pulmonary circulation.

ANATOMY

In contrast to systemic arteries that carry blood from the left ventricle to the rest of the body, the pulmonary arteries are relatively thin-walled vessels that normally do not need to withstand particularly high pressures. The pulmonary trunk, which is the outflow from the right ventricle, divides almost immediately into the right and left main pulmonary arteries, which subsequently divide into smaller and smaller branches. By the time the vessels are considered arterioles, the outer diameter is less than approximately 0.1 mm. An important feature of the smaller pulmonary arteries is the presence of smooth muscle within the walls, which is responsible for the vasoconstrictive response to various stimuli, particularly hypoxia.

The pulmonary capillaries form an extensive network of channels coursing through alveolar walls. They are in close proximity to alveolar gas, separated only by alveolar epithelial cells and a small amount of interstitium present in some regions of the alveolar wall (see Figs. 8–1 and 8–2). The design of this capillary system is extraordinarily well-suited to the requirements of gas exchange, as it contains an enormous effective surface area of contact between pulmonary capillaries and alveolar gas. The pulmonary veins, responsible for transporting oxygenated blood from the pulmonary capillaries to the left atrium, progressively combine into larger and larger vessels, until four major pulmonary veins enter the left atrium.

The bronchial arteries, which are actually part of the systemic circulation, provide nutrient blood flow to the bronchi. Generally, a single bronchial artery of variable origin (upper right intercostal, right subclavian, or internal mammary artery) supplies the right lung. Two bronchial arteries, usually arising from the thoracic aorta, supply the left lung. Communication between the bronchial and pulmonary circulations occurs at the level of the terminal respiratory units, and the blood originating in the bronchial arteries drains back to the heart primarily via the pulmonary veins.

An extensive network of lymphatic channels is also located primarily within the connective tissue sheaths around small vessels and airways. Though these channels do not generally course through the interstitial tissue of the alveolar walls, they are in close enough proximity to be effective at removing liquid and some solutes that constantly pass into the interstitium of the alveolar wall.

PHYSIOLOGY

Though the pulmonary circulation handles the same cardiac output from the right ventricle as the systemic circulation handles from the left, the former operates under much lower pressures and has substantially less resistance to flow than the latter. The systolic and diastolic pressures in the pulmonary artery are normally approximately 25 and 10 mm Hg, respectively, in contrast to 120 and 80 mm Hg in the systemic arteries. The pulmonary resistance can be calculated then according to the following formula:

$$R = \frac{\text{change in pressure}}{\text{flow}}$$

The change or drop in pressure across the pulmonary circuit is the mean pulmonary artery pressure minus the mean left atrial pressure. Left atrial pressure is difficult to measure directly, but a reasonably accurate indirect assessment can be made by measuring the "back pressure" in the pulmonary artery when forward flow has been occluded. A special catheter designed for this purpose, called a *pulmonary artery balloon occlusion catheter* or *Swan-Ganz catheter*, has had wide clinical application for such pressure measurements.

Assuming mean pulmonary artery (PA) and left atrial (LA) pressures of 15 and 6 mm Hg, respectively, along with a cardiac output of 6 L per min, the pulmonary resistance would be (15 – 6)/6 mm Hg per L per min, or 1.5 mm Hg per L per min. This resistance is approximately one-tenth that found in the systemic circulation.

Pulmonary vascular resistance = (mean PA pressure − mean LA pressure)/cardiac output; LA pressure is indirectly determined from occluded PA pressure.

Under conditions of increased cardiac output (e.g., exercise), the pulmonary circulation is actually able to decrease its resistance and handle the extra flow with only a minimal increase in pulmonary artery pressure. Two mechanisms appear to be responsible—recruitment of new vessels and, to a lesser extent, distension of previously perfused vessels. Under normal resting conditions, some of the pulmonary vessels are essentially receiving no blood flow but are capable of carrying part of the pulmonary blood flow should the pressure increase. Additionally, since pulmonary vessels have relatively thin walls, they are distensible and can enlarge their diameter under increased pressure to accommodate additional blood flow. With a means for increasing the total cross-sectional area of the pulmonary vasculature on demand, the pulmonary circulation is capable of lowering its resistance when the need for increased flow arises.

When cardiac output increases, recruitment and distension of pulmonary vessels prevent a significant increase in pulmonary artery pressure.

Distribution of Pulmonary Blood Flow

The relatively low pressures in the pulmonary artery have important implications for the way blood flow is distributed in the lung. In the upright position, blood going to the upper zones of the lung is flowing against gravity and must be under sufficient pressure in the pulmonary artery to make this anti-gravitational journey. Since the top of the lung is approximately 15 cm above the level of the main pulmonary arteries, a pressure of 15 cm water is required to achieve perfusion of the apices. The mean pulmonary artery pressure of 15 mm Hg (approximately 19 cm water) is normally just sufficient to achieve flow to this region. In contrast, flow to the lower lung zones, i.e., below the level of the main pulmonary arteries, is assisted by gravity. Therefore, in the upright individual, gravity provides a normal gradient of blood flow from the apex to the base of the lung, with the base receiving substantially greater flow than the apex (see Fig. 1–4). As we discussed in Chapter 1, this distribution of blood flow in the lung has major implications for the manner in which ventilation and perfusion are matched.

The distribution of blood flow in the lung can be measured quite conveniently with radioactive isotopes. A particularly useful technique involves intravenous injection of labeled particles, specifically macroaggregates of albumin, that are of sufficient size to lodge in the pulmonary capillaries. An external counter over the lung can then sense the distribution of lodged particles and hence the distribution of blood flow to the lung. This technique, when performed in the upright individual,

The distribution of blood flow within the lung is strongly influenced by gravity.

not only confirms the expected vertical gradient of blood flow in the lung but also detects regions of decreased or absent perfusion in disease states, as discussed in Chapter 3.

Pulmonary Vascular Response to Hypoxia

Pulmonary vasoconstriction occurs in response to alveolar hypoxia; this protective mechanism reduces blood flow to poorly ventilated alveoli, minimizing ventilation-perfusion mismatch.

An important physiologic feature of the pulmonary circulation is its response to hypoxia. When alveoli in an area of lung contain gas with a low P_{O_2}, generally less than 60 to 70 torr, the vessels supplying that region of lung undergo vasoconstriction. This response occurs primarily at the level of the small arteries or arterioles and serves as a protective mechanism for decreasing perfusion to poorly ventilated alveoli. Hence ventilation-perfusion mismatch is decreased, and areas of low ventilation-perfusion ratio, which contribute hypoxemic blood, are minimized.

When there are localized regions of lung with a low P_{O_2}, then the vasoconstrictive response is also localized. Under these circumstances, the overall pulmonary vascular resistance does not increase significantly. However, with a generalized decrease in P_{O_2}, as in many forms of lung disease or in subjects exposed to high altitude, pulmonary vasoconstriction is generalized. In this circumstance, pulmonary vascular resistance and pulmonary artery pressure are both increased. What would be a protective response in the case of localized disease is thus detrimental in the case of generalized disease and widespread alveolar hypoxia.

There is one circumstance in which such generalized pulmonary vasoconstriction in response to alveolar hypoxia is most beneficial, namely in the fetus. In utero, the alveoli receive no aeration, making the entire lung hypoxic. As a result, there is marked pulmonary vasoconstriction, accompanied by very high pulmonary vascular resistance and diversion of blood away from the lung. Instead, blood preferentially goes through the ductus arteriosus from the pulmonary artery to the aorta, and through the foramen ovale from the right to the left atrium.

At birth, when the first few breaths are taken, oxygen flows into the alveoli, and the pulmonary vasoconstriction is reversed. As a result of this pulmonary vasodilation (as well as constriction of the ductus arteriosus), right ventricular output now passes through the lungs, where the blood is oxygenated. Interestingly, the hypoxic vasoconstriction that persists throughout adult life is probably directly related to this important fetal response.

The mechanism of hypoxic vasoconstriction remains unknown. There are probably some local influences of alveolar hypoxia on the vessel wall, but whether neural or humoral factors make an additional contribution is uncertain.

Other Aspects of Pulmonary Vascular Physiology

An additional stimulus for pulmonary vasoconstriction is a low blood pH. Though this effect is less important than the effect of hypoxia, the two stimuli do appear to have a synergistic effect on increasing pulmonary vascular resistance. Any effect of P_{CO_2} on the pulmonary vasculature appears to be negligible; though hypercapnia may increase pulmonary vascular resistance, the effect is apparently mediated by changes in blood pH.

A low pH in blood is an additional stimulus for pulmonary vasoconstriction.

Another important aspect of pulmonary vascular physiology relates to fluid movement from pulmonary capillaries into the interstitium of the alveolar wall. Since abnormalities in fluid transport across the capillaries are most important in the adult respiratory distress syndrome and respiratory failure, we have elected to discuss this topic in Chapter 27.

Finally, although transport of blood between the heart and the lungs is the most obvious function of the pulmonary vasculature, these vessels have additional nonrespiratory, metabolic functions. A substantial amount of evidence shows that the pulmonary circulation has an important role in the inactivation of certain circulating bioactive chemicals. For example, serotonin (5-hydroxytryptamine) and bradykinin are primarily inactivated in the lung, probably at the level of the vascular endothelium. In addition, angiotensin I, an inactive decapeptide, is converted to the active octapeptide angiotensin II by angiotensin converting enzyme, which is produced by pulmonary vascular endothelial cells. Though the metabolic functions of the pulmonary vasculature are certainly important in modifying the effects of these substances, it is not known whether derangements in these functions are important consequences of diseases affecting the vasculature.

REFERENCES

Bergofsky, E. H.: Mechanisms underlying vasomotor regulation of regional pulmonary blood flow in normal and disease states. Am. J. Med. 57:378–394, 1974.

Fishman, A. P.: Hypoxia on the pulmonary circulation: how and where it acts. Circ. Res. 38:221–231, 1976.

Heistad, D. D., and Abboud, F. M.: Circulatory adjustments to hypoxia. Circulation 61:463–470, 1980.

Murray, J. F.: The Normal Lung: The Basis for Diagnosis and Treatment of Pulmonary Disease. Philadelphia, W. B. Saunders Co., 1976.

Robin, E. D.: Some basic and clinical challenges in the pulmonary circulation. Chest 81:357–363, 1982.

West, J. B.: Respiratory Physiology—The Essentials. 2nd ed. Baltimore, Williams & Wilkins, 1979.

13

Pulmonary Embolism

Pulmonary embolism is clearly one of the most important disorders affecting the pulmonary vasculature. Not only is it found in more than 60 percent of autopsies in which careful search is made, but it is also widely misdiagnosed, both in terms of overdiagnosis when not present and underdiagnosis when present.

The term pulmonary embolism refers to the movement of a blood clot from a systemic vein through the right side of the heart to the pulmonary circulation, where it lodges in one or more branches of the pulmonary artery. The clinical consequences of this common problem are quite variable, ranging from none to sudden death, depending on the size of the embolus and the medical condition of the patient. Though pulmonary embolism is intimately associated with the development of a thrombus elsewhere in the circulation, we will focus in this chapter on the pulmonary manifestations of thromboembolic disease, not on the clinical effects or diagnosis of the clot at the site of formation.

ETIOLOGY AND PATHOGENESIS

We have mentioned that a thrombus or blood clot is the material that travels to the pulmonary circulation in pulmonary embolic disease. However, it is important to note that other material can travel via the vasculature to the pulmonary arteries, including tumor cells or fragments, fat, amniotic fluid, and a variety of foreign materials that can be introduced into the circulation. We will not consider these additional, much less common types of pulmonary emboli in this chapter.

In the vast majority of cases, the lower extremities are the source of thrombi that embolize to the lungs. Though these thrombi frequently originate in the veins of the calf, propagation of the clots to the veins of the thigh is necessary to produce sufficiently large thrombi for clinically important embolism. Rarely, pulmonary emboli originate in the arms, pelvis, or right-sided chambers of the heart, but these several sources combined probably account for less than 5 percent of all pulmonary emboli.

Thrombi in the deep veins of the lower extremities are the usual source of pulmonary emboli.

It is commonly said that the following three factors potentially contribute to the genesis of venous thrombosis: (1) alteration in the mechanism of blood coagulation, i.e., hypercoagulability; (2) damage to the endothelium of the vessel wall; and (3) stasis or stagnation of blood flow. In practice, many specific risk factors for thromboemboli have been identified, including immobilization (e.g., bed rest, prolonged sitting during travel, immobilization of an extremity after fracture), the postoperative state, congestive heart failure, obesity, underlying carcinoma, the post-partum state, and chronic deep venous insufficiency.

It is important to note that not all thrombi resulting in embolic disease are clinically apparent. In fact, only about 50 percent of patients with pulmonary emboli have previous clinical evidence of venous thrombosis in the lower extremities or elsewhere.

PATHOLOGY

The pathologic changes that result from occlusion of a pulmonary artery depend to a large extent upon the location of the occlusion and the presence of other underlying disorders that compromise oxygen supply to the pulmonary parenchyma. There are two major consequences of vascular occlusion seen in the lung parenchyma distal to the site of occlusion. First, if minimal or no other oxygen supply reaches the parenchyma, either from the airways or from the bronchial arterial circulation, then frank necrosis of lung tissue (pulmonary infarction) will result. According to one estimate, only 10 to 15 percent of all pulmonary emboli result in pulmonary infarction. It has sometimes been said that compromise of two of the three oxygen sources to the lung—pulmonary artery, bronchial artery, and alveolar gas—is necessary before infarction results.

Second, when the integrity of the parenchyma is maintained and infarction does not result, often hemorrhage and edema are seen in lung tissue supplied by the occluded pulmonary artery. The name congestive atelectasis has often been applied to this process of parenchymal hemorrhage and edema without infarction.

Embolic occlusion of a vessel may lead to infarction or congestive atelectasis of the lung parenchyma.

With either pulmonary infarction or congestive atelectasis, the pathologic process generally extends to the visceral pleural surface, and corresponding radiographic changes are therefore often pleura-based. In some cases, pleural effusion may also result. As part of the natural history of infarction, there is generally contraction of the infarcted parenchyma and the eventual formation of a scar. With congestive atelectasis but no infarction, resolution of the process and resorption of the blood may leave few or no pathologic sequelae.

In many cases, neither of these pathologic changes occurs, and relatively little alteration of the distal lung parenchyma appears, presumably because of incomplete occlusion or sufficient nutrient oxygen from other sources. Frequently, the thrombus quickly fragments or undergoes a process of lysis, with smaller fragments moving progressively distally in the pulmonary arterial circulation. Whether or not this rapid process of clot dissolution occurs is also important in determining the pathologic consequences of pulmonary embolism.

With clots that do not fragment or lyse, there is generally a slower process of organization in the vessel wall and eventual recanalization. Webs may form within the arterial lumen and may sometimes be detected on pulmonary arteriogram or on pathologic examination as the only evidence for prior embolic disease.

PATHOPHYSIOLOGY

When a thrombus migrates to and lodges within a pulmonary vessel, a variety of consequences ensue. These relate not only to mechanical obstruction of one or more vessels but also to the secondary effects of various mediators released from the thrombus. We will first discuss the effects of mechanical occlusion of the vessels and then consider how chemical mediators contribute to the clinical effects.

When a vessel is occluded by an embolus and forward blood flow through the vessel stops, perfusion of pulmonary capillaries normally supplied by that vessel ceases. If ventilation to the corresponding alveoli continues, then the ventilation is wasted, i.e., the region of lung serves as dead space. As we discussed in Chapter 1, assuming that minute ventilation remains constant, increasing the dead space automatically decreases alveolar ventilation and hence CO_2 excretion. However, despite the potential for CO_2 retention in pulmonary embolic disease, hypercapnia is not a consequence of pulmonary embolus, mainly because patients routinely increase their minute ventilation after an embolus and more than compensate for the increase in dead space. In fact, the usual consequence of a pulmonary embolus is hyperventilation and hypocapnia, not hypercapnia. However, if minute ventilation is fixed, e.g., in an unconscious or anesthetized patient whose ventilation is controlled by a mechanical ventilator, then a rise in PCO_2 may result from a relatively large pulmonary embolus.

Pulmonary emboli are associated with hypocapnia, resulting from an increase in overall minute ventilation.

In addition to creating an area of dead space, another potential consequence of mechanical occlusion of one or more vessels is an increase in pulmonary vascular resistance. As we discussed earlier, the pulmonary vascular bed is capable of both recruitment and distension of vessels. Experimentally, we do not find an increase in resistance or pressure in the pulmonary vasculature until about 50 to 70 percent of the vascular bed is occluded. The experimental model is somewhat different from the clinical setting though, since release of chemical mediators may cause vasoconstriction and additional compromise of the pulmonary vasculature.

When there has been even further limitation of the vascular bed by the combination of mechanical occlusion and the effects of chemical mediators, the pulmonary resistance and pulmonary artery pressure may rise so high that the right ventricle cannot cope with the acute increase in workload. As a result, the forward output of the right ventricle may diminish, blood pressure may fall, and the patient may have a syncopal (fainting) episode or go into hypotensive shock. There may also be "backward" failure of the right ventricle, which is most apparent acutely with elevation of systemic venous pressure, reflected on physical examination by distension of jugular veins.

The hemodynamic consequences of an acute pulmonary embolus depend to a large extent on the presence of pre-existing emboli or pulmonary vascular disease. When there have been prior emboli, the right ventricular wall has already thickened (hypertrophied), and higher pressures can be maintained. On the other hand, adding an additional embolus to an already compromised pulmonary vascular bed may act as "the straw that broke the camel's back" and induce decompensation of the right ventricle.

Besides the direct mechanical effects of vessel occlusion, thrombi appear to release chemical mediators that have secondary effects on both airways and blood vessels of the lung. The exact source and nature of the chemical mediators are not entirely clear. Platelets that adhere to the thrombus are presumably an important source of such mediators as histamine, serotonin, and prostaglandins. Bronchoconstriction, largely at the level of small airways, appears to be an important effect of mediator release and is thought to be an explanation for the hypoxemia that so commonly accompanies pulmonary embolism. Constriction of small airways to regions of lung that are uninvolved with emboli and have maintained blood flow leads to regions of ventilation-perfusion mismatch (low ventilation-perfusion ratio) and to hypoxemia. Whether this is the entire explanation for the hypoxemia of pulmonary embolism is unknown; however, it is at least a contributing factor.

Bronchoconstriction of small airways, induced by chemical mediators released from the thrombus, may be an important mechanism of hypoxemia in pulmonary embolism.

As we mentioned earlier, the chemical mediators also affect the pulmonary vasculature. Vasoconstriction of pulmonary arteries and arterioles compounds the loss of vascular bed by clot and adds to the likelihood of major vascular compromise.

Three additional features of the pathophysiology of pulmonary embolism are worth mentioning. First, as a result of vascular compromise to one or more regions of lung, synthesis of the surface-active material surfactant by alveoli in the affected region is compromised. Consequently, alveoli may be more likely to collapse, and liquid may more likely leak into alveolar spaces. Second, hypocapnia appears to have the effect of inducing secondary bronchoconstriction of small airways. With the hypocapnia that occurs in pulmonary embolus, and particularly with the low alveolar PCO_2 in dead space regions of lung, secondary bronchoconstriction results. Both of these mechanisms, along with the small airway constriction induced by chemical mediators, may contribute to the volume loss or atelectasis that is frequently observed on chest roentgenograms of patients with pulmonary embolism.

Finally, as we mentioned in Chapter 12, a variety of bioactive substances are inactivated in the lung. Whether pulmonary embolism disturbs some of these nonrespiratory, metabolic functions of the lung is not at all clear, and whether clinical consequences might ensue from such a potential disturbance is totally unknown.

CLINICAL FEATURES

Most frequently, pulmonary embolism develops in the setting of one of the risk factors previously mentioned. Commonly, the embolus does not produce any significant symptoms, and the entire episode goes unnoticed by the patient and the physician. When the patient is symptomatic, acute onset of dyspnea is the most common complaint. Much less common is pleuritic chest pain or hemoptysis. Patients occasionally present with syncope, particularly in the setting of a massive embolus, defined as the obstruction of two or more lobes (or their equivalent).

Symptoms of pulmonary embolism:
1. dyspnea
2. pleuritic chest pain
3. hemoptysis
4. syncope

On physical examination, the most common findings are tachycardia and tachypnea. The chest examination may be entirely normal or show a variety of nonspecific findings, such as decreased air entry, localized rales, or wheezing. With pulmonary infarction extending to the pleura, a pleural friction rub may be heard, as may findings of a pleural effusion. Cardiac examination may show evidence of acute right ventricular overload, i.e., acute cor pulmonale, in which case the pulmonic component of the second heart sound (P_2) is increased, a right-sided S_4 is heard, and a right ventricular heave may be present. If the right ventricle actually fails, a right-sided S_3 may be heard, and jugular veins may also be distended. Examination of the lower extremities may reveal changes suggesting a thrombus, including tenderness, swelling, or a cord (palpable clot within a vessel). However, since only approximately 50 percent of patients with emboli arising from leg veins have clinical evidence of deep venous thrombosis, absence of these findings should not be surprising.

DIAGNOSTIC EVALUATION

The initial diagnostic evaluation of the patient with suspected pulmonary embolism generally includes a chest roentgenogram and measurement of arterial blood gases. The radiographic findings in acute pulmonary embolism are quite variable. Most frequently, the radiograph is normal. When the film is not normal, the abnormalities are often nonspecific, including areas of atelectasis or elevation of a hemidiaphragm, indicating volume loss. This volume loss, as we discussed earlier, may be related to decreased ventilation to the involved area as a result of small airway constriction and possibly loss of surfactant. In addition, if the patient has pleuritic chest pain, he or she may try to avoid pain by breathing more shallowly, which also contributes to atelectasis.

Occasionally, there is a localized area of decreased perfusion on the chest radiograph, corresponding to the region in which the vessel has been occluded. This finding is called "Westermark's sign" but is very difficult to read unless prior radiographs are available for comparison. With a large proximal embolus, there may occasionally be enlargement of a pulmonary artery near the hilum as a result of distension of the vessel by the clot itself. There may also be an apparent abrupt termination of the vessel, though this is usually difficult to see on a plain chest radiograph.

Both congestive atelectasis and infarction may appear as an opacified region on the roentgenogram. Classically, the density is shaped like a truncated cone, fanning out toward and reaching the pleural surface. This finding, called a "Hampton's hump," is also relatively infrequent. Finally, pleural disease, in the form of an effusion, may also be seen as an accompaniment of pulmonary embolic disease.

Arterial blood gases characteristically show hypoxemia and a respiratory alkalosis, i.e., hypocapnia. Since the P_{CO_2} is decreased, the arterial P_{O_2} appears higher than it would if hyperventilation were not present. However, if the alveolar-arterial oxygen difference ($AaDo_2$) is calculated, it is found to be increased. Occasionally, the P_{O_2} is normal, so that the presence of a normal P_{O_2} does not exclude the diagnosis of pulmonary embolism.

Characteristic arterial blood gases in pulmonary embolic disease:
1. decreased P_{O_2}
2. decreased P_{CO_2}
3. increased pH

The major screening test for pulmonary embolism is the perfusion lung scan, described in Chapter 3. Because of the obstruction to blood flow, the scan demonstrates absence of perfusion to the region of lung supplied by the occluded vessel (Fig. 13–1). If the scan is normal, pulmonary embolism is, for all practical purposes, excluded. Abnormalities, however, do not automatically indicate the presence of embolic disease. False positive lung scans are common because local decreases in blood flow may result from primary disease of the parenchyma or the airways. A ventilation scan, involving inhalation of a xenon radioisotope, is often added, since if regions of decreased blood flow are secondary to airways disease, there should be corresponding abnormalities on the ventilation scan. If parenchymal disease, such as a pneumonia, is the cause of a perfusion defect, then there should be a corresponding abnormality on the chest roentgenogram.

high sensitivity

sensitivity not v. high

to rule out airway ds as cause for decr. blood flow

pneumonia interstitial should be seen on CXR

Obviously, interpretation of the perfusion lung scan is a complicated process and depends on the clinical setting, the results of chest

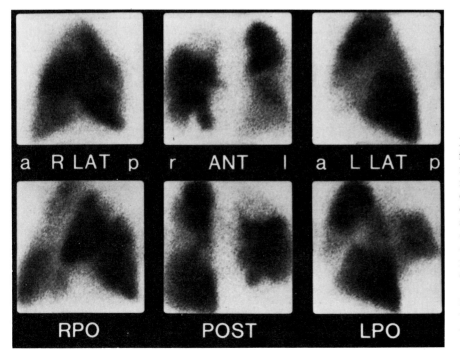

Figure 13–1. Positive perfusion scan demonstrating multiple perfusion defects in a patient with pulmonary emboli. The six views of a complete scan are shown: anterior (ANT), posterior (POST), right and left lateral (R LAT and L LAT), and right and left posterior obliques (RPO and LPO). a = anterior; p = posterior; r = right; l = left. Compare with normal scan in Figure 3–10. (Courtesy of Dr. Henry Royal.)

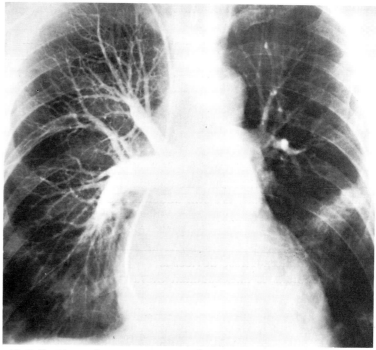

Figure 13–2. Positive pulmonary angiogram showing occlusion of the vessel supplying the left lower lobe. The area of density in the left mid-lung probably represents a pulmonary infarct. (Courtesy of Dr. Morris Simon.)

use all information to come up w/ probable % that it is PE

Major techniques for diagnosis of pulmonary emboli include ventilation-perfusion lung scanning and pulmonary angiography.

roentgenogram, and frequently the findings of a ventilation lung scan. Since the perfusion scan is often not definitive, a probability is placed on the likelihood of pulmonary embolism, taking into account the size and number of defects and the presence or absence of corresponding abnormalities on the radiograph and the ventilation lung scan.

When lung scanning is not conclusive, one frequently must pursue the diagnostic work-up with a more invasive procedure, pulmonary angiography, also discussed in Chapter 3. Though angiography is generally considered the "gold standard" for diagnosis of embolic disease, it also has pitfalls in interpretation and is not entirely without risk. Nevertheless, it is frequently useful, and the finding of a filling defect within a vessel or an abrupt cut-off is considered diagnostic of a pulmonary embolus (Fig. 13–2).

Since venous thrombosis in the leg veins is the most common source of pulmonary emboli, methods for diagnosis of the primary thrombus are also clinically important when considering pulmonary embolic disease. However, consideration of the individual diagnostic techniques for venous thrombosis is beyond the scope of this discussion.

TREATMENT

The standard treatment for a pulmonary embolus involves the use of anticoagulant therapy, initially heparin and then a coumarin derivative (warfarin), the latter usually given for weeks to months. However, the rationale for the use of anticoagulants is to prevent formation of new thrombi or propagation of old ones (in the legs), not to dissolve clots that have already embolized to the lungs.

Recently, there has been a great deal of interest in the use of thrombolytic agents, either streptokinase or urokinase, for treatment of pulmonary emboli. These agents, which may actually lyse recent blood clots, must be given within the first several days of the embolic event in order to be effective. Specific subgroups of patients are most likely to benefit from thrombolytic therapy, namely those patients with massive pulmonary embolus and those with hemodynamic compromise as a result of vascular occlusion. When one of these agents is used, treatment is generally continued for 24 to 48 hours and is followed by standard anticoagulant therapy. The usefulness and indications for this particular mode of therapy are still under active assessment.

In some circumstances, treatment of pulmonary embolism involves placement of a filtering device into the inferior vena cava, with the goal of trapping thrombi from the lower extremities en route to the pulmonary circulation. These devices are used most frequently if there are contraindications to anticoagulant therapy, such as bleeding problems, or if the patient already has such limited pulmonary vascular reserve that an additional clot to the lungs would be fatal.

Finally, no discussion of the treatment of pulmonary embolism is complete without a consideration of prophylactic methods used in the high-risk patient to prevent deep venous thrombosis. The most common prophylaxis is heparin administered subcutaneously in low dosage, which has proved to be effective and relatively nontoxic in particular groups of high-risk patients. It is now often administered to patients about to undergo thoracic or abdominal surgery and to a variety of other high-risk patients who are at bed rest in the hospital.

Options for therapy of pulmonary embolism:
1. anticoagulation (heparin, warfarin)
2. thrombolysis (streptokinase, urokinase)
3. inferior vena caval filter

REFERENCES

Reviews

Moser, K. M.: Pulmonary embolism. Am. Rev. Respir. Dis. 115:829–852, 1977.

Moser, K. M.: Venous thromboembolism: three simple decisions. Chest 83:117–121; 256–260, 1983.

Rosenow, E. C., III, Osmundson, P. J., and Brown, M. L.: Pulmonary embolism. Mayo Clin. Proc. 56:161–178, 1981.

Sasahara, A. A., Sharma, G. V. R. K., Barsamian, E. M., Schoolman, M., and Cella, G.: Pulmonary thromboembolism: diagnosis and treatment. JAMA 249:2945–2950, 1983.

Sharma, G. V. R. K., Tow, D. E., Parisi, A. F., and Sasahara, A. A.: Diagnosis of pulmonary embolism. Ann. Rev. Med. 28:159–166, 1977.

Specific Aspects

Bell, W. R., Simon, T. L., and DeMets, D. L.: The clinical features of submassive and massive pulmonary emboli. Am. J. Med. 62:355–360, 1977.

Dantzker, D. R. and Bower, J. S.: Alterations in gas exchange following pulmonary thromboembolism. Chest 81:495–501, 1982.

Goldhaber, S. Z., Hennekens, C. H., Evans, D. A., Newton, E. C., and Godleski, J. J.: Factors associated with correct antemortem diagnosis of major pulmonary embolism. Am. J. Med. 73:822–826, 1982.

McNeil, B. J.: A diagnostic strategy using ventilation-perfusion studies in patients suspect for pulmonary embolism. J. Nucl. Med. 17:613–616, 1976.

Robin, E. D.: Overdiagnosis and overtreatment of pulmonary embolism: the emperor may have no clothes. Ann. Intern. Med. 87:775–781, 1977.

Sharma, G. V. R. K., Cella, G., Parisi, A. F., and Sasahara, A. A.: Thrombolytic therapy. N. Engl. J. Med. 306:1268–1276, 1982.

Sherry, S.: Low-dose heparin for the prophylaxis of pulmonary embolism. Am. Rev. Respir. Dis. 114:661–666, 1976.

14

Pulmonary Hypertension

Elevation of intravascular pressure within the pulmonary circulation is the hallmark of pulmonary hypertension. In this chapter, we are specifically referring to elevated pulmonary arterial pressure (above approximately 30 to 35 torr systolic, 15 to 20 torr diastolic), though in some cases an elevation in pulmonary venous pressure is an important forerunner of pulmonary arterial hypertension. Since pulmonary hypertension has a number of causes that act by several different mechanisms, we have elected to organize this chapter into an initial consideration of features relevant to pulmonary hypertension in general, followed by discussion of a few of the important specific causes of pulmonary hypertension.

Before we proceed with this discussion, clarification of a few items is in order. First, as we mentioned, pulmonary hypertension merely refers to the elevation of pulmonary vascular pressure; it may be acute or chronic, depending upon the causative factors. In some cases, chronic pulmonary hypertension is punctuated by further acute elevations in pressure, often as a result of exacerbations of the underlying disease. Second, the development of right ventricular hypertrophy is the consequence of pulmonary hypertension, whatever the primary cause of the latter. When pulmonary hypertension is due to disorders of any part of the respiratory apparatus (airways, parenchyma and blood vessels, chest wall, respiratory musculature, or the central nervous system controller), the term *cor pulmonale* is used to refer to the resulting right ventricular hypertrophy. This term is not used to describe the right ventricular changes occurring as a consequence of primary cardiac disease or of increased flow to the pulmonary vascular bed.

PATHOGENESIS

A number of factors contribute to the pathogenesis of pulmonary arterial hypertension, both acutely and chronically. As we mentioned in Chapter 13, occlusion of a sufficient cross-sectional area of the pulmonary arteries by material within the vessels, such as pulmonary emboli, is obviously an important factor. Acutely, with massive pulmonary emboli occluding more than one-half to two-thirds of the vasculature, pulmonary arterial pressure is elevated. In the acute setting, the right ventricle may dilate as a response to its increased workload, since there is insufficient time for hypertrophy. In the chronic setting, multiple and recurrent pulmonary emboli may elevate pulmonary arterial pressures over a time period sufficient for right ventricular hypertrophy to occur.

Factors contributing to pulmonary arterial hypertension:
1. occlusion of vessels by emboli
2. primary thickening of arterial walls
3. loss of vessels by scarring or destruction of alveolar walls
4. pulmonary vasoconstriction (from hypoxia, acidosis)
5. increased pulmonary vascular flow (left-to-right shunt)
6. elevated left atrial pressure

Diminution of cross-sectional area as an outcome of primary disease of the pulmonary arterial walls is a second potential contributing factor to pulmonary hypertension. As we will discuss, thickening of the arterial and arteriolar walls occurs in such disorders as primary pulmonary hypertension and progressive systemic sclerosis (scleroderma). Compromise of the pulmonary vasculature and increased resistance to flow may be so pronounced in these primary disorders of the vessel wall that the level of pulmonary hypertension is quite severe.

The total cross-sectional area of the pulmonary vascular bed is also compromised by primary parenchymal disease, with loss of blood vessels from either a scarring or a destructive process affecting the alveolar walls. Both interstitial lung disease and emphysema can affect the pulmonary vasculature via this mechanism, though obviously the underlying pathology in the parenchyma appears quite different. With these diseases, it is common for pulmonary arterial pressure to be relatively normal at rest but elevated with exercise because of insufficient recruitment or distension of vessels to handle the increase in cardiac output.

A fourth and most important mechanism of pulmonary hypertension is vasoconstriction in response to hypoxia and, to a lesser extent, acidosis. The importance of this mechanism is related to its potential reversibility when a normal Po_2 and pH are achieved. In several causes of cor pulmonale, particularly chronic obstructive lung disease with Type B physiology, hypoxia is the single most important factor leading to pulmonary hypertension and is also potentially the most treatable. As we mentioned in Chapter 12, acidosis, either respiratory or metabolic, causes pulmonary vasoconstriction and, though it is less important than hypoxia, may augment the vasoconstrictive response to hypoxia.

When flow through the pulmonary vascular bed is increased, as in patients with congenital intracardiac (left-to-right) shunts, the vasculature is initially able to handle the augmented flow without any anatomic changes in the arteries or arterioles. However, over a prolonged period of time, there is thickening of the vessel walls, and pulmonary arterial resistance increases. Eventually, as a result of the high pulmonary resistance, right-sided cardiac pressures may become so elevated that the intracardiac shunt reverses in direction. This conversion to a right-to-left shunt is commonly called Eisenmenger's syndrome, and it is a potentially important consequence of an atrial or ventricular septal defect or a patent ductus arteriosus.

A final and very common mechanism of pulmonary arterial hypertension is elevation of pressure distally, either in the left atrium or left ventricle, and progressive elevation of the "back-pressure" first in the pulmonary capillaries and then in the pulmonary arterioles and arteries. As is the case with pulmonary hypertension eventually induced by increased flow in the pulmonary vasculature, here too the initial elevation in pressure is not accompanied by anatomic changes in the pulmonary arteries. Eventually, however, structural changes are seen, and measured pulmonary vascular resistance may be substantially increased. The major disorders that result in pulmonary hypertension by this final mechanism are mitral stenosis and chronic left ventricular failure.

PATHOLOGY

In many ways, the pathologic findings in the pulmonary vessels of patients with pulmonary hypertension are similar, regardless of the underlying etiology. In this section, we will specifically focus on these general changes.

Pathologic features of pulmonary hypertension:
1. intimal hypertrophy and medial hyperplasia of small arteries and arterioles
2. eventual obliteration of the lumen of small arteries/arterioles
3. thickening of the wall of larger (elastic) pulmonary arteries
4. right ventricular hypertrophy (with or without dilatation)

The most prominent abnormalities are frequently seen in vessels of the pulmonary arterial tree whose diameter is less than 1 mm, namely the small muscular arteries (0.1 to 1 mm) and the arterioles (less than 0.1 mm). The muscular arteries show hypertrophy of the media, composed of smooth muscle, and hyperplasia of the intimal layer lining the vessel lumen. In the arterioles, a significant muscular component to the vessel wall is normally not present, but with pulmonary hypertension these vessels undergo "muscularization" of their walls (Fig. 14–1A). Additionally, there is proliferation of the arteriolar intima. As a result of these changes, the luminal diameter is significantly decreased, and the pulmonary vascular resistance is elevated. Ultimately, the lumen may be completely obliterated, and the overall number of small vessels is greatly diminished.

When pulmonary hypertension becomes marked, additional changes are commonly seen in the larger (elastic) pulmonary arteries (Fig. 14–1B). These vessels, which normally have much thinner walls than vessels of comparable size in the systemic circulation, develop thickening of the wall, particularly in the media. They also develop the types of atherosclerotic plaques that are generally seen only in the higher pressure systemic circulation.

The cardiac consequences of pulmonary hypertension are seen pathologically as changes in the right ventricular wall. The magnitude of the changes depends primarily upon the severity and chronicity of the pulmonary hypertension rather than the nature of the underlying disorder. The major finding is concentric hypertrophy of the right

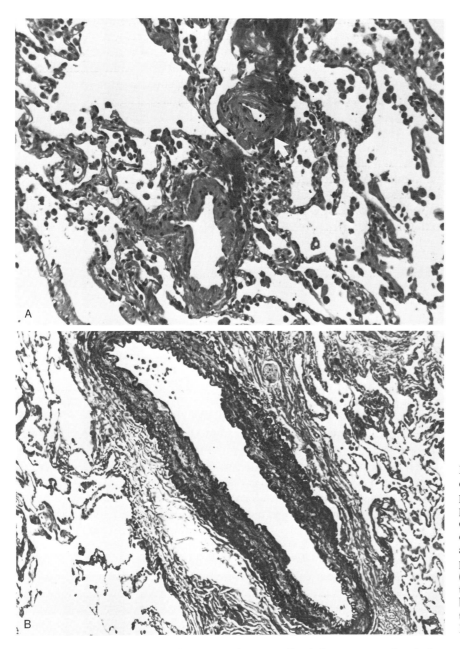

Figure 14–1. Histologic changes in pulmonary hypertension. *A*, Moderate-power photomicrograph demonstrating the thickened wall of a pulmonary arteriole (arrow). *B*, Low-power photomicrograph (elastic tissue stain) showing the thickened wall of a branch of the pulmonary artery. (Courtesy of Dr. Earl Kasdon.)

ventricular wall. If the right ventricle actually fails as a result of the chronic increase in workload, then dilatation of the right ventricle is also observed.

PATHOPHYSIOLOGY

The pathophysiologic changes in pulmonary hypertension are by definition characterized by alterations in pressure within the pulmonary circulation. If the primary component of the vascular change occurs at the level of the pulmonary arteries or arterioles, as is true of cor pulmonale, then the pulmonary arterial pressures (both systolic and diastolic) rise, while the pulmonary capillary pressure (reflecting back-pressure from the left atrium) remains normal. If, on the other hand, the pulmonary arterial hypertension is secondary to pulmonary venous and pulmonary capillary hypertension, as is the case with mitral stenosis or left ventricular failure, then the pulmonary capillary pressure is obviously also elevated above its normal level.

As pulmonary hypertension progresses, the right ventricular systolic pressure rises in conjunction with the increase in pulmonary arterial systolic pressure. The cardiac output usually remains normal early in the course of the process. When the right ventricle fails, the right ventricular end-diastolic pressure rises, and the cardiac output may decrease as well. The right atrial pressure also rises, which may be apparent on physical examination of the neck veins by an elevation in the jugular venous pressure.

CLINICAL FEATURES

Clinical features of pulmonary hypertension:
1. Symptoms—dyspnea, substernal chest pain, fatigue, syncope
2. Physical signs—loud P_2, prominent parasternal (RV) impulse, right-sided S_4; also, right-sided S_3, jugular venous distension, peripheral edema in case of RV failure.

Although the overall constellation of symptoms in patients with pulmonary hypertension depends upon the underlying disease, there are certain characteristic complaints that can be attributed to the pulmonary hypertension itself. Dyspnea is frequently observed, but in many patients it is difficult to know the primary etiology of this symptom. Patients may have substernal chest pain that is difficult, if not impossible, to distinguish from classical angina pectoris, particularly since the pain is frequently also related to exertion. It has been presumed that the chest pain is related to the increased workload of the right ventricle and to right ventricular ischemia, as opposed to the more frequent ischemia of the left ventricle associated with coronary artery disease. In many cases, as a result of an inability to increase cardiac output with exercise, patients may experience exertional fatigue or even syncope.

Physical examination shows several features that are more related to the cardiac consequences of pulmonary hypertension than to the actual disease of the pulmonary vessels. Pulmonary hypertension itself does not cause any changes on examination of the lungs, though patients with underlying lung disease obviously often have findings related to their primary disease. On cardiac examination, patients frequently exhibit an accentuation of the component of the second heart sound due to pulmonic valve closure (P_2), which is attributable to high pressure in the pulmonary artery. With right ventricular hypertrophy, there is often a prominent lift or heave of the region immediately to the left of the lower sternum, corresponding to a prominent right ventricular impulse during systole. As the right atrium contracts and empties its contents into the poorly compliant, hypertrophied right ventricle, a presystolic gallop (S_4) originating from the right ventricle may be heard. When the right ventricle fails, a mid-diastolic gallop (S_3) in the parasternal region is frequently heard, the jugular veins become distended, and peripheral edema may develop. Occasionally, one hears murmurs of pulmonic or tricuspid valve insufficiency.

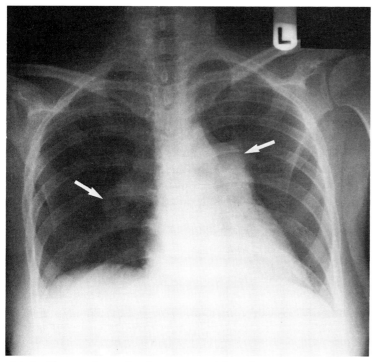

Figure 14–2. Chest radiograph of a patient with pulmonary hypertension due to pulmonary vascular disease associated with scleroderma. The central pulmonary arteries (arrows) are large bilaterally, but they rapidly taper off distally.

DIAGNOSTIC FEATURES

Most often, the status of the pulmonary vessels is initially assessed by chest radiography. With mild pulmonary hypertension originating at the arterial or arteriolar level, frequently no abnormalities are seen. As the pulmonary arterial hypertension becomes more significant, the central (hilar) pulmonary arteries increase in size, and the vessels often rapidly taper off, so that the distal vasculature appears attenuated (Fig. 14–2). With hypertrophy of the right ventricle, the cardiac silhouette may enlarge. This feature is most apparent on the lateral radiograph, which shows bulging of the anterior cardiac border.

When pulmonary hypertension is a consequence of either increased flow to the pulmonary vasculature (as in congenital heart disease with initial left-to-right shunting) or increased back-pressure from the pulmonary veins and pulmonary capillaries (as in mitral stenosis or left ventricular failure), the findings are significantly altered. In the case of congenital heart disease with left-to-right shunting, pulmonary blood flow is prominent, until there is reversal of the left-to-right shunt. When there is elevation of pulmonary venous pressure from mitral stenosis or left ventricular failure, the chest radiograph often shows "redistribution" of blood flow from lower to upper lung zones, accompanied by evidence of interstitial or alveolar edema.

Perfusion lung scanning is frequently a valuable adjunct in the assessment of patients with pulmonary hypertension. In particular, focal perfusion defects may suggest recurrent pulmonary emboli as a likely etiology for the elevation in pulmonary arterial pressure.

Pulmonary function tests may demonstrate underlying restrictive or obstructive disease; tests may also show decrease in diffusing capacity from loss of the pulmonary vascular bed.

Pulmonary function tests in evaluating the patient with pulmonary hypertension are useful primarily to look for underlying airflow obstruction (from chronic obstructive lung disease) or restricted lung volumes (from interstitial lung disease). As a result of the pulmonary hypertension itself and loss of the pulmonary vascular bed, the diffusing capacity may be decreased and often is the only additional abnormality noted.

Arterial blood gases are most useful for determining whether hypoxemia or acidosis plays a role in the pathogenesis of the pulmonary hypertension. Arterial Po_2 may also be mildly decreased as a result of the pulmonary vascular disease itself, apparently because of non-uniform distribution of disease and ventilation-perfusion mismatch.

An electrocardiogram may aid in the diagnosis of pulmonary hypertension by demonstrating right ventricular hypertrophy. Description of the specific findings is beyond the scope of this chapter but may be found in standard textbooks of cardiology or electrocardiography.

Definitive quantitation of the degree of pulmonary hypertension is made by cardiac catheterization. In many circumstances, such evaluation is not deemed to be necessary. However, in other circumstances, particularly in the evaluation of suspected primary pulmonary hypertension, measurements of right ventricular, pulmonary artery, and pulmonary capillary pressures are important in making the diagnosis and assessing severity of the disease.

SPECIFIC DISORDERS ASSOCIATED WITH PULMONARY HYPERTENSION

Primary Pulmonary Hypertension

Often, primary pulmonary hypertension appears in young women, is associated with Raynaud's syndrome, and has a poor prognosis.

Primary pulmonary hypertension is a disease of unknown etiology found most commonly in women between the ages of 20 and 40. Though there has been at least one outbreak of pulmonary hypertension attributed to a particular drug (an appetite suppressant named aminorex, now no longer available), the majority of cases cannot be attributed to any exogenous agent. It is well recognized that chronic and recurrent pulmonary embolization can closely mimic primary pulmonary hypertension. Consequently, the latter diagnosis cannot be made until the presence of chronic thromboemboli has been excluded.

The fact that patients with this disease frequently have Raynaud's syndrome (vasospasm of digital vessels upon exposure to cold) may indicate that vasospasm of pulmonary arteries plays a role in the initial pathogenesis of this disorder. Alternatively, since Raynaud's syndrome is often associated with an underlying connective tissue disease, we may infer that primary pulmonary hypertension is related to the general category of connective tissue diseases. Interestingly, patients with scleroderma occasionally develop a process of obliteration of pulmonary vessels, unassociated with interstitial lung disease, that closely resembles primary pulmonary hypertension.

The prognosis of primary pulmonary hypertension is generally considered to be poor; patients frequently die within several years of diagnosis. However, recent data suggest that a subgroup of patients has relatively stable disease with a much more favorable prognosis than has been generally accepted. For treatment, a number of vasodilators have been used in an attempt to reduce pulmonary arterial pressure, but the results have been inconsistent at best. Unfortunately, even when there is some vasodilation of pulmonary vessels, use of these agents is limited by dilation of systemic blood vessels and subsequent systemic arterial hypotension.

Pulmonary Hypertension Secondary to Airway or Parenchymal Lung Disease

The most common causes of cor pulmonale appear to be chronic obstructive lung disease and interstitial lung disease. In the former category, patients with Type B physiology, i.e., those with a prominent component of chronic bronchitis who are considered "blue bloaters," are particularly susceptible to development of pulmonary hypertension. Hypoxia is the single most important etiologic factor in these patients. Additional contributory factors include (1) respiratory acidosis, which may worsen vasoconstriction; (2) secondary polycythemia, a consequence of chronic hypoxemia, which further increases pulmonary artery pressures as a result of increased blood viscosity; and (3) loss of pulmonary vascular bed due to coexistent emphysema.

Any of the interstitial lung diseases, when relatively severe, may also be associated with cor pulmonale. In these patients, the major contributing factors appear to be (1) loss of vascular bed as a result of the scarring process in the alveolar walls and (2) hypoxia.

In both obstructive and interstitial disease, important therapy can be offered, namely correction of alveolar hypoxia and hypoxemia by administration of supplemental oxygen. In these patients, the goal is to maintain arterial Po_2 at a level greater than approximately 60 torr, above which hypoxic vasoconstriction is largely eliminated. Other forms of therapy aimed more specifically at the underlying disease have been discussed in Chapters 6, 10, and 11.

In addition to these two categories of lung disease, it is important to recognize that other disorders of the respiratory apparatus associated with hypoxemia and hypercapnia may be complicated by development of cor pulmonale. Specifically, disorders of control of breathing, of the chest bellows, or of the neural apparatus controlling the chest bellows, may each be complicated by cor pulmonale. These disorders will be discussed in more detail in Chapters 18 and 19.

Obstructive disease, interstitial disease, and a variety of neural, muscular, and chest wall diseases may produce pulmonary hypertension and cor pulmonale.

Pulmonary Arterial Hypertension Associated with Pulmonary Venous Hypertension

Mitral stenosis and chronic left ventricular failure are the two disorders most frequently associated with pulmonary venous, and subsequently pulmonary arterial, hypertension. These disorders do not fall into the category of cor pulmonale, since the underlying problem resulting in pulmonary hypertension is clearly of cardiac, not pulmonary, origin.

With pulmonary venous hypertension, the pathology and many of the clinical and diagnostic features are different in a relatively predictable way. Pathologically, dilated and tortuous capillaries and small veins may result from high pressures in the pulmonary veins and capillaries, along with chronic extravasation of red blood cells into the pulmonary parenchyma. In the process of handling the interstitial and alveolar hemoglobin, macrophages may become loaded with hemosiderin, a breakdown product of hemoglobin. These macrophages can be detected by appropriate staining of sputum for iron. Not infrequently, the alveolar walls have a fibrotic response, presumably secondary to the long-standing extravasation of blood, so that a component of interstitial lung disease with fibrosis may be seen.

Long-standing pulmonary venous hypertension is associated with extravasation of erythrocytes into the pulmonary parenchyma, hemosiderin-laden macrophages, and a fibrotic interstitial response.

As we mentioned earlier in the discussion of radiographic abnormalities, the presence of pulmonary venous hypertension adds several features to the chest radiograph, including redistribution of blood flow to the upper lobes and interstitial and alveolar edema. In addition, there are frequently Kerley B lines, small horizontal lines extending to the pleura at both lung bases, reflecting thickening of, or fluid in, lymphatics in interlobular septae, a consequence of interstitial edema.

Radiographic evidence of pulmonary venous hypertension:
1. redistribution of blood flow to upper zones
2. interstitial and alveolar edema
3. Kerley B lines

Treatment of these disorders certainly revolves around attempts to "correct" the cardiac disease, or at least to decrease pulmonary venous and capillary pressures. The potential reversibility of the pulmonary arterial hypertension depends upon the chronicity of the disease and the degree to which the venous hypertension can be alleviated.

REFERENCES

General Reviews

Heath, D., and Smith, P.: Pulmonary vascular disease. Med. Clin. North Am. 61:1279–1307, 1977.
Rounds, S., and Hill, N. S.: Pulmonary hypertensive diseases. Chest 85:397–405, 1984.

Primary Pulmonary Hypertension

Edwards, W. D., and Edwards, J. E.: Clinical primary pulmonary hypertension: three pathologic types. Circulation 56:884–888, 1977.
Fishman, A. P.: Primary pulmonary hypertension: more light or more tunnel? Ann. Intern. Med. 94:815–817, 1981.
Hermiller, J. B., et al.: Vasodilators and prostaglandin inhibitors in primary pulmonary hypertension. Ann. Intern. Med. 97:480–489, 1982.
Packer, M., Greenberg, B., Massie, B., and Dash, H.: Deleterious effects of hydralazine in patients with pulmonary hypertension. N. Engl. J. Med. 306:1326–1331, 1982.
Rich, S., and Brundage, B. H.: Primary pulmonary hypertension: current update. JAMA 251:2252–2254, 1984.
Walcott, G., Burchell, H. B., and Brown, A. L., Jr.: Primary pulmonary hypertension. Am. J. Med. 49:70–79, 1970.

Pulmonary Hypertension Associated with Cardiac Disease

Cortese, D. A.: Pulmonary function in mitral stenosis. Mayo Clin. Proc. 53:321–326, 1978.
Dalen, J. E., et al.: Early reduction of pulmonary vascular resistance after mitral-valve replacement. N. Engl. J. Med. 277:387–394, 1967.
Dexter, L.: Pulmonary vascular disease in acquired and congenital heart disease. Arch. Intern. Med. 139:922–928, 1979.

Cor Pulmonale

Fishman, A. P.: Chronic cor pulmonale. Am. Rev. Respir. Dis. 114:775–794, 1976.
Wynne, J. W.: The treatment of cor pulmonale. JAMA 239:2283–2285, 1978.

15

Pleural Disease

As we progress from the lung itself to other structures that are part of the process of respiration, an obvious area to consider is the adjacent pleura. In clinical medicine, this region is important not only because diseases of the lung commonly cause secondary abnormalities in the pleura, but also because the pleura is an important site of disease in its own right. Not infrequently, pleural disease is a manifestation of a multisystem process, either inflammatory, immune, or malignant in nature.

In this chapter, we will first discuss the anatomy of the pleura, followed by a few physiologic principles particularly relevant for fluid formation and absorption by the pleura. We will then proceed to a discussion of two types of abnormalities affecting the pleura—liquid in the pleural space (pleural effusion) and air in the pleural space (pneumothorax). Though we are unable to give a comprehensive treatment of all the disorders affecting the pleura, we will try to cover the major categories and to give the reader an understanding of the way in which different factors interact in the production of pleural disease. The primary malignancy of the pleura, called mesothelioma, will not be discussed in this chapter but rather in Chapter 21, which deals with neoplastic disease.

ANATOMY

When we use the term *pleura*, we are actually referring to the thin lining layer on the outer surface of the lung (*visceral pleura*), the corresponding lining layer on the inner surface of the chest wall (*parietal pleura*), and the space between them (the *pleural space*) (Fig. 15–1). Since the visceral and parietal pleural surfaces normally touch each other, the space between them is only a potential space, containing just a few milliliters of serous fluid. When air or a larger amount of fluid accumulates in the pleural space, the visceral and parietal pleural surfaces are separated, and the fact that there is a space between the lung and the chest wall becomes more apparent.

It is important to note that the pleura lines not only those surfaces of the lung that are in direct contact with the chest wall but also the diaphragmatic and mediastinal borders of the lung. As expected, these surfaces are called the *diaphragmatic* and *mediastinal pleura*, respectively (Fig. 15–1). Visceral pleura also separates the lobes of the lung from each other, so that the major and minor fissures are defined by two apposing visceral pleural surfaces.

Each of the two pleural surfaces, visceral and parietal, is a thin membrane, the surface of which consists of specific lining cells called *mesothelial cells*. Beneath the mesothelial cell layer is a thin layer of connective tissue. Blood vessels and lymphatic vessels course throughout the connective tissue and are quite important in the dynamics of liquid formation and resorption in the pleural space. There are also some sensory nerve endings in the parietal and diaphragmatic pleura, which are apparently responsible for the characteristic "pleuritic chest pain" arising from the pleura.

The blood vessels supplying the parietal pleural surface originate from the systemic arterial circulation, primarily the intercostal arteries. In contrast, the visceral pleura is supplied by vessels originating from the pulmonary artery. Depending on their location, the lymphatics that drain the pleural surfaces transport their fluid contents to different lymph nodes. Ultimately, any liquid transported by the lymphatic

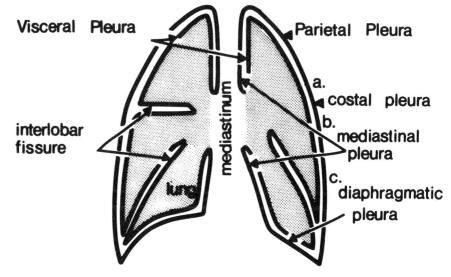

Figure 15–1. Anatomic features of the pleura. The pleural space is located between the visceral and parietal pleural surfaces. The pleura lines not only the surfaces of the lung in contact with the chest wall (costal pleura) but also the mediastinal and diaphragmatic borders (mediastinal and diaphragmatic pleura, respectively). (From Lowell, J. R.: Pleural Effusions: A Comprehensive Review. Baltimore, University Park Press, 1977, p. 7. Reproduced with permission.)

channels finds its way to the right lymphatic or thoracic ducts, which empty into the systemic venous circulation.

PHYSIOLOGY

At both the parietal and visceral pleural surfaces, liquid and solutes can potentially filter out of the capillaries and into the pleural space. Several different forces promote fluid filtration or resorption, and the net movement of fluid between the pleural capillaries and the pleural space depends on the magnitude of these counterbalancing forces. For capillaries adjacent to a pericapillary space, the hydrostatic pressure in the capillary promotes movement of fluid out of the vessel and into the pericapillary space, while the colloid osmotic pressure (the osmotic pressure exerted by protein drawing in fluid) hinders movement of liquid out of the capillary. Likewise, hydrostatic and colloid osmotic pressures in the pericapillary space comprise the opposing forces acting on liquid within the pericapillary region.

The effect of these forces is summarized in the Starling equation, which describes the movement of fluid between vascular and extravascular compartments of any part of the body, not just the pleura. According to this equation,

$$\text{Fluid movement} = K[(P_c - P_{is}) - \sigma (COP_c - COP_{is})]$$

where K = filtration coefficient (a function of the permeability of the pleural surface), P = hydrostatic pressure, COP = colloid osmotic pressure, σ is a measure of capillary permeability to protein (called the reflection coefficient), and the subscripts "c" and "is" refer to the capillary and the pericapillary interstitial space, respectively. In this case, the pericapillary interstitial space is essentially the pleural space, and P_{is} and COP_{is} therefore refer to intrapleural pressure and the colloid osmotic pressure of pleural fluid, respectively.

When applying these concepts to the pleura, the visceral and parietal pleurae must be considered individually, and the Starling equation must be applied separately for movement of fluid between each of these surfaces and the pleural space. If we substitute values obtained by direct measurement or by estimation into this equation, we find that there is a net pressure of approximately 9 cm H_2O favoring movement of fluid from the parietal pleura to the pleural space. In contrast, the net pressure for filtering fluid from the visceral pleura to the pleural space is approximately -10 cm H_2O. Since this latter pressure is negative, the driving pressure is actually in the direction favoring resorption of fluid by the visceral pleura from the pleural space.

The explanation for the difference in driving pressure at the parietal versus the visceral pleural surface revolves around the hydrostatic pressure in the pleural capillaries. Whereas the blood supply to the parietal pleura originates from the high-pressure systemic arterial circulation, the visceral pleura is supplied by the low-pressure pulmonary arterial circulation. Thus, the hydrostatic pressure in the arterial side of parietal pleural capillaries is relatively high and favors filtration

The Starling equation can be applied to the pleural surfaces.
P_c *of parietal pleura = 30 cm H_2O*
P_c *of visceral pleura = 11 cm H_2O*
P_{is} *(mean intrapleural pressure) = -5 cm H_2O*
COP_c *= 32 cm H_2O*
COP_{is} *= 6 cm H_2O*
σ *= 1, K = 1*
Fluid movement at parietal pleura
= [30 - (-5)] - 1 (32 - 6)
= 9 cm H_2O
Fluid movement at visceral pleura
= [11 - (-5)] - 1 (32 - 6)
= -10 cm H_2O

of fluid into the pleural space. On the other hand, the low hydrostatic pressure in the arterial side of visceral pleural capillaries is not sufficient to overcome colloid osmotic pressure in the capillary blood. Accordingly, fluid moves from the pleural space into the visceral pleural capillaries.

In summary, there is a driving force for fluid to be filtered from the parietal pleura into the pleural space and then resorbed by the visceral pleura. Over the course of a day, it has been estimated that approximately 5 to 10 L of fluid pass through the pleural space because of these pressure gradients.

Pleural fluid is filtered from the parietal pleura into the pleural space and reabsorbed by the visceral pleura and pleural lymphatics.

In addition to the resorption of fluid from the pleural space by the visceral pleura, there is also movement of fluid and solutes out of the pleural space and into pleural lymphatics. The lymphatics are particularly important for removing protein in disorders in which there is leakage of proteins from both parietal and visceral pleural surfaces into the pleural space. It has been estimated that the lymphatics are normally responsible for clearing approximately 250 to 500 ml of liquid over a 24 hour period.

PLEURAL EFFUSION

In the normal individual, resorption of pleural fluid maintains pace with pleural fluid formation so that fluid does not accumulate. However, a variety of diseases affect the forces governing pleural fluid filtration or resorption, resulting in fluid formation exceeding fluid removal, i.e., development of pleural effusion(s). We will first discuss the pathogenesis (dynamics) of fluid accumulation and then proceed with a consideration of some of the etiologies, clinical features, and diagnostic approaches to pleural effusions.

Pathogenesis of Pleural Fluid Accumulation

In theory, a change in the magnitude of any of the factors outlined in the Starling equation can cause sufficient imbalance of pleural fluid dynamics to result in pleural fluid accumulation. In practice, it is easiest to divide these changes into the following two categories: (1) alteration of the permeability of the pleural surface, i.e., changes in the filtration coefficient (K) and the reflection coefficient (σ), so that the pleura is more permeable to fluid and to larger molecular weight components of blood; and (2) alteration in the driving pressure, encompassing a change in hydrostatic or colloid osmotic pressures of the parietal or visceral pleura, without any change in pleural permeability.

The most common types of disease causing a change in the filtration and reflection coefficients are inflammatory or neoplastic diseases involving the pleura. In these circumstances, the pleural surface is more permeable to proteins, so that the accumulated fluid has a relatively high protein content. This type of fluid, due to a change in permeability and associated with a relatively high protein content, is termed an *exudate*.

Table 15–1. MAJOR CAUSES OF PLEURAL EFFUSION

Transudate
    Increased hydrostatic pressure
        Congestive heart failure
    Decreased plasma oncotic pressure
        Cirrhosis
        Nephrotic syndrome
Exudate
    Inflammatory
        Infection (TB, bacterial pneumonia)
        Pulmonary embolus (infarction)
        Connective tissue disease (lupus, rheumatoid arthritis)
        Adjacent to subdiaphragmatic disease (pancreatitis, subphrenic
            abscess)
    Malignant

In contrast, an increase in hydrostatic pressure within pleural capillaries (e.g., as might be seen in congestive heart failure), or a decrease in plasma colloid osmotic pressure (as in hypoproteinemia), would be expected to result in accumulation of fluid with a low protein content, since the pleural barrier is still relatively impermeable to proteins. This type of fluid, due to a change in the driving pressure (without increased permeability) and associated with a low protein content, is termed a *transudate*.

Exudates are due to increased permeability of the pleural surface; transudates are due to changes in pleural hydrostatic or colloid osmotic pressures.

Etiologies of Pleural Effusion

The numerous causes of pleural fluid accumulation are best divided into transudative and exudative categories (Table 15–1). As we will discuss, this distinction is generally easy to make and is most important in guiding the physician along the best route for further evaluation. Transudative fluid usually implies that the pathologic process is not one primarily involving the pleural surfaces, whereas exudative fluid often suggests that the pleura is affected by the disease process causing the effusion.

Transudative Pleural Fluid

Most frequently, transudative pleural fluid is associated with congestive heart failure and elevation of hydrostatic pressure in the pleural capillaries. It is difficult to say whether pulmonary venous hypertension (with left-sided heart failure) or systemic venous hypertension (with right-sided failure) is the more important factor. Pleural effusion is particularly likely when both ventricles have failed and pulmonary and systemic venous hypertension coexist.

Patients with hypoproteinemia have decreased plasma colloid osmotic pressure, and they may develop pleural fluid because hydrostatic pressure in pleural capillaries is now less opposed by the osmotic pressure provided by plasma proteins. The most common circumstances resulting in hypoproteinemia and pleural effusion(s) are liver disease (with decreased hepatic synthesis of protein) or nephrotic syndrome (with excessive renal losses of protein). Interestingly, in both cases, patients often have simultaneous fluid in the peritoneum (ascites).

Leakage of the ascitic fluid through breaks or defects in the diaphragm, or transport via diaphragmatic lymphatics, probably also contributes to the formation of pleural fluid.

Exudative Pleural Fluid

Exudative pleural fluid generally implies an increase in the permeability of the pleural surfaces, so that protein and fluid more readily enter the pleural space. Though a wide variety of processes can result in exudative pleural effusions, the two main etiologic categories are inflammatory and neoplastic disease. The inflammatory processes often originate within the lung but extend to the visceral pleural surface. Infection (especially bacterial pneumonia or tuberculosis) and pulmonary embolus (often with infarction) are two common examples. In the case of pneumonia extending to the pleural surface, an associated pleural effusion is called a *parapneumonic effusion*. When the effusion itself harbors organisms (or has an exuberant inflammatory response with many thousands of neutrophils), then the effusion is called an *empyema*. Though infection within the pleural space commonly is secondary to a pneumonia, empyema may also result from infection introduced through the chest wall, as in trauma or surgery involving the thorax.

In tuberculosis, there may be rupture of a subpleural focus of infection into the pleural space, after which an inflammatory response of the pleura ensues (with or without growth of the tubercle bacilli within the pleural space). In some cases, the pulmonary focus is not apparent, and pleural involvement is the major manifestation of tuberculosis within the thorax.

Other forms of inflammatory disease affecting the pleura primarily involve the pleural surface as opposed to the lung. Several of the connective tissue diseases, particularly systemic lupus erythematosus and rheumatoid arthritis, are associated with pleural involvement that is independent of changes within the pulmonary parenchyma. Inflammatory processes below the diaphragm, such as pancreatitis or a subphrenic abscess, are often accompanied by "sympathetic" pleural inflammation and development of an exudative pleural effusion. In this circumstance, transport of fluid from the abdomen via diaphragmatic lymphatics or through defects in the diaphragm is probably important in the pathogenesis of pleural fluid accumulation.

Malignancy may cause pleural effusion by several mechanisms, but the resulting fluid is generally exudative in nature. Commonly, malignant cells are found on the pleural surface, arriving there either by direct extension from an intrapulmonary malignancy or by hematogenous (bloodstream) dissemination from a distant source. In other cases, lymphatic channels or lymph nodes are blocked by foci of tumor, so that the normal lymphatic clearance mechanism for protein and fluid from the pleural space is impaired. In these latter cases, malignant cells are generally not found on examination of the pleural fluid.

A host of other disorders may have pleural effusion as a clinical manifestation. The list includes such varied processes as hypothyroidism, benign ovarian tumors (Meigs' syndrome), asbestos exposure, and primary disorders of the lymphatic channels, just to name a few. More detailed discussion of the various disorders with potential for pleural fluid accumulation may be found in references listed at the end of this chapter.

Clinical Features

A patient with pleural fluid may or may not have symptoms due to the pleural disease. Whether or not symptoms are present depends on the size of the effusion(s) as well as the nature of the underlying process. The inflammatory processes affecting the pleura frequently result in pleuritic chest pain, i.e., a sharp pain aggravated by respiration. When an effusion is quite large, patients may experience dyspnea resulting from compromise of the underlying lung. With small or moderate-sized effusions, a patient with otherwise normal lungs generally does not experience dyspnea just from the presence of fluid in the pleural space. When the pleural fluid has an inflammatory nature or is frankly infected, fever is also commonly found.

On physical examination of the chest, the region overlying the effusion is dull to percussion. Breath sounds are also usually decreased in this region as a result of decreased transmission of sound through the fluid medium in the pleura. At the upper level of the effusion, egophony may sometimes be heard as a manifestation of increased transmission of sound resulting from compression (atelectasis) of the underlying lung parenchyma. A scratchy, pleural friction rub may be present, particularly with an inflammatory process involving the pleural surfaces.

Common clinical features with pleural effusion(s): Symptoms—pleuritic chest pain, dyspnea, fever Physical signs—dullness, ↓ breath sounds, egophony at upper level, pleural friction rub

Diagnostic Approach

The PA and lateral chest roentgenograms are clearly most important in the initial evaluation of the patient with suspected pleural effusion (Fig. 15–2). With a small effusion, one sees blunting of the normally sharp angle between the diaphragm and the chest wall (costophrenic angle). Often this blunting is first apparent on inspection of the posterior costophrenic angle on the lateral roentgenogram, since this is the most dependent area of the pleural space. With a larger effusion, a homogeneous opacity of liquid density appears and is most obvious at the lung base(s) when the patient is upright. The fluid may also track along the lateral chest wall, forming a meniscus.

When certain inflammatory effusions persist over a period of time, fluid may no longer be free-flowing within the pleural space, as fibrous bands of tissue (loculations) form within the pleura. In such circumstances, fluid is not necessarily positioned as one would expect from the effects of gravity, and atypical appearances may be found. In order to detect whether fluid is free-flowing, or whether small costophrenic angle densities represent pleural fluid, a lateral decubitus chest radiograph may be extremely useful. In this view, the patient lies on his or her side, and free-flowing fluid shifts position to line the most dependent part of the pleural space (Fig. 15–3).

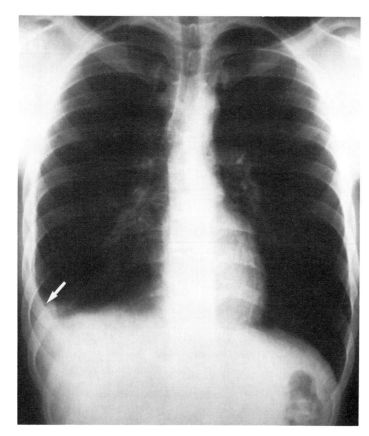

Figure 15–2. Chest radiograph demonstrating a small right pleural effusion. The right costophrenic angle is blunted by the effusion (arrow). The curvature of a lateral rib overlies the meniscus of the pleural fluid.

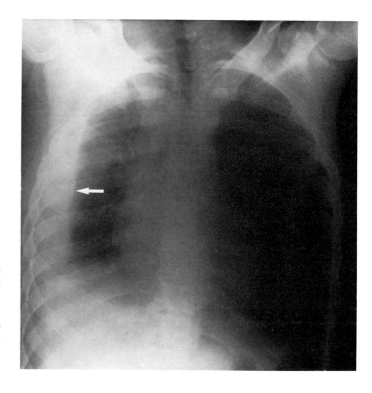

Figure 15–3. Right lateral decubitus chest radiograph of the patient shown in Figure 15–2. With the patient lying on his right side, pleural fluid (arrow) flows freely to the dependent part of the pleural space adjacent to the right lateral chest wall. The film is shown upright for convenience of comparison with Figure 15–2.

Another technique frequently used to evaluate the presence and location of pleural fluid is ultrasonography. When pleural fluid is present, a characteristic echo-free space can be detected between the chest wall and lung. Ultrasound is particularly useful in locating a small effusion not apparent on physical examination and in guiding the physician to a suitable site for thoracentesis.

When pleural fluid is present and the etiologic diagnosis is uncertain, sampling the fluid by thoracentesis (withdrawal of fluid by a needle or catheter) allows determination of the cellular and chemical characteristics of the fluid. These features define whether it is transudative or exudative and frequently give other clues about etiology. Though different criteria have been used at various times to determine whether an effusion is a transudate or exudate, the most common criteria now include the levels of protein and the enzyme lactic dehydrogenase (LDH) within the fluid, both in absolute numbers and relative to the corresponding values in serum. Exudative fluid has high levels of protein and/or LDH, whereas transudative fluid is associated with low levels of both.

An exudative effusion is defined by one or more of the following:
1. Pleural fluid/serum protein ratio >0.5
2. Pleural fluid/serum LDH ratio >0.6
3. Pleural fluid LDH >2/3 × upper limit of normal serum LDH

Pleural fluid obtained by thoracentesis is also routinely analyzed for absolute numbers and types of cellular constituents, for bacteria (by stains and cultures), and for glucose level. In many cases, amylase level and pH of the pleural fluid are also measured. Special slides are prepared for cytologic examination, and a search for malignant cells is made. Detailed discussion of the findings in different disorders may also be found in the references listed at the end of this chapter.

In some cases, pleural tissue is sampled by pleural biopsy, generally performed with a relatively large cutting needle inserted through the skin of the chest wall. Histologic examination of this tissue is most useful for demonstrating granulomas of tuberculosis or implants of tumor cells from a malignant process.

Pulmonary function tests are generally not part of the routine evaluation of patients with pleural effusion. However, it is worth noting that a significant effusion may impair lung expansion sufficiently to cause a restrictive pattern (with decreased lung volumes) on pulmonary function testing.

Treatment

The treatment of pleural effusion depends entirely on the nature of the underlying process and is usually directed at this process rather than at the effusion itself. In cases in which there is a high likelihood that the effusion will eventuate in extensive fibrosis or loculation of the pleural space, e.g., with an empyema or a hemothorax (blood in the pleural space, often secondary to trauma), the fluid is drained with a catheter or a relatively large-bore tube inserted into the pleural space.

In other cases in which there are recurrent large effusions, especially due to malignancy, the fluid is drained with a large-bore tube, and an irritating agent (e.g., tetracycline) is instilled via the tube into the pleural space to induce inflammation and to cause the visceral and parietal pleural surfaces to become adherent. This process of sclerosis eliminates the pleural space and, if effective, prevents recurrence of pleural effusion on the side that the procedure was performed.

PNEUMOTHORAX

Air is not normally present between the visceral and parietal pleural surfaces. However, air can be introduced into the pleural space by a break in the surface of either pleural membrane, thus creating a *pneumothorax*. Since pressure within the pleural space is subatmospheric, air readily enters the space if there is any communication with air at atmospheric pressure.

Etiology and Pathogenesis

A pneumothorax can be due to a break in the parietal pleura (e.g., from trauma, needle or catheter insertion) or in the visceral pleura (e.g., from rupture of a subpleural air pocket, necrosis of lung adjacent to the pleura).

When a pneumothorax is created by the entry of air through the chest wall and the parietal pleura, the most common etiologies are (1) trauma (such as a knife or gunshot wound) and (2) introduction of air (either intentionally or unintentionally) via a needle or catheter inserted through the chest wall and into the pleural space. On the other hand, air may enter the pleura through a break in the visceral pleura, allowing communication between the airways or alveoli and the pleural space. Examples of the latter circumstance include rupture of a subpleural air pocket (such as a bleb, cyst, or bulla) into the pleural space, or necrosis of the lung adjacent to the pleura by a destructive pneumonia or neoplasm.

In some cases, a reason for the pneumothorax is apparent, i.e., one can identify an underlying abnormality in the lung or a form of lung disease known to be associated with subpleural air pockets (emphysema or interstitial lung disease with honeycombing and subpleural cysts) or destruction of lung tissue adjacent to the pleural surface (necrotizing pneumonia or neoplasm). Pneumothorax in these clinical settings is said to be secondary to the known lung disease.

In contrast, other patients do not have a defined abnormality of the lung adjacent to the pleura and are therefore said to have a *primary* or *spontaneous pneumothorax*. Even in this latter circumstance, there are frequently small subpleural pockets of air (blebs) that have gone unrecognized clinically and on routine radiographic examination. With a spontaneous pneumothorax, it is believed that air may dissect through the alveolar wall to interstitial tissue and along lobular septae to the subpleural surface. The resulting subpleural bleb ruptures (either soon thereafter or at a later time) into the pleural space, creating a pneumothorax. This pathogenesis may be important not only in patients without any known respiratory disease who develop a spontaneous pneumothorax, but also in patients with asthma who have a normal chest radiograph but then develop a "spontaneous" pneumothorax during the course of an acute asthmatic attack. In the asthmatic patient, air trapping and distension of alveoli promote tracking of air through tissue of the lung parenchyma and development of a "spontaneous" pneumothorax.

Patients who are receiving positive pressure to their tracheobronchial tree and alveoli, e.g., with mechanical ventilation, are also subject to development of a pneumothorax. In this case, as a result of positive pressure, a pre-existing subpleural bleb may rupture, or air may track from alveoli through tissue of the lung parenchyma to the subpleural region, as just described.

Pathophysiology

The pathophysiologic consequences of a pneumothorax are quite variable, ranging from none to the development of acute cardiovascular collapse. The size of the pneumothorax, i.e., the amount of air within the pleural space, is an important determinant of the clinical effects. Because the lung is enclosed within a relatively rigid chest wall, accumulation of a substantial amount of pleural air is accompanied by collapse of the underlying lung parenchyma. In extreme cases, air in the pleural space occupies almost the entire hemithorax, and the lung is totally collapsed and functionless until the air is resorbed or removed.

Air in the pleural space is generally under atmospheric or subatmospheric pressure. In some cases, the air may be under positive pressure, creating a *tension pneumothorax*. This tension within the pleural space is believed to occur as a result of a "check-valve" mechanism, by which air is free to enter the pleural space during inspiration, but the site of entry is closed during expiration. Therefore, only one-way movement of air into the pleural space is permitted, the intrapleural pressure increases, and the underlying lung collapses further. When pleural pressure is sufficiently high, the mediastinum and trachea may be shifted away from the side of the pneumothorax, but more importantly the positive pressure inhibits venous return to the superior and inferior venae cavae. As a result of decreased blood flow into the right atrium and ventricle, cardiac output and blood pressure fall, and emergency treatment is necessary to release the air under tension and reverse the cardiovascular collapse. A particularly important risk factor for the development of a tension pneumothorax is positive pressure ventilation with a mechanical ventilator. When a pneumothorax occurs in this situation, the ventilator may continue to introduce air under high pressure through the site of rupture in the visceral pleura.

For most cases of pneumothorax, once the site of entry into the pleural space is closed, the air is spontaneously resorbed. The reason is that the partial pressure of air in a pneumothorax is higher than the partial pressure of gas in surrounding venous or capillary blood. For example, air within the pleural space might have a pressure a few torr below atmospheric, or approximately 755 to 758 torr. In contrast, gas pressures in mixed venous blood are approximately as follows: $P_{O_2} = 40$ torr, $P_{CO_2} = 46$ torr, $P_{N_2} = 573$ torr, and $P_{H_2O} = 47$ torr. The total gas pressure in mixed venous blood is therefore 706 torr, which is approximately 50 torr below that of air in, the pleural space. Consequently, there is a gradient for diffusion of gas from the pleural space into mixed venous blood. With continued diffusion of gas in this direction, the size of the pneumothorax is slowly reduced, the gas pressures within the pleural space are maintained, and the gradient favoring absorption of gas continues until all the air is resorbed. Obviously, when a pneumothorax is causing significant clinical problems, the physician need not wait for spontaneous resorption of the air but can actively remove the air with a needle, catheter, or tube inserted into the pleural space.

Clinical Features

In many cases, the clinical setting is appropriate for the development of a pneumothorax, e.g., the patient may have predisposing underlying lung disease or may be receiving positive pressure ventilation with a mechanical ventilator. Interestingly, in the group of patients who develop a spontaneous pneumothorax, there is a striking predominance of males. In addition, the patients are often young adults and frequently are tall and thin.

Clinical features of pneumothorax:
Symptoms—chest pain, dyspnea
Physical signs—asymmetric (decreased) breath sounds, hyper-resonance, tracheal deviation (tension), ↓ blood pressure (tension)

The most common complaints at the time of pneumothorax are the acute onset of chest pain and/or dyspnea. However, some may be totally asymptomatic, particularly if the pneumothorax is small. On physical examination, the findings depend to a large extent on the size of the pneumothorax. Because of decreased transmission of sound, breath sounds and tactile fremitus are diminished or absent. With a significant amount of air in the pleural space, there may be increased resonance to percussion over the affected lung.

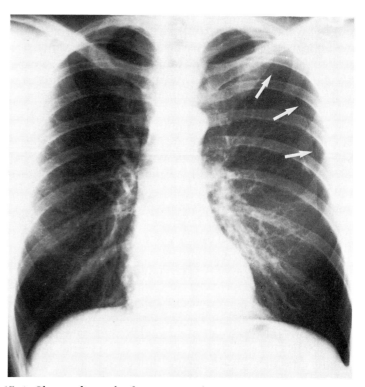

Figure 15–4. Chest radiograph of a patient with a spontaneous pneumothorax on the left. Arrows point to the visceral pleural surface of the lung. Beyond the visceral pleura is air within the pleural space; no lung markings can be seen in this region.

When the pneumothorax is under tension, the patient is often in acute distress, and a decrease in blood pressure or even frank cardiovascular collapse may be present. Palpation of the trachea frequently demonstrates deviation away from the side of the pneumothorax.

Diagnostic Approach

The diagnosis of pneumothorax is made or confirmed by chest roentgenogram. The characteristic finding is a curved line representing the edge of the lung (the visceral pleura) separated from the chest wall. Between the edge of the lung and the chest wall, the pleural space is lucent, and none of the normal vascular markings of the lung are seen in this region (Fig. 15–4 and 15–5). When the pneumothorax is small, separation of the visceral and parietal pleura appears only at the apex of the lung, where the pleural air generally accumulates first. If the pneumothorax is substantial, the lung loses a ·significant amount of volume and therefore has a greater density than usual.

When both fluid and air are present in the pleural space (*hydropneumothorax*), the fluid no longer appears as a meniscus tracking up along the lateral chest wall. Rather, the fluid falls to the most dependent part of the pleural space and appears as a liquid density with a perfectly horizontal upper border (Fig. 15–5). Finally, when gas in the pleural

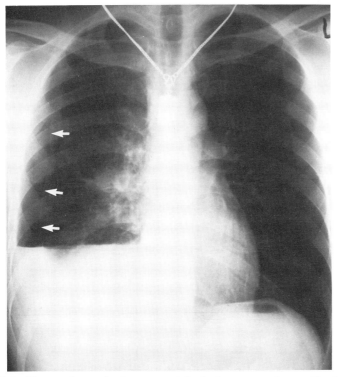

Figure 15–5. Chest radiograph showing a right hydropneumothorax. The horizontal line in the lower right hemithorax is the interface between air and liquid in the pleural space. Arrows point to the visceral pleura above the level of the effusion. There is air in the pleural space between the visceral pleura and the chest wall.

space is under tension, there is often evidence for structures (e.g., trachea and mediastinum) being "pushed" away from the side of the pneumothorax.

Treatment

The treatment of a pneumothorax is determined by its size as well as by the ensuing clinical consequences. With a small pneumothorax causing few symptoms, it is best to wait for spontaneous resolution of the pneumothorax. When the pneumothorax is large or the patient has significant clinical sequelae, the air is best removed, usually by a catheter or large-bore tube inserted into the pleural space. Occasionally, patients have recurrent spontaneous pneumothoraces, requiring obliteration of the pleural space by any one of a number of methods.

If a patient has hemodynamic compromise because of a tension pneumothorax, a needle, catheter, or tube must immediately be inserted to relieve the pressure. When this is performed, one can readily hear the sound of air under pressure escaping from the pleural space. The most important results of decompression are improvement in cardiac output and an increase in arterial blood pressure, since venous return is no longer compromised.

REFERENCES

General Reviews

Light, R. W.: Pleural Diseases. Philadelphia, Lea & Febiger, 1983.

Pleural Effusion

Black, L. F.: The pleural space and pleural fluid. Mayo Clin. Proc. 47:493–506, 1972.
Chernow, B., and Sahn, S. A.: Carcinomatous involvement of the pleura. Am. J. Med. 63:695–702, 1977.
Leff, A., Hopewell, P. C., and Costello, J.: Pleural effusion from malignancy. Ann. Intern. Med. 88:532–537, 1978.
Light, R. W.: Management of parapneumonic effusions. Arch. Intern. Med. 141:1339–1341, 1981.
Light, R. W.: Pleural effusions. Med. Clin. North Am. 61:1339–1352, 1977.
Light, R. W., MacGregor, M. I., Luchsinger, P. C., and Ball, W. C., Jr.: Pleural effusions: the diagnostic separation of transudates and exudates. Ann. Intern. Med. 77:507–513, 1972.
Lowell, J. R.: Pleural Effusions: A Comprehensive Review. Baltimore, University Park Press, 1977.
Wallach, H. W.: Intrapleural tetracycline for malignant pleural effusions. Chest 68:510–512, 1975.
Weese, W. C., Shindler, E. R., Smith, I. M., and Rabinovich, S.: Empyema of the thorax then and now. Arch. Intern. Med. 131:516–520, 1973.

Pneumothorax

Killen, D. A., and Gobbel, W. G., Jr.: Spontaneous Pneumothorax. Boston, Little, Brown, 1968.
Lichter, I., and Gwynne, J. F.: Spontaneous pneumothorax in young adults: a clinical and pathological study. Thorax 26:409–417, 1971.
Ruckley, C. V., and McCormack, R. J. M.: The management of spontaneous pneumothorax. Thorax 21:139–144, 1966.

Mediastinal Disease

The mediastinum is defined as the region of the thoracic cavity located between the two lungs. Included within the mediastinum are numerous structures, ranging from the heart and the great vessels (aorta, superior and inferior vena cava) to lymph nodes and nerves. The physician dealing with diseases of the lung is confronted with mediastinal disease in two major ways—either because of a chest radiograph demonstrating an abnormal mediastinum, or because of symptoms similar to those originating from primary pulmonary disease. In this chapter, we will obviously not attempt to cover all of the disorders affecting mediastinal structures, since diseases of the heart and great vessels lie in the realm of the cardiologist. Rather, we will first describe some of the anatomic features of the mediastinum and then proceed with a discussion of two of the most common clinical problems relating to the mediastinum—mediastinal masses and pneumomediastinum.

ANATOMIC FEATURES

The mediastinum is bounded superiorly by bony structures of the thoracic inlet and inferiorly by the diaphragm. Laterally, the mediastinal pleura on each side serves as a membrane separating the medial aspect of the lung (with its visceral pleura) from the structures contained within the mediastinum.

The mediastinum is most frequently divided into three anatomic regions – anterior, middle, and posterior (Table 16–1). This division is particularly useful for characterizing mediastinal masses, since specific etiologies often have a predilection for one particular compartment over the others. Normal structures located within or coursing through each of the compartments may serve as the origin of a mediastinal mass. Consequently, knowledge of the structures contained within each of the three regions is quite important for the clinician evaluating a patient with a mediastinal mass.

It is easiest to visualize the borders of the three mediastinal compartments on a lateral chest roentgenogram, as shown in Figure 16–1. The anterior compartment extends from the sternum to the anterior border of the pericardium. Included within this region are the thymus, lymph nodes, and loose connective tissue.

The borders of the middle mediastinum are the anterior and posterior pericardium. This region includes the heart, pericardium, and great vessels as well as the trachea, lymph nodes, and phrenic nerves. The upper portion of the vagus nerve also courses through the middle mediastinum.

Finally, the posterior mediastinum extends from the posterior pericardium to the vertebral column. This compartment normally includes the esophagus and descending aorta as well as the chain of sympathetic nerves and the lower portion of the vagus nerves. In addition, some lymph nodes and loose connective tissue may be found in this region.

Table 16–1. MEDIASTINAL COMPARTMENTS: ANATOMY AND PATHOLOGY

Compartment	Borders	Normal Structures	Masses
Anterior	Anterior—sternum Posterior—pericardium, ascending aorta, brachiocephalic vessels	Lymph nodes Connective tissue Thymus (remnant in adults)	Thymoma Germ cell neoplasm Carcinoma Lymphoma Thyroid enlargement (intrathoracic goiter)
Middle	Anterior—anterior pericardium, ascending aorta, brachiocephalic vessels Posterior—posterior pericardium	Pericardium Heart Vessels—ascending aorta, venae cavae, main pulmonary arteries Trachea Lymph nodes Nerves—phrenic, upper vagus	Carcinoma Lymphoma Pericardial cyst Bronchogenic cyst Benign lymph node enlargement (granulomatous disease)
Posterior	Anterior—posterior pericardium Posterior—vertebral column	Vessels—descending aorta Esophagus Nerves—sympathetic chain, lower vagus Lymph nodes Connective tissue	Neurogenic tumors Diaphragmatic hernias Lymphoma

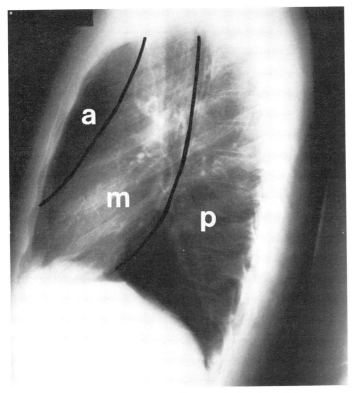

Figure 16–1. Lateral chest roentgenogram showing the borders of the three mediastinal compartments. a = anterior; m = middle; p = posterior.

MEDIASTINAL MASSES

Etiologies

Since there is a predilection for certain types of mediastinal masses to occur in specific mediastinal compartments, it is easiest to consider separately masses occurring in each of the three anatomic regions. However, it is important to remember that there is still a fair amount of overlap, i.e., many types of mediastinal masses are not exclusively limited to the compartment in which they most frequently are found. A summary of the types of mediastinal masses, arranged by anatomic compartment, can be found in Table 16–1.

Anterior Mediastinal Masses

The major types of anterior mediastinal mass are thymoma, germ cell tumor, carcinoma, lymphoma, and thyroid gland enlargement. Thymomas, or tumors of the thymus gland, are the most common type of neoplasm originating in the anterior compartment. They may be either benign or malignant in behavior, depending more on whether they are well encapsulated rather than on any particular histologic features. Thymomas are notable for their association with a variety of systemic syndromes. The best known and most common of these is

Myasthenia gravis is frequent in patients with thymoma.

myasthenia gravis, which is found in 10 to 50 percent of patients with thymic tumors. Myasthenia is characterized clinically by muscle weakness and pathophysiologically by a decreased number of acetylcholine receptors at neuromuscular junctions. The latter is frequently due to antibodies against the acetylcholine receptor.

Germ cell tumors are believed to originate from primitive germ cells that probably underwent abnormal migration during an early developmental period. Several types of germ cell tumors have been described. The most common of these is the teratoma, a tumor composed of ectodermal, mesodermal, and endodermal derivatives. The types of tissue seen are clearly foreign to the area from which the tumor arose and may include such elements as skin, hair, cartilage, and bone. As is true of thymomas, these tumors may be either benign or malignant in behavior, approximately 80 percent being described as benign. Other less common germ cell tumors that may arise in the mediastinum include seminomas and choriocarcinomas.

Carcinomas are another relatively frequent cause of a mediastinal mass. In many cases, the mediastinal involvement is secondary to a primary neoplasm found elsewhere, particularly in the lung. In occasional cases, no other tumor is apparent, and the patients are felt to have a primary carcinoma originating in the mediastinum. Carcinomatous involvement of the mediastinum is not limited to the anterior mediastinum but is also common in the middle mediastinal compartment.

Lymphoma may involve the mediastinum either as part of a disseminated process, in which the mediastinum is only one locus of the disease, or as a primary mediastinal mass without other clinically apparent tissue involvement. Hodgkin's disease, particularly the nodular sclerosis subtype, is well described as presenting solely with a mediastinal mass, though other forms of non-Hodgkin's lymphoma may also have a similar presentation. Like carcinoma, lymphoma involving the mediastinum is most common in either the anterior or middle mediastinal compartments.

Thyroid tissue may be the origin of a mediastinal mass, usually as a result of extension from thyroid tissue in the neck. Since these masses are generally not functional, the patients do not have clinical or laboratory evidence of hyperthyroidism. Only rarely do these masses of thyroid origin prove to be malignant.

There are a variety of less common neoplasms that may present in the anterior mediastinum, including parathyroid tumors and tumors of fatty or connective tissue origin. Given the infrequency of these tumors, they will not be discussed in this section.

Lymphoma and carcinoma commonly affect anterior or middle compartments; mediastinal disease may be isolated or part of more widespread involvement.

Middle Mediastinal Masses

In the middle mediastinum, carcinomas and lymphomas may be found, as we already mentioned in the discussion of anterior mediastinal masses. In addition, the middle mediastinum is frequently the location of benign cysts originating from structures found within this region. For example, fluid-filled pericardial or bronchogenic cysts originate from the pericardium and the tracheobronchial tree, respectively. However, these cysts are generally self-contained and usually do not directly communicate with either the pericardium or the airways.

Benign enlargement of lymph nodes in the middle mediastinum, often associated with enlarged hilar nodes, is commonly found in granulomatous diseases, particularly sarcoidosis and tuberculosis.

Posterior Mediastinal Masses

The posterior mediastinum is characteristically the location of tumors of neurogenic origin. These tumors may arise from a variety of nerve elements found in either peripheral nerves, the sympathetic nervous system chain, or paraganglionic tissue. Examples include neurilemmomas (arising from the sheath of Schwann), ganglioneuromas and neuroblastomas (respectively, benign and malignant lesions arising from the sympathetic nervous system), and pheochromocytomas. Diaphragmatic hernias, either congenital or acquired, are frequently posterior, with the herniated intra-abdominal organ appearing as a mediastinal mass.

Clinical Features

Almost half of the patients with a mediastinal mass have no symptoms, and the mass is first detected on an incidentally performed chest roentgenogram. In the other patients, symptoms are frequently chest pain, cough, and dyspnea. Occasionally, there may be evidence of esophageal or superior vena caval compression, giving rise to difficulty swallowing (dysphagia) or to facial and upper extremity edema due to impairment of venous return (superior vena cava syndrome). As we mentioned earlier, thymic tumors may present with muscle weakness characteristic of myasthenia gravis. Finally, a variety of systemic symptoms may be related to the presence of a lymphoma or other malignancy, or to hormone production by hormonally active mediastinal tumors.

Diagnostic Approach

The initial diagnostic test in almost all cases is the chest roentgenogram, which generally demonstrates the mass and allows determination of its location within the mediastinum (Fig. 16–2). Further characterization of the mass can be made by a variety of other techniques, but computed tomographic (CT) scanning has emerged as the most valuable of these. The CT scan is particularly useful for defining the cross-sectional appearance of the lesion, its density, and its relationship to other structures within the mediastinum.

CT scanning is useful in the evaluation of mediastinal masses.

However, the definitive diagnosis of the type of mediastinal mass rests with the examination of tissue by histopathologic techniques. Tissue is frequently obtained by either mediastinoscopy, in which a rigid scope is inserted into the mediastinum via an incision at the suprasternal notch, or by exploration of the mediastinum by a surgical approach that is anterior and adjacent to the sternum (parasternal mediastinotomy). In some patients, aspiration or biopsy of the mass by a needle inserted percutaneously may provide sufficient tissue to make a diagnosis. In many cases the patient has a more extensive procedure allowing biopsy and removal of the mass at the same time.

Techniques for biopsy of a mediastinal mass:
1. mediastinoscopy
2. parasternal mediastinotomy
3. percutaneous needle aspiration or biopsy

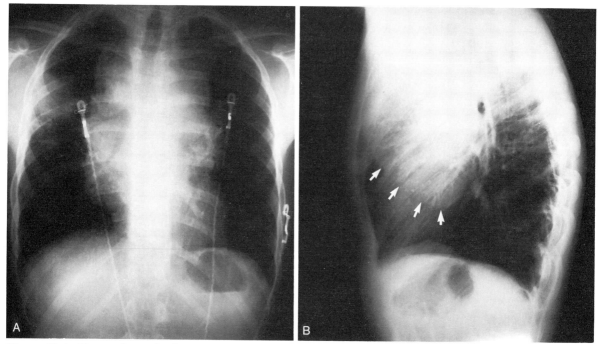

Figure 16–2. Chest radiograph of a patient with a large mediastinal mass. The mass, proven at surgery to be a germ cell tumor (seminoma), involves both anterior and middle mediastinal compartments. Posteroanterior (*A*) and lateral (*B*) views. Arrows outline the inferior border of the mass on the lateral view.

Treatment

Treatment of the various mediastinal masses depends to a large extent upon the nature of the lesion. In many cases, complete removal of the mass by surgery is the preferred procedure. Since benign lesions may enlarge and compress vital mediastinal structures, excision of the mass is frequently indicated. In addition, there may be complicating hemorrhage or infection of a benign lesion and eventually even malignant transformation of an initially benign tumor.

In the case of malignant tumors, treatment depends on the type of tumor and the presence or absence of invasion of other mediastinal structures. Since surgical removal of the malignant lesion is often not indicated or not possible, chemotherapy and radiotherapy are frequently the primary forms of treatment.

PNEUMOMEDIASTINUM

Normally, free air is not present within the mediastinum. When air enters the mediastinum for any of a number of reasons, a *pneumomediastinum* is said to be present.

Etiology and Pathogenesis

There are three major sources of air entry to the mediastinum: (1) through the skin and chest wall, as one commonly sees in the setting of penetrating trauma; (2) from a tear or defect in the esophagus or the trachea, allowing air to enter the mediastinum directly from either of these structures; and (3) from the alveoli. In the latter circumstance, an increase in intra-alveolar pressure may induce air entry into interstitial tissues of the alveolar wall. This interstitial air may then dissect alongside the wall of blood vessels coursing through the interstitium. Once air tracks back proximally, it may eventually enter the mediastinum at the site of origin of the vessels in the mediastinum.

Probably the most commonly occurring pathogenesis of pneumomediastinum is the one just described. In some cases, the reason for the increase in intra-alveolar pressure is obvious, e.g., severe coughing, vomiting, or straining. In patients receiving assisted ventilation with a mechanical ventilator, the positive pressure produced by the ventilator may initiate alveolar rupture and a pneumomediastinum. Asthmatics may also develop a pneumomediastinum, presumably related to the development of high intra-alveolar pressure behind an obstructed bronchus. In other circumstances, the immediate cause of the pneumomediastinum is not apparent, and the patient truly has a "spontaneous" pneumomediastinum.

Sources of air entry in pneumomediastinum:
1. external (penetrating trauma)
2. tracheal or esophageal tear
3. alveolar rupture and tracking of air proximally

Pathophysiology

With the accumulation of air in the mediastinum, we might expect an increase in pressure causing a decrease in venous return to the great veins with resulting cardiovascular compromise. However, when pressure builds up within the mediastinum, air usually dissects further along fascial planes into the neck, allowing release of the pressure and preventing disastrous cardiovascular complications. In addition, an increase in mediastinal pressure sometimes results in rupture of the mediastinal pleura and escape of air into the pleural space.

Once air has entered the soft tissues of the neck, the patient is said to have *subcutaneous emphysema.* If there is continued entry of air from the mediastinum into the neck, the air dissects further over soft tissues of the chest and abdominal walls to produce more extensive subcutaneous emphysema.

Because of the escape route available for mediastinal air and the opportunity for decompression, major cardiovascular complications are quite uncommon. The development of subcutaneous emphysema, though unsightly, is also usually without major clinical sequelae.

Mediastinal air often results in subcutaneous emphysema.

Clinical Features

At its onset, patients with a pneumomediastinum often experience relatively sudden substernal chest pain. There may also be dyspnea and rarely cardiovascular compromise and hypotension. In some cases, the patient is not symptomatic from the pneumomediastinum, and the problem is detected on chest radiograph, e.g., in a film obtained during the course of an asthmatic attack.

Physical examination may reveal a crunching or clicking sound synchronous with the heartbeat on cardiac auscultation. If the patient has subcutaneous emphysema associated with the pneumomediastinum, popping and crackling sounds (crepitations) may be both heard and felt when pressure is applied to the affected skin and subcutaneous tissue.

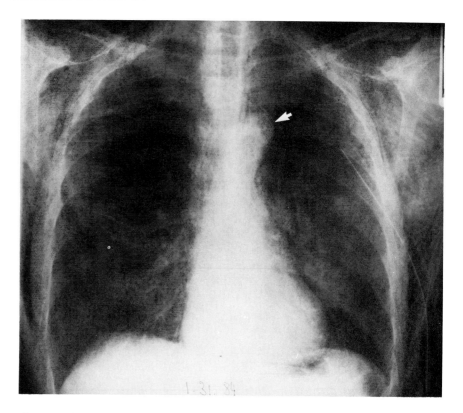

Figure 16–3. Chest radiograph demonstrating a pneumomediastinum and air in the subcutaneous tissues (subcutaneous emphysema). There are numerous radiolucent stripes outlining the mediastinal structures; these stripes represent air within the mediastinum. The arrow points to air around the aortic arch.

Diagnostic Approach

The chest radiograph is the most important study in documenting a pneumomediastinum. Gas may be seen within the mediastinal tissues and is usually visible as one or more radiolucent stripes alongside and parallel to the heart border or the aorta (Fig. 16–3).

Treatment

No treatment is generally necessary for pneumomediastinum, even when accompanied by subcutaneous emphysema. The air is usually resorbed spontaneously over a period of time. When pneumomediastinum is a consequence of tracheobronchial or esophageal rupture, surgery may be necessary for repair of the underlying tear. In the rare circumstance when pressure builds up within the mediastinum, an incision or tube may be necessary to allow escape of air from the mediastinum and release of the pressure.

REFERENCES

Crowe, J. K., Brown, L. R., and Muhm, J. R.: Computed tomography of the mediastinum. Radiology 128:75–87, 1978.

Hyson, E. A., and Ravin, C. E.: Radiographic features of mediastinal anatomy. Chest 75:609–613, 1979.

Maunder, R. J., Pierson, D. J., and Hudson, L. D.: Subcutaneous and mediastinal emphysema: pathophysiology, diagnosis, and management. Arch. Int. Med. 144:1447–1453, 1984.

McLoud, T. C., and Meyer, J.E.: Mediastinal metastases. Radiol. Clin. North Am. 20:453–468, 1982.

Silverman, N. A., and Sabiston, D. C., Jr.: Mediastinal masses. Surg. Clin. North Am. 60:757–777, 1980.

Anatomic and Physiologic Aspects of Neural, Muscular, and Chest Wall Interactions with the Lungs

Respiratory Control
　　Organization of Respiratory Control
　　　The Respiratory Generator
　　　Input from Other Regions of the CNS
　　　Chemoreceptors
　　　Input from Other Receptors
　　Ventilatory Responses to Hypercapnia and Hypoxia
　　Ventilatory Response to Other Stimuli
Respiratory Muscles

　　　The movement of gas into and out of the lungs requires the action of a pump that is capable of creating negative intrathoracic pressure, expanding the lungs, and initiating airflow with each inspiration. This pump-like action is provided by the respiratory muscles, including the diaphragm, working in conjunction with the chest wall. However, the muscles themselves do not have any rhythmic activity in the way that cardiac muscle does, and they must be driven by rhythmic impulses provided by a "controller."

　　　In this chapter, we will discuss anatomic and physiologic features of the controlling system and the respiratory muscles in order to provide background for the discussion in the subsequent two chapters. In those chapters, disorders affecting respiratory control, respiratory musculature, and the chest wall will be considered. Whereas much of the physiology and many of the clinical problems we will discuss here and in the next two chapters do not directly involve the lungs, they are so closely intertwined with respiratory function and dysfunction that they are appropriately considered in a textbook of pulmonary disease.

RESPIRATORY CONTROL

Though the process of breathing is a normal rhythmic activity that occurs without conscious effort, it involves an intricate controlling mechanism at the level of the central nervous system. The CNS transmits signals to the respiratory muscles, initiating inspiration approximately 12 to 20 times per minute. Remarkably, this controlling system is normally able to respond to varied needs of the individual, appropriately increasing ventilation during exercise and maintaining arterial blood gases within a narrow range.

In this section, we will first describe the structural organization of neural control of ventilation and then proceed to consider how various stimuli may interact with and adjust the output of the respiratory controller. Finally, we will briefly discuss the way in which the output of the controller can be quantified and how these techniques have proved useful in the evaluation of patients with a variety of clinical disorders.

Organization of Respiratory Control

The basic organization of the respiratory control system is outlined in Figure 17–1. Crucial to this system is the central nervous system "generator," from which signals originate that travel down the spinal cord to the various respiratory muscles. The inspiratory muscles, including the diaphragm and the external intercostal muscles, respond to the signals by contracting and initiating inspiration. This process will be described in more detail when we consider the muscles themselves later in this chapter.

As a result of inspiratory muscular contraction, the diaphragm descends, the chest wall expands, and air flows from the mouth through the tracheobronchial tree to the alveolar spaces. Gas exchange in the

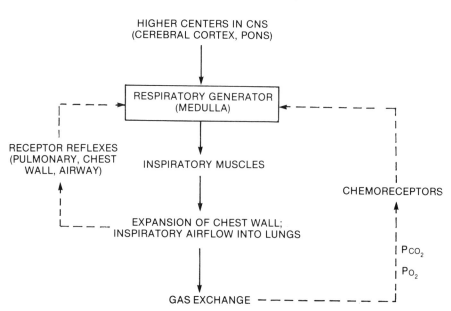

Figure 17–1. Schematic diagram depicting organization of the respiratory control system. The dotted lines show feedback loops affecting the respiratory generator.

distal parenchyma allows movement of O_2 into the blood and a corresponding release of CO_2.

Though this sequence of events sounds relatively straightforward, it is complicated by an intricate feedback system that adjusts or "fine tunes" the output of the generator to achieve the desired effect. If there is an inadequate response of the respiratory muscles to the generator's signal, as judged by a variety of respiratory "reflexes," then the generator increases its output to compensate for the lack of expected effect. If the arterial blood gases deviate from the desired level, then chemosensors for O_2 and CO_2 alter their input to the respiratory generator, ultimately affecting its output. Additionally, input from other regions of the central nervous system, particularly the cerebral cortex and the pons, can adjust the net output of the generator.

The Respiratory Generator

Considering the obvious importance of the respiratory generator in this scheme of respiratory control, it is of interest to define its anatomy and its mode of action in more detail. Much of the work clarifying the location of the respiratory generator involved animal experiments with transections at various levels of the central nervous system and assessment of the subsequent effects on ventilation. Since transection between the brain and brainstem does not significantly alter ventilation, the generator apparently resides somewhere at the level of the brainstem or lower and does not require interaction with higher cortical centers. When transections are made at various points within the brainstem, the breathing pattern is substantially altered, but ventilation is not eliminated. It is only when a transection is made between the medulla and the spinal cord that ventilation ceases, indicating that the respiratory generator resides within the medulla.

Although we have been referring to the respiratory center (or the generator) as a single region, it appears that more than one network of neurons within the medulla is involved in initiating and coordinating respiratory activity. According to a widely held model, one group of neurons is responsible for initiating inspiration and regulating its speed as a result of the intensity of neuronal activity. Another group of neurons controls the "switching off" of inspiration and hence determines the onset of expiration.

A central respiratory generator within the medulla controls activity of the respiratory muscles.

Therefore, we may distinguish two aspects of ventilatory control—the degree of inspiratory drive or central inspiratory activity, which regulates the inspiratory flow rate, and the timing mechanism, which controls the termination of inspiration. These two determining factors act in concert to set the respiratory rate and tidal volume, and thus the minute ventilation and the specific pattern of breathing.

Input from Other Regions of the CNS

Even though the medullary respiratory center does not require additional input to drive ventilation, it does receive other information that contributes to a regular pattern of breathing and to more precise ventilatory control. For example, input from the pons appears to be necessary for a normal, coordinated breathing pattern. When the influence of the <u>pons</u> is lost, irregularities in the breathing pattern ensue.

In addition to pathways involved in the "automatic" or involuntary control of ventilation, the cerebral cortex exerts a conscious or voluntary control over ventilation. Interestingly, the automatic control of ventilation may be disturbed while conscious control remains intact. In these cases, during wakefulness the cerebral cortex exerts sufficient voluntary control over ventilation to maintain normal arterial blood gases. During periods when the patient is dependent upon automatic ventilatory control, e.g., during sleep, marked hypoventilation or apnea may occur. This rare condition has been termed *Ondine's curse* after a mythological tale in which the suitor of Neptune's daughter was cursed to lose automatic control over all bodily functions.

Chemoreceptors

As shown in Figure 17–1, maintenance of arterial blood gases is the final goal of ventilatory control, and an important feedback loop exists to adjust respiratory center output if blood gases are not maintained at the desired level. Elevation of the P_{CO_2} (hypercapnia) and depression of the P_{O_2} (hypoxemia) are both capable of stimulating ventilation. In each case, one or more chemoreceptors "sense" alterations in P_{CO_2} or P_{O_2} and accordingly vary their input to the medullary respiratory center.

Changes in P_{CO_2} are sensed primarily at a central chemoreceptor in the medulla.

The primary sensor for CO_2 is located near the ventrolateral surface of the medulla and is called the *central chemoreceptor*. Even though it is located in the medulla, the central chemoreceptor is clearly separate from the medullary respiratory center and should not be confused with it. The central chemoreceptor actually does not appear to respond directly to blood P_{CO_2} but rather to the pH of the extracellular fluid (ECF) surrounding the chemoreceptor. The pH, in turn, is determined by the level of bicarbonate ion as well as P_{CO_2}. The feedback loop for CO_2 can be summarized as follows:

Increased arterial blood P_{CO_2} → increased brain ECF P_{CO_2} → decreased brain ECF pH → decreased pH at central chemoreceptor → stimulation of central chemoreceptor → stimulation of medullary respiratory center → increased ventilation → decreased arterial blood P_{CO_2}.

The primary sensors for O_2 are not located in the central nervous system but rather in two *peripheral chemoreceptors*, called the carotid body and aortic body chemoreceptors. The carotid chemoreceptors, which are quantitatively much more important than aortic chemoreceptors, are located just beyond the bifurcation of each common carotid artery into internal and external branches. The aortic chemoreceptor, on the other hand, is found between the pulmonary artery and the arch of the aorta.

The major sensors for P_{O_2} are the peripheral (carotid and aortic body) chemoreceptors.

These chemoreceptors are sensitive to changes in P_{O_2}, with hypoxia stimulating chemoreceptor discharge. The peripheral chemoreceptors also have a minor role in sensing P_{CO_2}, but they are clearly much less important for this purpose than the central chemoreceptors. Peripheral chemoreceptor discharge is transmitted back to the central nervous system by cranial nerves—the glossopharyngeal in the case of the

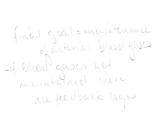

carotid bodies and the vagus nerve for the aortic bodies. The information is ultimately transmitted to the medullary respiratory center, so that its output is augmented as a result of hypoxemia.

Input from Other Receptors

In addition to chemoreceptor effects, we must consider input that originates from receptors in the lung (including the airways) and is carried via the vagus nerve to the central nervous system. Stretch receptors, located within the smooth muscle of airway walls, respond to changes in lung inflation; as the lung is inflated, receptor discharge increases. In animals, this stretch receptor reflex (known as the Hering-Breuer reflex) is responsible for apnea that occurs as a result of lung inflation. In contrast, conscious human adults do not readily demonstrate the Hering-Breuer reflex, and the role of the stretch receptors in ventilatory control is not entirely clear. Presumably, they contribute to the "switching off" of inspiration, i.e., initiation of expiration, after a critical level of inspiratory inflation has been reached.

Irritant receptors, located superficially along the lining of airways, may also initiate tachypnea, usually in response to some noxious stimulus, such as a chemical or irritating dust. Juxtacapillary or J receptors are found within the pulmonary interstitium, adjacent to capillaries. One of their effects is to cause tachypnea, and they may be responsible for the respiratory stimulation caused by inflammatory processes or accumulation of fluid within the pulmonary interstitium.

Finally, receptors in the chest wall, particularly in the intercostal muscles, appear to play a role in the fine tuning of ventilation. The muscle spindles are part of a reflex arc that adjusts the output of respiratory muscles if the desired degree of muscular work has not been achieved.

Ventilatory Responses to Hypercapnia and Hypoxia

Two of the stimuli for ventilation that have been best studied are well-defined chemical ones, hypercapnia and hypoxia. As we mentioned above, hypercapnia is sensed primarily (but not exclusively) by the central chemoreceptor, and the actual stimulus appears to be the pH of brain extracellular fluid. In contrast, hypoxia stimulates ventilation by acting upon peripheral chemoreceptors, carotid much more than aortic.

When arterial P_{O_2} is held constant, ventilation increases in adults by approximately 3 L per min for each mm Hg rise in arterial P_{CO_2}. This relatively linear response, the magnitude of which varies considerably among individuals, is shown in Figure 17–2. It can also be appreciated from Figure 17–2 that the response to increments in P_{CO_2} also depends upon the P_{O_2}; at a lower P_{O_2}, the response to hypercapnia is heightened.

With chronic hypercapnia, the ventilatory response to further increases in P_{CO_2} is diminished. The reason that CO_2 responsiveness is blunted is relatively straightforward. When CO_2 retention persists over days, the kidneys excrete less bicarbonate, and plasma and tissue

Ventilatory responsiveness to CO_2 is blunted in patients with chronic hypercapnia.

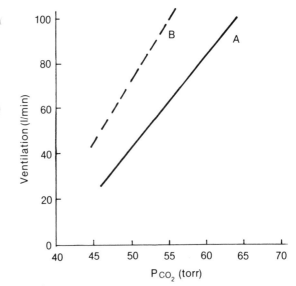

Figure 17-2. Ventilatory response to progressive elevation of P_{CO_2} in a normal individual. The solid line (A) shows the response when the simultaneous P_{O_2} is high (hyperoxic conditions); the dotted line (B) shows the heightened response when simultaneous P_{O_2} is low (hypoxic conditions).

bicarbonate levels rise. The elevated bicarbonate can then buffer more successfully any acute changes in P_{CO_2}, so that brain ECF pH changes less for any given increment in P_{CO_2}.

With hypoxemia, there is not the same linear relationship between alterations in partial pressure and ventilation. Rather, the ventilatory response is relatively small until the P_{O_2} falls to approximately 60 torr,

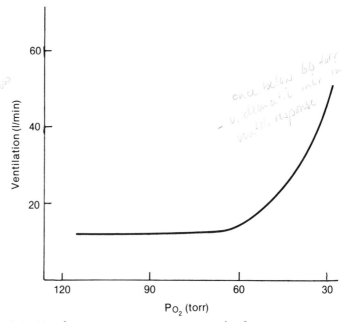

Figure 17-3. Ventilatory response to progressively decreasing P_{O_2} in a normal individual (with P_{CO_2} kept constant). Ventilation does not rise significantly until the P_{O_2} falls to approximately 60 torr.

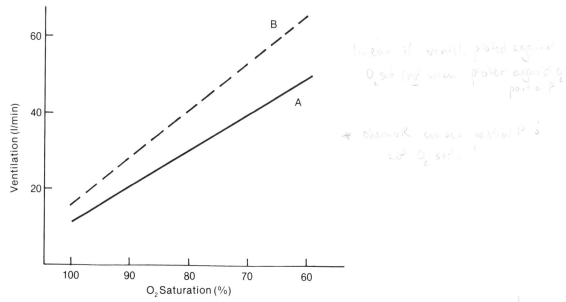

Figure 17–4. Ventilatory response to hypoxia, plotted using O_2 saturation rather than PO_2. The relationship between ventilation and O_2 saturation during progressive hypoxia is linear. The solid line (A) shows the response when measured at a normal PCO_2; the dotted line (B) shows the augmented response at an elevated PCO_2.

below which ventilatory increases are much more dramatic (Fig. 17–3). The curvilinear relationship between PO_2 and ventilation can be made linear if ventilation is plotted against O_2 saturation instead of partial pressure (Fig. 17–4). However, despite the linear relationship between ventilation and O_2 saturation, it is actually the partial pressure of O_2, not the content or saturation, that is sensed by the chemoreceptor.

The PCO_2 also has an effect on a subject's response to hypoxia. The sensitivity to hypoxia is increased as the PCO_2 is raised, or decreased as the PCO_2 is lowered (Fig. 17–4). This feature is important to consider when testing for responsiveness to hypoxia. As the subject hyperventilates in response to a low PO_2, the PCO_2 drops, and ventilation is stimulated less than it would be if the PCO_2 were unchanged. Therefore, the PCO_2 is best kept constant, so that the conditions for testing are actually "isocapnic" hypoxia.

When the clinician suspects a disorder of ventilatory control, quantitation of the ventilatory response to hypercapnia or hypoxia may be performed. However, there is a wide range of responses to these stimuli even in seemingly normal individuals. This fact must obviously be taken into account when ventilatory response data are interpreted.

Ventilatory Response to Other Stimuli

One of the most important times for a rapid and appropriate increase in ventilation is in response to a change in metabolic requirements. For example, with the metabolic needs of exercise, a normal individual can increase ventilation from a resting value of 5 L per min to 60 L per min or more, without any demonstrable change in arterial blood gases. According to one popular theory, the initial rapid increase in ventilation at the onset of exercise is due to a neural stimulus, though the origin is not clear. After the initial rapid augmentation in ventilation, there is a later and slower rise that is probably due to a blood-borne chemical stimulus. However, there are many unanswered questions about the remarkably appropriate way that ventilation is capable of responding to the demands of exercise.

Another important ventilatory response is that to alterations in acid-base status. With excess metabolic acid production, i.e., metabolic acidosis, ventilation increases as the pH is lowered, and the elimination of additional CO_2 aids in returning the pH toward normal. However, the mechanism of this ventilatory response has not been agreed upon. Chemoreceptors appear to be important, but there is debate about the relative contributions of peripheral and central chemoreceptors to the ventilatory response.

RESPIRATORY MUSCLES

The purpose of signals emanating from the respiratory generator is to initiate inspiratory muscle activity. Though the primary inspiratory muscle is clearly the diaphragm, other muscle groups contribute to optimal movement of the chest wall under a variety of conditions and needs. Notable among these other inspiratory muscle groups are the external intercostals and the accessory muscles, including sternocleidomastoid, trapezius, and scalene muscles. However, we must also not forget that there are additional muscles whose activity aids in coordinating upper airway activity during inspiration. Proper functioning of these muscles maintains patency of the upper airway, whereas dysfunction may be important in the pathogenesis of certain clinical disorders associated with upper airway obstruction.

During inspiration, contraction of the diaphragm and shortening of its muscle fibers are known to occur. Since each hemidiaphragm is a dome-shaped sheet of muscle attached at the midline and at the lateral chest wall, contraction acts to flatten out the upward-directed dome and to cause descent of the diaphragm (Fig. 17–5). In addition, the manner in which the diaphragm is inserted onto the lateral ribs and the orientation of the muscle fibers of the diaphragm cause the lower rib cage to be elevated (and thus expanded) with inspiratory contraction. Therefore, when the diaphragm contracts, abdominal contents are pushed downward (increasing intra-abdominal pressure), the chest wall expands, intrathoracic pressure is lowered, and air flows into the lungs. With normal resting breathing, the most apparent inspiratory motion is the outward movement of the abdomen, resulting from diaphragmatic descent and increased abdominal pressure.

The external intercostals appear to aid inspiration somewhat by increasing the anteroposterior diameter of the thorax, but their overall contribution to inspiration is much less than that of the diaphragm. Accessory muscle groups are generally not used for resting breathing in normal individuals, but they may substantially contribute to inspiratory muscle activity in the face of high work loads (particularly in

The diaphragm is the major muscle of inspiration; the less important external intercostals and accessory muscles may increase their role in disease states.

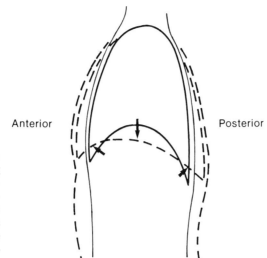

Figure 17–5. Diaphragmatic motion during breathing. In going from expiration (solid lines) to inspiration (dotted lines), the diaphragm contracts and becomes flatter, while the chest wall is lifted upward. The arrows indicate the direction of diaphragmatic motion during contraction.

disease states). External intercostals and accessory muscles may also be important in "stabilizing" the chest wall during inspiration and allowing diaphragmatic contraction to result in maximal intrathoracic pressure and volume changes.

An important determinant of the efficacy of diaphragmatic contraction is the initial shape and length of the diaphragm. For any muscle, the strength of contraction is decreased when its initial length is less, and the diaphragm is no exception. Therefore, at high lung volumes, the diaphragm is lower and foreshortened before its active contraction, so that the strength of contraction is diminished. Additionally, the radius of curvature affects the amount of pressure generated by muscular contraction. According to the Laplace relationship, the pressure generated for a given contractile tension is inversely proportional to the radius of curvature. At high lung volumes, the diaphragm is flatter, the radius of curvature is greater, and the effective pressure generated is therefore again diminished. The importance of these factors will become apparent in our discussion of diaphragmatic function in obstructive lung disease, in which resting lung volume may be abnormally high.

The effectiveness of diaphragmatic contraction is decreased at high resting lung volumes, when the diaphragm is flatter and shorter.

In contrast to inspiration, expiration is a relatively passive process whereby the lung and chest wall return to the resting position. However, when breathing is deep and forceful, or when there is increased airways resistance during expiration, the action of expiratory muscles may be important in aiding expiratory airflow. In particular, abdominal muscles (rectus and transverse abdominis, internal and external obliques) and internal intercostals are important in this role.

In summary, the normal operation of the respiratory apparatus depends upon a signal generated by the respiratory center and eventually translated into an efficient pattern of respiratory muscle contraction. Though feedback and control systems insure the optimal functioning of this system, this finely coordinated mechanism may fail in numerous ways. It will be the goal of Chapters 18 and 19 to examine clinically important dysfunction occurring at various levels of this complex system.

REFERENCES

Respiratory Control

Berger, A. J., Mitchell, R. A., and Severinghaus, J. W.: Regulation of respiration. N. Engl. J. Med. 297:92–97; 138–143; 194–201, 1977.

Cherniack, N. S.: The clinical assessment of the chemical regulation of ventilation. Chest 70:274–281, 1976.

Cherniack, N. S., Nochomovitz, M. L., and Altose, M. D.: Disorders of respiratory control. *In* Simmons, D. H. (ed.): Current Pulmonology. Vol. 4. New York, John Wiley & Sons, 1982, pp. 189–214.

Hedemark, L. L., and Kronenberg, R. S.: Chemical regulation of respiration. Chest 82:488–494, 1982.

Lopata, M., and Lourenco, R. V.: Evaluation of respiratory control. Clin. Chest Med. 1:33–45, 1980.

Mitchell, R. A.: Neural regulation of respiration. Clin. Chest Med. 1:3–12, 1980.

Mitchell, R. A., and Berger, A. J.: Neural regulation of respiration. Am. Rev. Respir. Dis. 111:206–224, 1975.

Respiratory Muscles

Derenne, J-P., Macklem, P. T., and Roussos, C.: The respiratory muscles: mechanics, control, and pathophysiology. Am. Rev. Respir. Dis. 118:119–133; 373–390; 581–601, 1978.

Guenter, C. A., and Whitelaw, W. A.: The role of diaphragm function in disease. Arch. Intern. Med. 139:806–808, 1979.

International Symposium on the Diaphragm. Am. Rev. Respir. Dis. 119 (Part 2 supplement):1–181, 1979.

Macklem, P. T.: Respiratory muscles: the vital pump. Chest 78:753–758, 1980.

Roussos, C., and Macklem, P. T.: The respiratory muscles. N. Engl. J. Med. 307:786–797, 1982.

Disorders of Ventilatory Control

The finely tuned system of ventilatory control described in the last chapter is altered in a variety of clinical circumstances. In some cases, a primary disorder of the nervous system may affect the neurologic network involved in ventilatory control and may therefore diminish the "drive" to breathe. In other instances, the controlling system undergoes a process of adaptation in response to primary lung disease and any alteration in function is therefore a secondary phenomenon.

In this chapter, we will consider both primary and secondary disturbances in ventilatory control. Of the secondary disorders, the one most commonly seen is that associated with chronic obstructive pulmonary disease, and we will therefore limit the discussion of secondary disorders of ventilatory control to this entity. We will also mention a common disturbance in the pattern of breathing, termed Cheyne-Stokes breathing, and will briefly discuss its pathogenesis. Finally, we will discuss ventilatory disorders associated with sleep, since a problem with ventilatory control may be crucial in the pathogenesis of sleep-related respiratory dysfunction.

PRIMARY NEUROLOGIC DISEASE

Several diseases of the nervous system alter ventilation, apparently by affecting regions involved in ventilatory control. However, the results are variable, depending on the particular type of disorder and region involved. In some cases, hyperventilation is prominent, whereas in others associated hypoventilation is significant. In a third category, the most apparent change is in the pattern of breathing.

Presentation with Hyperventilation

Many acute disorders of the central nervous system are associated with hyperventilation.

With certain acute disorders of the central nervous system, hyperventilation (i.e., decreased PCO_2 and respiratory alkalosis) is relatively common. Acute infections (meningitis or encephalitis), strokes, and trauma affecting the central nervous system are notable examples. The exact mechanism of hyperventilation in these situations is not known with certainty.

Presentation with Hypoventilation

At the other extreme, some patients present with hypoventilation, presumably resulting from a primary insult to the nervous system that affects centers involved with control of breathing. In such circumstances, patients have an elevated PCO_2, but since the clinical problems are generally not acute ones, the pH has returned toward normal as a result of renal compensation, i.e., retention of bicarbonate. When no specific etiology or prior event can be found to explain the hypoventilation, the patient is said to have *idiopathic hypoventilation* or *primary alveolar hypoventilation*. Other patients have had a significant insult to the nervous system at some time in the past, such as encephalitis, and chronic hypoventilation is presumably a sequela of the past event.

Patients with these syndromes of hypoventilation are characterized by depressed ventilatory responses to the chemical stimuli of hypercapnia and hypoxia. Measurement of arterial blood gases generally reveals an elevation in arterial PCO_2 accompanied by a decrease in PO_2, the latter being primarily due to hypoventilation. As in other disorders associated with these blood gas abnormalities, cor pulmonale may result and may be the manner in which patients with these syndromes present. The term *Ondine's curse*, which we mentioned in Chapter 17, has often been applied to many such patients with alveolar hypoventilation—specifically when automatic control of ventilation is impaired, but voluntary control remains intact.

Treatment of alveolar hypoventilation due to depressed central respiratory drive:
1. pharmacologic (e.g., progesterone)
2. electrical stimulation of phrenic nerve
3. assisted ventilation

Treatment of alveolar hypoventilation has generally centered around two modalities, either drugs (most commonly the hormone progesterone) or electrical stimulation of the phrenic nerve. Progesterone is well known to be a respiratory stimulant and in some cases may improve respiratory drive and decrease CO_2 retention. As another approach, the diaphragm may be induced to contract by repetitive electrical stimulation of the phrenic nerve, which can be achieved by intermittent current applied to an implanted electrode. An alternative to these two modes of therapy involves assisting ventilation, especially at night, with any of several assist devices. These provide either positive pressure to the airway or negative pressure around the chest, thus augmenting minute ventilation without altering the patient's own respiratory drive.

Abnormal Patterns of Breathing

Besides disturbances in overall alveolar ventilation, patients with neurologic disease may demonstrate abnormal patterns of breathing. The term *ataxic breathing* is applied to a grossly irregular breathing pattern observed with certain lesions in the medulla that presumably separate the medullary respiratory center from higher brainstem control sites normally having input into the medulla. In contrast, certain lesions in the pons result in a breathing pattern characterized by a prolonged inspiratory pause; this pattern is termed *apneustic breathing*.

Another type of abnormal breathing pattern is termed *Cheyne-Stokes breathing*. Unlike the other patterns mentioned above, Cheyne-Stokes breathing is quite common and warrants a special section to describe it and discuss what is known about its pathogenesis.

CHEYNE-STOKES BREATHING

Cheyne-Stokes breathing is the term applied to a pattern of cyclic breathing in which periods of gradually increasing ventilation alternate with periods of gradually decreasing ventilation (even to the point of apnea). This type of ventilation is schematized in Figure 18–1. It has been known for many years that two main types of disorders are associated with this type of breathing—congestive heart failure and some forms of central nervous system disease. How these two etiologic factors give rise to this pattern of breathing has been a subject of great interest.

Central to the pathogenesis of Cheyne-Stokes ventilation is a defect in the feedback nature of ventilatory control. Normally, the controlling system is able to adjust its output to compensate for arterial blood gases that differ from the ideal or desired state. For example, with an elevated arterial P_{CO_2}, the central chemoreceptor signals the medullary respiratory center to increase its output in order to augment ventilation and restore P_{CO_2} to normal. Similarly, the peripheral chemoreceptor responds to hypoxemia by increasing its output, signal-

Common etiologies of Cheyne-Stokes ventilation are congestive heart failure and some forms of central nervous system disease.

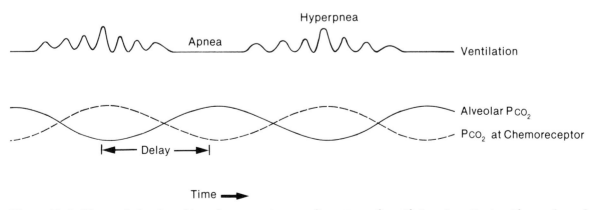

Figure 18–1. Cheyne-Stokes breathing, demonstrating a cyclic pattern of ventilation. In patients with a prolonged circulation time, the delay between the signal to the chemoreceptor (P_{CO_2} at the chemoreceptor) and ventilatory output (reflected by alveolar P_{CO_2}) is shown.

ing the medullary respiratory center to augment ventilation and restore P_{O_2} to normal.

However, there are times when this feedback system may fail and actually "backfire," especially if there is a delayed response to the signal or if it responds more than necessary and overshoots the mark. This defect in the feedback process appears to be at work in Cheyne-Stokes breathing. We will touch upon a few aspects of recent theories proposed to explain Cheyne-Stokes ventilation, but for further discussion the interested reader is referred to references at the end of this chapter.

In the case of congestive heart failure, it has generally been proposed that a prolonged circulation time results in an abnormal delay between events in the lung and the sensing of P_{CO_2} changes by the central chemoreceptor. Hence, medullary respiratory output is out of phase with gas exchange at the lungs, and oscillations in ventilation occur as the central chemoreceptor and the medullary respiratory center make belated attempts to maintain a stable P_{CO_2} (see Fig. 18–1).

With central nervous system disease leading to Cheyne-Stokes ventilation, it has been proposed that a heightened dependence on hypoxic (as opposed to hypercapnic) chemosensitivity leads to an "instability" of respiratory control. Unlike the situation with hypercapnia, in which there is a relatively linear response of ventilation to changes in arterial P_{CO_2}, the response to hypoxia is alinear. Hence, for the same drop in P_{O_2}, the increment in ventilation is larger at a lower absolute P_{O_2} (see Fig. 17–3). At a relatively high initial P_{O_2}, the system is likely not to respond to small changes in P_{O_2} but is then apt to overshoot as the P_{O_2} falls further. This instability of the respiratory control system results in a widely oscillating output from the respiratory center and thus in the observed cyclic pattern of ventilation.

CONTROL ABNORMALITIES SECONDARY TO LUNG DISEASE

Ventilatory control mechanisms often respond to various forms of primary lung disease by altering respiratory center output. Either stimulation of peripheral chemoreceptors by hypoxemia or stimulation of receptors by diseases affecting the pulmonary interstitium can induce the respiratory center to increase its output, resulting in a respiratory alkalosis. On the other hand, many patients with chronic obstructive lung disease are found to have CO_2 retention, implying that the ventilatory control mechanism is reset to operate at a higher setpoint for P_{CO_2}. In this discussion, we will focus on the latter circumstance, since ventilatory control abnormalities are of particular clinical importance in the setting of chronic obstructive lung disease.

As we mentioned in Chapter 6, some patients with COPD (Type A pathophysiology) do not generally demonstrate CO_2 retention, whereas others (Type B) are often characterized by hypercapnia. When responsiveness to increased levels of P_{CO_2} is measured in the hypercapnic patients, it is apparent that their ventilatory response is diminished. However, these patients with chronic, compensated respiratory acidosis have higher levels of plasma (as well as CSF) bicarbonate because of bicarbonate retention by the kidneys. Therefore, for any increment in P_{CO_2}, the effect on pH at the medullary chemoreceptor is attenuated by the increased buffering capacity available. A "chicken and egg" question then becomes important: Is the CO_2 retention secondary to an underlying ventilatory control abnormality in these patients, or is the diminution in ventilatory sensitivity merely secondary to chronic CO_2 retention? Though this question remains unanswered, there is some evidence to suggest that familial factors may be important, and that patients with lower respiratory sensitivity (on a genetic basis) may be the ones more likely to develop CO_2 retention.

Whatever the answer to this question, there is a clinically important corollary to this depression in CO_2 sensitivity, irrespective of the cause of CO_2 retention. When oxygen is administered to the chronically hypoxemic and hypercapnic patient, the P_{CO_2} may rise even further. At the extreme, if very high levels of inspired oxygen are administered, substantial depression in ventilation may result, to the point of life-threatening CO_2 retention. This phenomenon is frequently ascribed to loss of sensitivity to CO_2 as a ventilatory stimulus, resulting from chronic CO_2 retention. Such patients are therefore thought to be primarily dependent on hypoxic drive as a ventilatory stimulus; when this stimulus is removed after administration of high levels of inspired oxygen, patients hypoventilate and may even become apneic.

Administration of O_2 to the chronically hypoxemic and hypercapnic patient may elevate P_{CO_2}.

However, it appears that this phenomenon is actually more complicated, since the degree of further CO_2 retention does not necessarily correlate with the depression in minute ventilation. It is now thought that other factors, including alteration in the pattern of breathing and in ventilation-perfusion relationships as a result of oxygen administration, may also contribute to this well-recognized clinical phenomenon.

SLEEP APNEA SYNDROME

As the final topic in this chapter, we will consider a relatively recently recognized disorder of respiration during sleep, the *sleep apnea syndrome*. Though the fundamental cause of this syndrome remains unknown, it is generally presumed to represent a disorder of ventilatory control, specifically control of upper airway muscles.

In the sleep apnea syndrome, patients have repetitive periods of apnea, i.e., cessation of breathing, occurring during sleep. A period of more than 10 seconds without airflow is generally considered to constitute an apneic episode, and patients with this syndrome often have hundreds of such episodes during the course of a night's sleep.

Types

Sleep apnea syndrome is commonly divided into several types—obstructive, central, and mixed—depending on the nature of the episodes. In obstructive apnea, the drive to breathe is still present during the apneic episode, but transient obstruction of the upper airway prevents inspiratory airflow. Inspiratory muscles are active during obstructive apnea; however, their attempts at initiating airflow are to no avail. In central apnea, there is no drive to breathe during

Categories of sleep apnea syndrome:
1. obstructive
2. central
3. mixed

the apneic period, i.e., no signal from the respiratory center to initiate inspiration. Hence, no respiratory muscle activity can be observed when airflow ceases. Frequently, patients have episodes of both obstructive and central apnea and thus are said to have a mixed picture. Since clinically significant episodes of obstructive apnea are more frequent than those of central apnea, we will focus on the pathophysiology, clinical features, complications, and treatment of obstructive apnea.

Clinical Features

Clinically, patients with sleep apnea syndrome may present because of (1) symptoms or signs that they (or a sleep partner) have noticed during the course of a night's sleep; (2) daytime symptoms; or (3) complications that arise from the repetitive apneic episodes. During sleep, patients with episodes of obstructive apnea are often noted to have a markedly deranged sleep pattern. Loud snoring is particularly prominent, and patients may often have obvious snorting and agitation as a result of trying to breathe against the obstructed airway. They may have violent movements during periods of obstruction; not uncommonly, the sleep partner complains of being hit or injured as a result of these violent movements. Upon awakening, patients often complain of a severe headache, presumably related to the derangements in gas exchange that occur during the apneic episodes.

With such a disordered pattern of sleep, it is not surprising that patients may be overly somnolent during the normal waking hours. It has been presumed that effective sleep deprivation is the main reason for the patient's hypersomnolence. However, a possible contributory role for an underlying central nervous system disorder is difficult to rule out. The degree of somnolence in these patients can be debilitating; patients commonly fall asleep while driving, eating, working, or doing a variety of other usual daytime activities. Patients are also often considered to have a personality disorder, partially because of their extreme hypersomnolence and partially because of psychologic changes that have presumably resulted from their disease.

Clinical features of sleep apnea syndrome:
1. disordered respiration during sleep
2. daytime hypersomnolence
3. cardiovascular complications

Secondary complications that ensue are primarily cardiovascular. During the episodes of apnea, patients frequently have a variety of cardiac arrhythmias or conduction disturbances, occasionally of life-threatening proportions. As a result of episodes of prolonged hypoxemia at night, pulmonary hypertension may result, and patients may even present with unexplained cor pulmonale. Systemic hypertension is also not an infrequent accompaniment of the disorder.

Pathophysiology

The pathophysiology of obstruction in sleep apnea syndrome has been only partially explained. The site of upper airway obstruction in most cases appears to be the oropharynx. The obstruction results from the loss of tone of pharyngeal muscles or the muscles that normally cause the tongue to protrude forward from the posterior pharyngeal wall (the genioglossus muscles). Obstruction is more likely to be a problem in patients who are obese (with short, fat necks) or in those with a small jaw (micrognathia) or a large tongue. However, many patients do not have any of these risk factors, and there are now data to suggest that familial factors may also be involved. Perhaps the automatic control of these upper airway muscles is abnormal during sleep, resulting in loss of tone and subsequent airway obstruction.

During an episode of central apnea, monitoring of chest wall motion reveals no movement, corresponding to cessation of airflow and a fall in oxygen saturation (Fig. 18–2A). With obstructive apnea, chest wall and abdominal movement can be detected during a fruitless attempt to move air through the obstructed airway. Airflow measured simultaneously is found to be absent (i.e., tidal volume = 0), and the

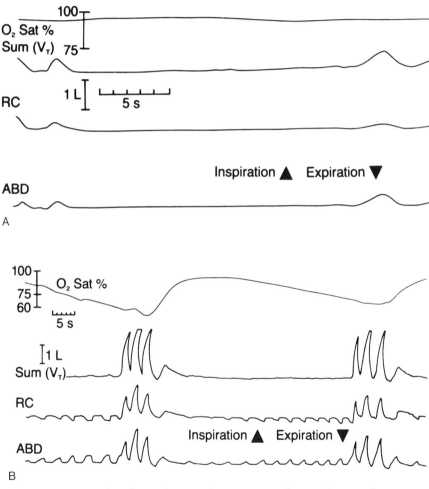

Figure 18–2. Examples of recordings in sleep apnea syndrome, showing O_2 saturation (O_2 Sat), rib cage (RC) and abdominal (ABD) movement, and tidal volume (V_T, monitored as the sum of rib cage and abdominal movements). *A*, Central sleep apnea. There is absence of abdominal, rib cage, and sum movements associated with a small fall in arterial oxygen saturation. *B*, Obstructive sleep apnea. Apneas at beginning and midportion of recording are marked by absence of sum movements (V_T) despite respiratory efforts. Note that when the diaphragm contracts and the upper airway is obstructed during attempted inspiration, the abdomen moves out (upward on tracing) while the rib cage moves paradoxically inward (downward). Each apnea shown is associated with a marked fall in O_2 saturation and is terminated by three deep breaths. (From Tobin, M. J., Cohn, M. A., and Sackner, M. A.: Arch. Intern. Med. 143:1221–1228, 1983. Reproduced with permission.)

oxygen saturation drops, often to profoundly low levels (Fig. 18–2B). When oxygen saturation drops significantly during sleep, disturbances in cardiac rhythm occur, and elevation of pulmonary artery pressure may be seen as a consequence of hypoxia-induced pulmonary vasoconstriction.

Treatment

In patients with central apnea, treatment generally revolves around the use of respiratory stimulants or even an electrical, implanted phrenic nerve pacemaker to stimulate the diaphragm. In obstructive apnea, some patients surprisingly may respond to respiratory stimulants, but often in severe cases a tube must be placed in the trachea (tracheostomy) to allow air to bypass the site of upper airway obstruction. With patients who are markedly obese, an attempt at significant weight loss is often made, occasionally with improvement in the number or severity of the apneic episodes. Despite the apparent drastic nature of tracheostomy as a form of treatment, the therapeutic response is often quite gratifying. Patients may have a dramatic reversal of their symptoms and a striking improvement in their lifestyle, which was previously limited by intractable daytime sleepiness.

REFERENCES

Primary Neurologic Disease

Farmer, W. C., Glenn, W. W. L., and Gee, J. B. L.: Alveolar hypoventilation syndrome: studies of ventilatory control in patients selected for diaphragm pacing. Am. J. Med. 64:39–49, 1978.

Garay, S. M., Turino, G. M., and Goldring, R. M.: Sustained reversal of chronic hypercapnia in patients with alveolar hypoventilation syndromes: long-term maintenance with noninvasive nocturnal mechanical ventilation. Am. J. Med. 70:269–274, 1981.

Mellins, R. B., Balfour, H. H., Turino, G. M., and Winters, R. W.: Failure of automatic control of ventilation (Ondine's curse). Medicine 49:487–504, 1970.

Reichel, J.: Primary alveolar hypoventilation. Clin. Chest Med. 1:119–124, 1980.

Cheyne-Stokes Breathing

Cherniack, N. S., and Fishman, A. P.: Abnormal breathing patterns. DM 21(7):1–45, 1975.

Cherniack, N. S., and Longobardo, G. S.: Cheyne-Stokes breathing: an instability in physiologic control. N. Engl. J. Med. 288:952–957, 1973.

Control Abnormalities Secondary to Lung Disease

Aubier, M., et al.: Effects of the administration of O_2 on ventilation and blood gases in patients with chronic obstructive pulmonary disease during acute respiratory failure. Am. Rev. Respir. Dis. 122:747–754, 1980.

Milic-Emili, J., and Aubier, M.: Some recent advances in the study of the control of breathing in patients with chronic obstructive lung disease. Anesth. Analg. (Cleve.) 59:865–873, 1980.

Mountain, R., Zwillich, C., and Weil, J.: Hypoventilation in obstructive lung disease: the role of familial factors. N. Engl. J. Med. 298:521–525, 1978.

Park, S. S.: Respiratory control in chronic obstructive pulmonary diseases. Clin. Chest Med. 1:73–84, 1980.

Sleep Apnea Syndrome

Cherniack, N. S.: Respiratory dysrhythmias during sleep. N. Engl. J. Med. 305:325–330, 1981.

Guilleminault, C., Cummiskey, J., and Dement, W. C.: Sleep apnea syndrome: recent advances. Adv. Intern. Med. 26:347–372, 1980.

Guilleminault, C., Tilkian, A., and Dement, W. C.: The sleep apnea syndromes. Ann. Rev. Med. 27:465–483, 1976.

Phillipson, E. A.: Control of breathing during sleep. Am. Rev. Respir. Dis. 118:909–939, 1978.

Tobin, M. J., Cohn, M. A., and Sackner, M. A.: Breathing abnormalities during sleep. Arch. Intern. Med. 143:1221–1228, 1983.

19

Disorders of the
Respiratory Pump

The chest wall, diaphragm, and related neuromuscular apparatus moving the chest wall act in concert to translate signals from the ventilatory controller into expansion of the thorax. Together, these structures constitute the respiratory pump, an obviously important system that may fail as a result of diseases affecting any of its parts. Since disorders of the respiratory pump include a wide variety of specific problems, we will limit ourselves to a discussion of those entities that are most common and most important clinically: (1) neuromuscular disease affecting the muscles of respiration (e.g., myasthenia gravis, Guillain-Barré syndrome, polio, amyotrophic lateral sclerosis), (2) diaphragmatic fatigue, and (3) diseases affecting the chest wall (e.g., kyphoscoliosis, obesity).

NEUROMUSCULAR DISEASE AFFECTING THE MUSCLES OF RESPIRATION

A number of neuromuscular diseases have in common the potential for affecting the muscles of respiration. In some cases, the underlying process is an acute and generally reversible one, e.g., Guillain-Barré syndrome, and the muscles of respiration are transiently affected for a variable period of time. In other cases, the neuromuscular damage is permanent, and any consequences that affect the muscles of respiration are unfortunately chronic and irreversible. We will first briefly define some specific neurologic disorders with respiratory sequelae and then proceed with a discussion of the pathophysiology and clinical consequences of these diseases as they relate to the respiratory system.

Specific Diseases

The major neuromuscular diseases that can affect the muscles of respiration are listed in Table 19–1; several are discussed here in more detail. *Guillain-Barré syndrome*, also called acute idiopathic polyneuritis, is a disorder that is presumed to have an immune basis and is characterized by demyelination of peripheral nerves. Frequently, patients have a history of a recent viral illness, followed by development of an ascending paralysis. Classically, weakness or paralysis starts symmetrically in the lower extremities and then progresses or ascends proximally to the upper extremities and trunk. In severe cases, respiratory muscle weakness or paralysis accompanies the more usual limb and trunk symptoms. Generally, the natural history of this disease leads to recovery, and permanent sequelae are frequently absent. When respiratory muscles are affected, respiratory failure often supervenes but is usually reversible over the course of weeks to months.

In *myasthenia gravis*, patients experience weakness and fatigue of voluntary muscles, most frequently those innervated by cranial nerves, but peripheral (limb) and potentially respiratory muscles are also affected. The primary abnormality is found at the neuromuscular junction, where transmission of impulses from nerve to muscle is impaired by a decreased number of receptors on the muscle for the neurotransmitter acetylcholine and by the presence of antibodies against these receptors. Though myasthenia is a chronic illness, the manifestations can often be kept under control by appropriate therapy, and individual episodes of respiratory failure are potentially reversible.

Poliomyelitis is a viral disease in which the polio virus attacks motor nerve cells of the spinal cord and brainstem. Both the diaphragm and intercostal muscles can be affected, with resulting weakness or paralysis and respiratory failure. Recovery of respiratory muscle function is generally the case in surviving patients, though occasional patients have chronic respiratory insufficiency from prior disease. Fortunately, new cases are quite rare, as the result of mass vaccination of the population.

Amyotrophic lateral sclerosis, often abbreviated ALS, is a degen-

Table 19–1. DISORDERS OF THE RESPIRATORY PUMP

Neuromuscular Diseases
    Gullain-Barré syndrome
    Myasthenia gravis
    Poliomyelitis
    Amyotrophic lateral sclerosis
    Quadriplegia
    Polymyositis
    Muscular dystrophy
Chest Wall Diseases
    Kyphoscoliosis
    Obesity
    Ankylosing spondylitis

erative disease of the nervous system that involves both upper and lower motor neurons. Commonly, muscles innervated by both cranial nerves and spinal nerves are affected. Clinically, patients develop progressive muscle weakness and wasting, eventually leading to profound weakness of respiratory muscles and death. Though the time course of the disease is variable from patient to patient, the natural history is one of irreversibility and progressive deterioration.

Pathophysiology and Clinical Consequences

Weakness of respiratory muscles is the hallmark of respiratory involvement by the neuromuscular diseases. Depending on the specific disease, chest wall (intercostal) muscles, diaphragm, and expiratory muscles of the abdominal wall are each affected to a variable extent.

Because of the impairment of inspiratory muscle strength, patients may be unable to maintain sufficient minute ventilation for adequate CO_2 elimination. Additionally, patients often alter their pattern of breathing, taking more shallow and more frequent breaths. Though this pattern of breathing may be easier and more comfortable for these patients, it is also less efficient, since a greater proportion of each breath is wasted on ventilating the anatomic dead space. Therefore, even if total minute ventilation is maintained, alveolar ventilation (and thus CO_2 elimination) is impaired by the altered pattern of breathing.

Features of neuromuscular disease:
1. altered pattern of breathing ($\uparrow$ rate, $\downarrow$ tidal volume)
2. ineffective cough
3. restrictive pattern on pulmonary function tests
4. decreased maximal inspiratory/expiratory pressures
5. $\uparrow$ P_{CO_2}, often with $\downarrow$ P_{O_2}

The respiratory difficulty developed by patients with neuromuscular disease is also complicated by weakness of expiratory muscles and an ineffective cough. Recurrent respiratory tract infections, accumulation of secretions, and areas of collapse or atelectasis thus contribute to the clinical problems posed by these patients.

Symptomatically, patients may be dyspneic and anxious; they may also have a feeling of suffocation. Often, the presence of generalized muscle weakness severely limits their activity and lessens the degree of dyspnea that would be present if they were capable of more exertion.

With severe neuromuscular disease, pulmonary function tests show a restrictive pattern of impairment. Though FRC is generally maintained, assuming no change in either lung or chest wall compliance, TLC is decreased as a result of inspiratory muscle weakness, and RV is frequently increased as a result of expiratory muscle weakness (see Fig. 19–1). We can actually quantitate the degree of muscle weakness by measuring the maximal inspiratory and expiratory pressures the patient is able to generate against a meter that registers pressure. Both maximal inspiratory pressure (MIP) and maximal expiratory pressure (MEP) may be significantly depressed.

In the setting of severe muscle weakness, arterial blood gases are most notable for the presence of alveolar hypoventilation, i.e., hypercapnia. Hypoxemia also occurs as a result of alveolar hypoventilation and the associated depression in alveolar P_{O_2}. When hypoventilation is the sole cause of hypoxemia, the alveolar-arterial oxygen difference is normal. However, complications of atelectasis, respiratory tract infections, and inadequately cleared secretions may add a component of ventilation-perfusion mismatch that further depresses P_{O_2} and increases the AaD_{O_2}.

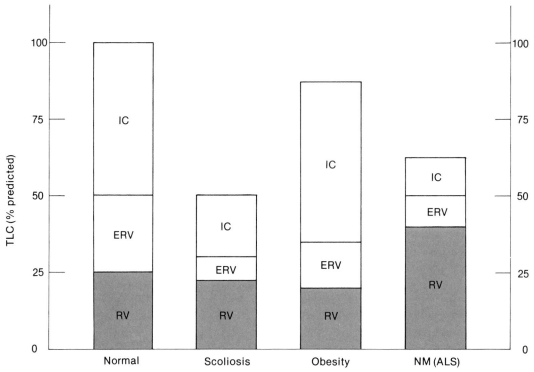

Figure 19–1. Examples of lung volumes (TLC and its subdivisions) in patients with chest wall and neuromuscular disease compared with those of a normal subject. Clear area represents vital capacity and its subdivisions, i.e., inspiratory capacity (IC) and expiratory reserve volume (ERV); shaded area represents residual volume (RV). (Adapted from Bergofsky, E. H.: Am. Rev. Respir. Dis. 119:643–669, 1979. Reproduced with permission.)

DIAPHRAGMATIC FATIGUE

Excluding cardiac muscle, the diaphragm is the single muscle used most consistently and repetitively throughout the course of a lifetime. Fortunately, it is well suited for sustained activity and for aerobic metabolism, and under normal circumstances the diaphragm does not become fatigued.

However, if the diaphragm is required to perform an excessive amount of work or if its energy supplies are limited, fatigue may develop and may contribute to respiratory dysfunction in certain clinical settings. For example, if a normal individual repetitively uses the diaphragm to generate 40 percent or more of its maximal force, fatigue develops and prevents this degree of effort from being sustained indefinitely. For patients with diseases that increase the work of breathing, particularly obstructive lung disease and diseases of the chest wall (to be described shortly), the diaphragm works at a level much closer to the point of fatigue. When a superimposed acute illness further increases the work of breathing, or when an intercurrent problem (e.g., depressed cardiac output, anemia, or hypoxemia) decreases the energy supply available to the diaphragm, then diaphragmatic fatigue may contribute to the development of hypoventilation and respiratory failure.

Inefficient diaphragmatic contraction is an additional factor that may contribute to diaphragmatic fatigue, especially in the patient with

Factors contributing to diaphragmatic fatigue:
1. increased work of breathing
2. decreased energy supply to diaphragm
3. inefficient diaphragmatic contraction

obstructive lung disease. When the diaphragm is flattened and fibers are shortened as a result of hyperinflated lungs, the force or pressure developed during contraction is less for any given level of diaphragmatic excitation (see Chapter 17). Therefore, a higher degree of stimulation is necessary to generate comparable pressure by the diaphragm, and increased energy consumption results.

Diaphragmatic fatigue is often difficult to detect, since the force generated by the diaphragm cannot be measured conveniently. Ideally, diaphragmatic fatigue is documented by measuring the pressure across the diaphragm (i.e., the difference between abdominal and pleural pressure, called the transdiaphragmatic pressure) during diaphragmatic stimulation or contraction. As an alternative to measurement of trans-diaphragmatic pressure, we can more easily assess the pattern of motion of the abdomen during breathing when the patient is supine. If diaphragmatic contraction is especially weak or absent, pleural pressure falls mainly as a result of contraction of other inspiratory muscles. The negative pleural pressure is transmitted across the relatively flaccid diaphragm to the abdomen, which then moves paradoxically inward during inspiration.

Diaphragmatic weakness can be demonstrated in the supine position by inward motion of the abdomen during inspiration.

Along with recent investigation of the role of diaphragmatic fatigue in respiratory failure, there have also been attempts to improve or reverse fatigue. Use of assisted ventilation with a mechanical ventilator to rest the diaphragm has been suggested as an important measure to reverse fatigue. Alternatively, use of aminophylline has recently been shown to increase the strength of diaphragmatic contraction and may therefore improve the function of the failing diaphragm.

DISEASES AFFECTING THE CHEST WALL

With certain diseases of the chest wall, the chest may be difficult to expand, and normal inspiration may therefore be impeded. These disorders are listed in Table 19–1 along with other disturbances of the respiratory pump. We will focus in this discussion on two specific disorders that pose the greatest clinical problems—kyphoscoliosis and obesity.

Kyphoscoliosis

Kyphoscoliosis is defined as an abnormal curvature of the spine in both the lateral and anteroposterior directions (Fig. 19–2). As a result of this deformity, the rib cage becomes stiffer and more difficult to expand, i.e., chest wall compliance is decreased. In patients with significant kyphoscoliosis, respiratory difficulties are common. In particularly severe cases, chronic respiratory failure is the unfortunate consequence. Though some cases of kyphoscoliosis are actually secondary to neuromuscular disease such as poliomyelitis, the majority of severe cases associated with respiratory impairment are idiopathic.

Several pathophysiologic features contribute to respiratory dysfunction in patients with kyphoscoliosis. A crucial underlying problem is the increased work of breathing resulting from the poorly compliant chest wall. To maintain even a normal minute ventilation, the work expenditure of the respiratory muscles is greatly increased. In addition,

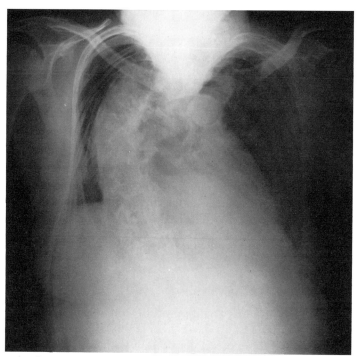

Figure 19-2. Chest radiograph of a patient with severe kyphoscoliosis. There is marked curvature of the spine and distortion of the chest wall.

however, patients decrease their tidal volume and increase respiratory frequency because of difficulty expanding the abnormally stiff chest wall. Consequently, the proportion of wasted ventilation rises, and alveolar ventilation falls unless total ventilation undergoes a compensatory increase. Hence, the high work of breathing acts in concert with the altered pattern of breathing to decrease alveolar ventilation and increase PCO_2.

Additionally, the marked distortion of the chest wall causes underventilation of some regions of lung, ventilation-perfusion mismatch, and hypoxemia. Therefore, there are frequently two causes for hypoxemia in kyphoscoliosis—hypoventilation and ventilation-perfusion mismatch.

A common complication of severe kyphoscoliosis is pulmonary hypertension and cor pulmonale. Hypoxemia and, to a lesser extent, hypercapnia are important for the development of pulmonary hypertension. However, increased resistance of the pulmonary vessels also results from compression and possibly from impaired development in regions where the chest wall is especially distorted. Long-standing pulmonary hypertension itself also causes structural changes in the vessels, with thickening of the walls of pulmonary arteries. This thickening is not acutely reversible even with correction of the hypoxemia.

Exertional dyspnea is probably the most common symptom experienced by patients with severe kyphoscoliosis and respiratory impairment. Unlike patients with neuromuscular disease, those with a chest wall deformity such as kyphoscoliosis have normal muscle strength and therefore are otherwise capable of normal levels of exertion. Patients with kyphoscoliosis also are not subject to the same difficulty in

Features of severe kyphoscoliosis:
1. increased work of breathing
2. altered pattern of breathing (↑ rate, ↓ tidal volume)
3. exertional dyspnea
4. ventilation-perfusion mismatch
5. ↑ PCO_2, often with ↓ PO_2
6. pulmonary hypertension, cor pulmonale
7. restrictive pattern on pulmonary function tests

generating an effective cough as patients with neuromuscular disease. Expiratory muscle function is preserved, an effective cough is maintained, and problems with secretions and recurrent respiratory tract infections are not prominent clinical features.

Pulmonary function tests in patients with kyphoscoliosis are notable for a restrictive pattern of impairment, with a decrease in the total lung capacity. Vital capacity is also significantly decreased, whereas residual volume tends to be relatively preserved. Functional residual capacity, determined by the outward recoil of the chest wall balanced by the inward recoil of the lung, is decreased, since the poorly compliant chest wall has a diminished propensity to recoil outward (Fig. 19–1).

As mentioned earlier, severe cases of kyphoscoliosis are generally characterized by hypercapnia and hypoxemia. The latter is usually due both to hypoventilation and to ventilation-perfusion mismatch. Chronic respiratory insufficiency and cor pulmonale are the end results of severe kyphoscoliosis, and the level of respiratory difficulty appears to correlate with the severity of the chest wall deformity.

Obesity

Obesity certainly has many consequences for health, and respiratory symptoms are but one aspect. It can produce a wide spectrum in severity of respiratory impairment, ranging from no symptoms to marked limitation in function. Surprisingly, the degree of obesity does not appear to correlate with the presence or severity of respiratory dysfunction. Some patients who are massively obese have no difficulty in comparison with much less obese patients who may be severely limited. In order to explain these discrepancies, we must invoke several factors that contribute to respiratory dysfunction; obesity is just one of these factors.

The problem of respiratory impairment in obesity was popularly known for years as the *Pickwickian syndrome* or *obesity-hypoventilation syndrome*. The name Pickwickian syndrome was applied because of the description of the fat boy, Joe, in Dickens' *Pickwick Papers*, who had many of the characteristics described in this syndrome. Specifically, Joe had features of massive obesity, somnolence, and peripheral edema, the latter presumably related to cor pulmonale and right ventricular failure. With the accumulation of more recent knowledge about the pathogenesis of respiratory impairment in obesity, the term Pickwickian syndrome has become less meaningful.

Obesity itself appears to exert two effects on the respiratory system. As a result of excess soft tissue, the chest wall becomes stiffer or less compliant, and thus more work is necessary for expansion of the thorax. In addition, the massive accumulation of soft tissue in the abdominal wall exerts pressure on abdominal contents, forcing the diaphragm up to a higher resting position.

In a fashion similar to that of kyphoscoliosis, the stiff chest wall results in lower tidal volumes and increased wasted or dead space ventilation. Therefore, in order to maintain adequate alveolar ventilation, overall minute ventilation must increase, unfortunately in the face of increased work of breathing. Some patients are able to compensate appropriately by increasing their overall minute ventilation, and P_{CO_2} remains normal. Others do not compensate fully, and hypercapnia is the necessary consequence.

Exactly what distinguishes these two types of patients is not really known. Perhaps patients in the latter group, to whom the term obesity-hypoventilation syndrome can be applied, started out with a central nervous system respiratory controller that was relatively hyporesponsive. Output of the controller might not have responded sufficiently to keep pace with increased ventilatory requirements, and CO_2 retention would then result. Once patients actually become hypercapnic, it is much more difficult to assess the innate responsiveness of the patient's ventilatory controller, since chronic hypercapnia, i.e., chronic respiratory acidosis with a compensatory metabolic alkalosis, blunts the responsiveness of the central chemoreceptor.

The high resting position of the diaphragm in obesity, occurring as a result of pressure from the obese abdomen, is associated with decreased expansion of the lung and actual closure of small airways and alveoli at the bases. The dependent regions are thus hypoventilated relative to their perfusion, and this ventilation-perfusion mismatch results in arterial hypoxemia.

An additional factor that contributes to the overall clinical picture in many massively obese patients is upper airway obstruction during sleep, i.e., the obstructive form of sleep-apnea syndrome. Presumably, soft tissue deposition in the neck and tissues surrounding the upper airway predisposes to episodes of complete upper airway obstruction during sleep. In a large percentage of cases, somnolence that occurs in patients who supposedly have the obesity-hypoventilation syndrome is probably related to the presence of obstructive sleep-apnea.

While obesity, depressed respiratory drive, and sleep-apnea syndrome contribute to respiratory dysfunction, exactly how they interact in individual patients is often difficult to assess. Since both sleep-apnea syndrome and depressed respiratory drive also occur in patients who are not obese, it is reasonable to view the three features in terms of a Venn diagram (Fig. 19–3). Probably the most marked symptoms and respiratory dysfunction are seen in patients who have all three problems and who are represented at the intersection of the three circles.

The symptoms that may occur in the obese patient can be associated with the increased work of breathing (e.g., dyspnea) or with

Features of obesity:
1. decreased chest wall compliance
2. high diaphragms (low FRC)
3. altered pattern of breathing (↑ rate, ↓ tidal volume)
4. ventilation-perfusion mismatch
5. variable ↑ P_{CO_2}, ↓ P_{O_2}
6. obstructive apnea (sometimes)

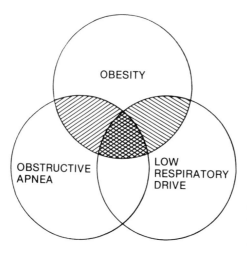

Figure 19–3. Venn diagram giving hypothetical indication of the way obesity interacts with obstructive apnea and low respiratory drive. In this schema, the overlap shown on the left includes obese, normocapnic patients with obstructive apnea. The overlap shown on the right includes hypercapnic obese patients without obstructive apnea. The overlap shown by the center crosshatching includes obese, hypercapnic patients with obstructive apnea.

the sleep-apnea syndrome (e.g., daytime somnolence, disordered sleep with profound snoring). Patients may also have clinical manifestations related to the complications of pulmonary hypertension, cor pulmonale, and right ventricular failure. These complications are largely related to arterial hypoxemia both during the day and at night, particularly if the patient has sleep-apnea syndrome.

Pulmonary function tests frequently demonstrate a restrictive pattern of dysfunction, with a decrease in the total lung capacity. As we mentioned earlier, the diaphragm is pushed up in the massively obese patient, reducing FRC. Since FRC in these patients is much closer to RV, spirometry shows ERV to be greatly reduced. This pattern of functional impairment is shown in Figure 19–1.

In most obese patients, arterial blood gases show a decrease in the Po_2 and an increase in the $AaDo_2$ as a consequence of high diaphragms, airway and alveolar closure, and ventilation-perfusion mismatch. If Pco_2 is not elevated, these patients are sometimes said to have "simple obesity." When the Pco_2 is elevated, the term obesity-hypoventilation syndrome is often used, and in these cases superimposed hypoventilation is an additional factor contributing to hypoxemia. Obviously, if the patient has sleep-apnea syndrome, arterial blood gases become even more deranged at night during episodes of apnea.

In the treatment of obese patients with respiratory dysfunction, weight loss is theoretically crucial. If weight loss is successful, many of the clinical problems may resolve. Unfortunately, attempts at significant weight loss are often futile, and one is forced to institute other modes of therapy. In patients who hypoventilate, respiratory stimulants, especially progesterone, have been used with some success. If the patient has obstructive sleep-apnea syndrome, a tracheostomy may be necessary if the clinical manifestations are sufficiently severe.

REFERENCES

Neuromuscular Disease Affecting the Muscles of Respiration

Derenne, J-P., Macklem, P. T., and Roussos, C.: The respiratory muscles: mechanics, control, and pathophysiology. Am. Rev. Respir. Dis. 118:581–601, 1978.

Luce, J. M., and Culver, B. H.: Respiratory muscle function in health and disease. Chest 81:82–90, 1982.

Moore, P., and James, O.: Guillain-Barré syndrome: incidence, management and outcome of major complications. Crit. Care Med. 9:549–555, 1981.

Roussos, C., and Macklem, P. T.: The respiratory muscles. N. Engl. J. Med. 307:786–797, 1982.

Diaphragmatic Fatigue

Aubier, M., De Troyer, A., Sampson, M., Macklem, P. T., and Roussos, C.: Aminophylline improves diaphragmatic contractility. N. Engl. J. Med. 305:249–252, 1981.

Belman, M. J., and Sieck, G. C.: The ventilatory muscles: fatigue, endurance and training. Chest 82:761–766, 1982.

Roussos, C., and Macklem, P. T.: The respiratory muscles. N. Engl. J. Med. 307:786–797, 1982.

Diseases Affecting the Chest Wall

Bergofsky, E. H.: Respiratory failure in disorders of the thoracic cage. Am. Rev. Respir. Dis. 119:643–669, 1979.

Kafer, E. R.: Respiratory and cardiovascular functions in scoliosis. Bull. Eur. Physiopathol. Respir. 13:299–321, 1977.

Libby, D. M., Briscoe, W. A., Boyce, B., and Smith, J. P.: Acute respiratory failure in scoliosis or kyphosis. Am. J. Med. 73:532–538, 1982.

Luce, J. M.: Respiratory complications of obesity. Chest 78:626–631, 1980.

Sutton, F. D., Zwillich, C. W., Creagh, C. E., Pierson, D. J., and Weil, J. V.: Progesterone for outpatient treatment of Pickwickian syndrome. Ann. Intern. Med. 83:476–479, 1975.

20

Lung Cancer: Etiologic and Pathologic Aspects

> **Etiology and Pathogenesis**
>   Smoking
>   Occupational Factors
>   Air Pollution
>   Genetic Factors
>   Parenchymal Scarring
> **Pathology**
>   Squamous Cell Carcinoma
>   Small Cell Carcinoma
>   Adenocarcinoma
>   Large Cell Carcinoma

Carcinoma of the lung, a public health problem of immense proportions, has been a source of great frustration to individual physicians and to the medical profession in general. Over the past several decades, its primary cause—cigarette smoking—has been identified without a shadow of a doubt. However, little headway has been made in either prevention (i.e., significant reduction in exposure to the major causative factor) or treatment of this devastating illness.

A few statistics are useful to put the magnitude of the problem into perspective. There are now well over 100,000 new cases of lung cancer diagnosed in the United States each year, and more than 100,000 individuals die annually as a result of this disease. Carcinoma of the lung is now the leading cause of cancer deaths among men, and it is soon about to surpass breast cancer as the leading cause among women as well. Overall, lung cancer is responsible for approximately 25 percent of all deaths due to cancer and approximately 5 percent of all deaths from any cause. It is a sobering thought to realize that during the past five years more Americans were killed by lung cancer than were killed in all the wars in the nation's history.

Unfortunately, the number of cases and the number of deaths related to lung cancer are dramatically increasing. Over the 25 years between 1950 and 1975, the death rate rose more than 200 percent. For no other form of cancer has the increase approached that seen with lung cancer. Yet our ability to treat carcinoma of the lung has not improved in any substantial way. Five-year survival has remained at 10 percent or less over the past 3 decades, making the prognosis of this disease still dismal in the vast majority of cases.

We will divide the discussion of carcinoma of the lung into two parts. In this chapter, we will consider what is known about the etiology of lung cancer and then describe pathologic aspects and classification of the different types of tumors. In Chapter 21, we will continue by discussing clinical aspects of the disease, including diagnostic and therapeutic considerations. Finally, we will conclude Chapter 21 with a brief discussion of two additional types of neoplastic disease affecting the respiratory system, bronchial carcinoid tumor (bronchial adenoma) and mesothelioma, along with a consideration of the common problem of the patient with a solitary pulmonary nodule.

ETIOLOGY AND PATHOGENESIS

For no other common cancer affecting man have the causative factors been worked out as well as for lung cancer. Cigarette smoking is clearly responsible for the vast majority of cases, and additional risk factors associated with occupational exposure have also been identified. After discussing these two major risk factors, we will briefly mention what is known about possible roles for air pollution and genetic factors in the causation of this disease. Finally, we will consider the importance of previous scarring within the pulmonary parenchyma, which has been implicated in the development of "scar carcinomas."

Smoking

A wealth of data now implicates cigarette smoking as the single most important risk factor for development of carcinoma of the lung. As might be expected, the duration of the smoking history, the number of cigarettes smoked each day, the depth of inhalation, and the amount of each cigarette smoked all correlate with the risk for development of lung cancer. As a rough but easy way to quantitate prior cigarette exposure, the duration of the smoking history in years can be multiplied by the number of packs smoked per day, giving the number of "pack-years" smoked.

Though the evidence incriminating smoking with lung cancer is incontrovertible, the responsible component of cigarette smoke has not been identified with certainty. Cigarette smoke consists of a gaseous phase and a particulate phase, and potential carcinogens have been found in both phases, ranging from nitrosamines to benzo[a]pyrene and other polycyclic hydrocarbons. Filters appear to decrease but certainly not eliminate the potential carcinogenic effects of cigarettes. There is also a substantially lower risk for lung cancer associated with cigar or pipe smoking, presumably related to the fact that cigar and pipe smoke is generally not inhaled.

The actual development of lung cancer as a result of smoking takes many years of exposure. However, histologic abnormalities prior to development of a frank carcinoma have been well documented in the

Histologic abnormalities in the bronchial epithelium induced by smoking precede the development of carcinoma.

bronchial epithelium of smokers. These changes, including loss of bronchial cilia, hyperplasia of bronchial epithelial cells, and nuclear abnormalities, may be the histologic forerunners of a true carcinoma. If a patient stops smoking, many of these precancerous changes are reversible. Epidemiologic studies have suggested that the risk for development of lung cancer actually reverts back to the level seen in nonsmokers after cessation of smoking for more than 10 to 15 years. Unfortunately, in many cases, malignant cells have already developed by the time the patient stops smoking, and it is merely a matter of time before the carcinoma becomes clinically apparent.

Occupational Factors

A number of potential environmental risk factors have now been identified, most of which occur with occupational exposure. Perhaps the most widely studied of the environmental or occupationally-related carcinogens is asbestos, which is a fibrous silicate used because of its properties of fire resistance and thermal insulation. As we mentioned in Chapter 10, building or repairing ships and working with insulation, construction, or brake linings are just a few of the many ways in which an individual may be exposed to asbestos.

The risk of lung cancer is markedly increased by the combined risk factors of asbestos exposure and smoking.

Carcinoma of the lung is the most likely malignancy to complicate asbestos exposure, though other tumors, especially mesothelioma (see Chapter 21), are also strongly associated with prior asbestos exposure. The risk for development of lung cancer is particularly high in a smoker exposed to asbestos, in which case these two risk factors probably have a multiplicative effect. Specifically, asbestos alone appears to confer a 5- to 10-fold increase in risk for lung cancer, whereas smoking alone is associated with an approximately 10-fold increased risk. Together, the two risk factors make the patient who smokes and has an asbestos exposure 50 to 100 times more likely to develop carcinoma of the lung than his or her nonsmoking, nonexposed counterpart. Like other forms of asbestos-related disease, there is a long time lapse before the development of the complication. In the case of lung cancer, more than 20 years generally elapse after exposure before the tumor becomes apparent.

Several other types of occupational exposure have now also been implicated in the subsequent development of lung cancer. As is the case with asbestos, there is generally a long latent period of at least two decades from the time of exposure until presentation of the tumor. Examples of these exposures include arsenic (in the manufacture of pesticides, glass, pigments, and paints), ionizing radiation (especially in uranium miners), haloethers (bis-chloromethyl ether and chloromethyl methyl ether in chemical industry workers), and polycyclic aromatic hydrocarbons (in petroleum, coal tar, and foundry workers), just to name a few.

Air Pollution

Though potential carcinogens (some of which are also found in cigarette smoke) have been identified in regions where the air is particularly polluted, the overall role of air pollution in lung cancer is unclear. However, it is reasonably well established that any risk associated with air pollution is small compared with the risk from smoking.

Genetic Factors

Why some heavy smokers develop lung cancer while others do not is a question that has great importance but no answer. We assume that genetic factors must make some individuals at higher risk for lung cancer after exposure to carcinogens. One theory has proposed that the enzyme aryl hydrocarbon hydroxylase, which can convert hydrocarbons to carcinogenic metabolites, is involved. This enzyme is induced by smoking, and it has been suggested that genetically determined inducibility of this enzyme by smoking may correlate with the risk for developing lung cancer. However, the data relating to this theory have been inconsistent, and it has thus not been universally accepted.

Presumably, other as yet unidentified genetic factors affect the susceptibility to environmental carcinogens. If we were able to identify such individuals at risk, we could perhaps make a particular effort to prevent their becoming exposed to the known environmental carcinogens.

Parenchymal Scarring

Scar tissue within the lung can be a locus for the subsequent occurrence of lung cancer, called a *scar carcinoma*. The scarring may be either localized (e.g., resulting from an old focus of tuberculosis or another infection) or diffuse (e.g., from pulmonary fibrosis, whether idiopathic or associated with a specific etiology). Most frequently, scar carcinomas of the lung are adenocarcinomas and often a specific subtype called bronchioloalveolar carcinoma. These cell types will be discussed in more detail in the next section of this chapter.

Though it is easy to consider carcinomas occurring within or adjacent to scar tissue as scar carcinomas, it also appears that adenocarcinomas of the lung may develop fibrotic areas within the tumor. Therefore, in some cases it may be impossible to know whether the scar preceded or followed development of the carcinoma.

PATHOLOGY

The term bronchogenic carcinoma is often used interchangeably with the term lung cancer, implying that lung cancers arise from bronchi or bronchial structures. Many if not most lung cancers do indeed originate within airways, but other tumors arise in the periphery of the lung, and their cell of origin is somewhat less clear. In this section, we will discuss the currently accepted classification of lung cancer and attempt to recount what is known about the histogenesis of the various types of tumors.

Major histologic categories of
lung cancer:
1. squamous cell carcinoma
2. small cell carcinoma
3. adenocarcinoma
4. large cell carcinoma

Almost all lung cancers fall within one of four histologic categories: (1) squamous cell carcinoma, (2) small cell carcinoma, (3) adenocarcinoma, and (4) large cell carcinoma. Within each of these four categories are several subcategories, which for our purposes are less important. However, we will mention two specific subcategories, bronchioloalveolar carcinoma (a type of adenocarcinoma) and oat cell carcinoma (a type of small cell carcinoma), since these pathologic diagnoses are frequently made and the terms often used in the clinical setting.

Each of the four major categories is associated with cigarette smoking. However, the statistical association between smoking and the individual cell types is greatest for squamous and small cell carcinomas, which are seen almost exclusively in smokers. Even though smoking also increases the risk for developing adenocarcinoma and large cell carcinoma, these cell types are also observed in nonsmokers.

Squamous Cell Carcinoma

Approximately one third of all bronchogenic carcinomas are of the squamous cell type. These tumors originate within the epithelial layer of the bronchial wall, in which a series of progressive histologic abnormalities result from chronic or repetitive cigarette smoke–induced injury.

Initially, there is metaplasia of the normal bronchial columnar epithelial cells, which are replaced by squamous epithelial cells. Over time these squamous cells become more and more atypical in appearance, until there is development of a well-localized carcinoma, i.e., carcinoma in situ. Eventually, the carcinoma extends beyond the bronchial mucosa and becomes frankly invasive. At this stage the tumor generally presents clinically, by producing either symptoms or radiographic changes. In some cases, detection of the carcinoma is made at the earlier in situ stage, usually by recognition of the malignant cells in a specimen of sputum obtained for cytologic examination.

Specific histologic features of squamous cell carcinoma allow the pathologist to make this diagnosis. These tumors are characterized by the presence of keratin as well as "squamous pearls" and intercellular bridges (Fig. 20–1).

Features of squamous cell
carcinomas:
1. generally arise in proximal
airways
2. may cause airway
obstruction, leading to distal
atelectasis or pneumonia
3. may cavitate
4. intrathoracic spread rather
than distant metastases

Squamous cell carcinomas tend to be located in relatively large or proximal airways, most commonly at the subsegmental, segmental, or lobar level. With growth of the tumor into the bronchial lumen, the airway may become obstructed, and the lung distal to the obstruction frequently collapses (i.e., becomes atelectatic) and may develop a postobstructive pneumonia. Sometimes, the tumor mass develops a cavity within it; this finding of cavitation is much more common with squamous cell than with other types of bronchogenic carcinoma.

Spread of squamous cell carcinoma beyond the airway usually involves (1) direct extension to the pulmonary parenchyma or to other neighboring structures or (2) invasion of lymphatics, with spread to local lymph nodes in the hilum or mediastinum. These tumors have a general tendency to remain within the thorax and to cause problems by intrathoracic complications rather than by distant metastasis. The overall prognosis in terms of the potential for five-year survival is better

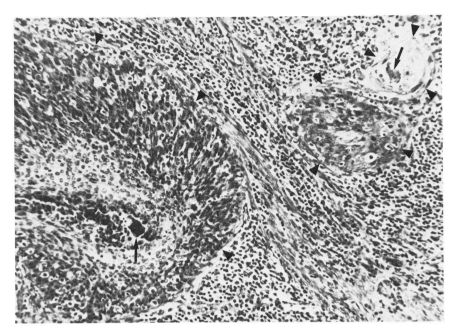

Figure 20–1. Low-power photomicrograph of squamous cell carcinoma. There are three foci of tumor, each highlighted by arrowheads. The intervening regions show connective tissue and inflammatory cells. Arrows point to two areas of keratin formation by the tumor. (Courtesy of Dr. Earl Kasdon.)

for patients with squamous cell carcinoma than for patients with any of the other cell types.

Small Cell Carcinoma

Small cell carcinoma, comprising approximately 20 percent of all lung cancers, consists of several subtypes, of which oat cell carcinoma is the most commonly encountered. Like squamous cell carcinoma, carcinomas within the small cell category also generally originate within the bronchial wall, most commonly at a proximal level. There is dispute about the cell of origin of small cell carcinoma. According to one popular (but unproven) theory, these tumors arise from a neurosecretory type of epithelial cell termed the Kulchitsky or K cell. These cells have the capacity for polypeptide production and are considered to be a type of APUD cell (i.e., capable of *a*mine *p*recursor *u*ptake and *d*ecarboxylation). Another popular and more recent theory suggests that small cell carcinomas, like other lung cancers, have an endodermal origin. The eventual cell type then depends on the pattern and degree of differentiation from the endodermal precursor cell.

In the most common or oat cell subtype, the malignant cells appear as small, darkly stained cells with sparse cytoplasm (Fig. 20–2). The local growth of the tumor often follows a submucosal pattern, but the tumor quickly invades lymphatics and submucosal blood vessels. Hilar and mediastinal nodes are involved early in the course of the disease and are frequently the most prominent aspect of the radiographic presentation.

Because of the rapid dissemination of small cell carcinoma, metastatic spread to distant sites is also a common early complication. Distant disease, which may be clinically occult at the time of presentation, often affects the brain, liver, bone (and bone marrow), and

Features of small cell (especially oat cell) carcinomas:
1. generally arise in proximal airways
2. commonly produce polypeptide hormones
3. hilar and mediastinal node involvement
4. early, distant metastatic disease

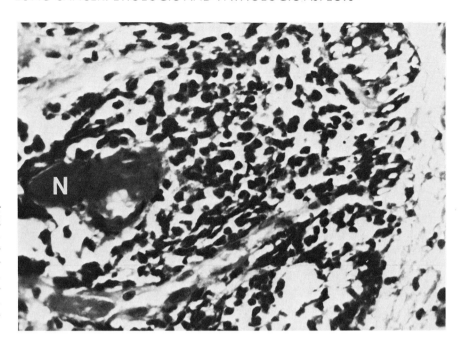

Figure 20–2. High-power photomicrograph of small cell (oat cell) carcinoma. The malignant cells have irregular, darkly stained nuclei and sparse cytoplasm. There is a small area of necrosis (N) within the tumor. (Courtesy of Dr. Earl Kasdon.)

adrenal glands. It is this propensity for early metastatic involvement that gives small cell carcinoma the worst prognosis among the four major categories of bronchogenic carcinoma.

Adenocarcinoma

Adenocarcinoma now appears to have reached or surpassed squamous cell carcinoma as the most frequent cell type, accounting for more than one third of all lung tumors. Since the majority of adenocarcinomas occur in the periphery of the lung, it is much harder to relate their origin to the bronchial wall. Nevertheless, many are thought to arise from cells comprising bronchial mucous glands, explaining the glandular or acinar nature of these tumors. Presumably, other cellular constituents of the lung may also be the site of origin of some adenocarcinomas, particularly ones that arise in the lung periphery. As we mentioned earlier in this chapter, adenocarcinomas frequently appear at a site of parenchymal scarring that is either localized or part of a diffuse fibrotic process.

The characteristic appearance defining adenocarcinoma is the tendency to form glands and to produce mucus (Fig. 20–3). In the bronchioloalveolar subcategory of adenocarcinoma, the malignant cells seem to grow and spread along the pre-existing alveolar walls, almost as though they were using the alveolar wall as a scaffolding for their growth (Fig. 20–4).

Features of adenocarcinomas:
1. often present as a solitary, peripheral pulmonary nodule
2. may arise in an old parenchymal scar
3. generally localized when presenting as a peripheral lung nodule
4. spread to hilar and mediastinal nodes and to distant sites

The usual presenting pattern of adenocarcinoma is a peripheral lung nodule or mass. Occasionally, the tumors can arise within a relatively large bronchus and may therefore present with complications of localized bronchial obstruction, as seen with squamous cell carcinoma. The bronchioloalveolar subcategory can present in several ways—as a nodule or mass lesion, as a localized infiltrate simulating a pneumonia, or as widespread parenchymal disease.

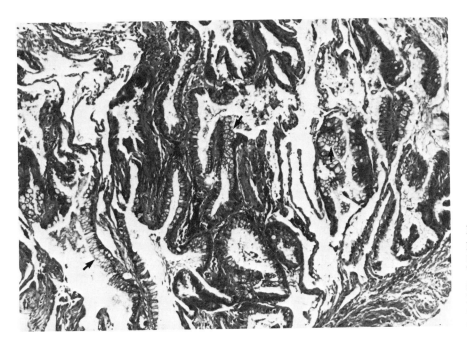

Figure 20–3. Low-power photomicrograph of an adenocarcinoma of the lung. The malignant cells form gland-like structures and produce mucus (arrows). (Courtesy of Dr. Earl Kasdon.)

Though adenocarcinoma may spread locally to adjacent regions of lung or to pleura, it also has a propensity for nodal involvement (hilar and mediastinal) and for distant metastatic spread. Like small cell carcinoma, it spreads to liver, bone, central nervous system, and adrenal glands. In comparison with small cell carcinoma, however, adenocarcinoma is more likely to be localized at the time of presentation, particularly when it presents as a solitary peripheral lung nodule. The overall prognosis for adenocarcinoma is not surprising given this behavior; its natural history and survival rates are intermediate between those of squamous cell and small cell carcinomas.

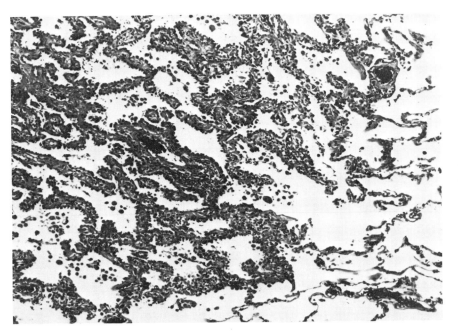

Figure 20–4. Low-power photomicrograph of bronchioloalveolar carcinoma. The tumor cells appear to be growing along the pre-existing alveolar walls. The lower right corner of the photograph shows normal alveolar walls, which can be contrasted with the areas of tumor. (Courtesy of Dr. Earl Kasdon.)

Large Cell Carcinoma

The final major cell type, large cell carcinoma, accounts for approximately 15 to 20 percent of all lung cancers. In a sense, it is the most difficult to define well, largely because the tumors are often defined by the characteristics they lack, i.e., specific features that would otherwise classify them as one of the other three cell types. It is also difficult to pinpoint the cell(s) of origin from which these tumors arise.

The behavior of these tumors is relatively similar to that of adenocarcinoma. They often appear in the periphery of the lung as mass lesions, though tending to be somewhat larger than adenocarcinomas. Their natural history is also similar to that of adenocarcinoma, both in terms of propensity for spread and overall prognosis.

For a summary of the distinguishing features of each cell type, Table 21–1 in Chapter 21 reiterates many of the points we have discussed so far.

REFERENCES

References for Chapters 20 and 21 are found at the end of Chapter 21.

Lung Cancer: Clinical Aspects

In this chapter, our goal is to extend the discussion of lung cancer into the clinical realm and to relate how the pathologic processes considered in Chapter 20 are encountered in a clinical setting. We will start by outlining the major clinical features of lung cancer and then proceed with a discussion of the diagnostic approach and general principles of management. We will conclude the chapter with a brief discussion of bronchial carcinoid tumors, malignant mesothelioma, and the clinical problem of the solitary pulmonary nodule.

CLINICAL FEATURES

Since lung cancer presumably starts with a single malignant cell, there must be a long period of repetitive divisions and doubling of cell number before the tumor becomes clinically apparent. During this preclinical period, it has been estimated that approximately 30 divisions take place before the tumor reaches 1 cm in diameter. This process most likely requires a number of years, during which time the patient and the physician are unaware of the tumor.

In general, the possibility of lung cancer is raised because of findings on chest radiograph or sputum cytology, or because of an assortment of symptoms that may ensue. We will focus here primarily on symptoms, saving chest radiography and sputum cytology for the section on diagnostic approach. The symptoms at the time of presentation may relate to the primary lung lesion itself, to metastatic disease (either in intrathoracic lymph nodes or at distant sites), or to what are commonly called "paraneoplastic syndromes."

Symptoms Relating to Primary Lung Lesion

Potential clinical problems with lung cancer:
1. symptoms from an endobronchial tumor—cough, hemoptysis
2. problems of bronchial obstruction—postobstructive pneumonia, dyspnea
3. pleural involvement—chest pain, pleural effusion, dyspnea
4. involvement of adjacent structures—heart, esophagus
5. complications of mediastinal involvement—phrenic or recurrent laryngeal nerve paralysis, SVC obstruction
6. distant metastases—brain, bone or bone marrow, liver, adrenals
7. ectopic hormone production—ACTH, ADH, (?) PTH
8. other paraneoplastic syndromes—neurologic, clubbing, hypertrophic osteoarthropathy
9. nonspecific systemic effects—anorexia, weight loss

Perhaps the most common symptoms developing in the patient with lung cancer are cough and hemoptysis. Since patients who develop bronchogenic carcinoma are generally smokers, they often dismiss their symptoms (particularly cough) as routine complications of smoking and chronic bronchitis. With tumors originating in large airways, such as squamous or small cell carcinoma, patients may also have problems related to bronchial obstruction, e.g., pneumonia behind the obstruction or shortness of breath secondary to occlusion of a major bronchus. In contrast, with tumors that arise in the periphery of the lung, including many adenocarcarcinomas and large cell carcinomas, patients tend not to have symptoms related to bronchial involvement and often present solely with findings on a routinely obtained chest radiograph.

When tumors involve the pleural surface, either by direct extension or by metastatic spread, patients may have chest pain, often pleuritic in nature, or dyspnea resulting from substantial accumulation of pleural fluid. Other adjacent structures, particularly the heart and esophagus, can be involved by direct invasion or extrinsic compression by the tumor; resulting complications include pericardial effusion, arrhythmias, and dysphagia.

Symptoms Relating to Nodal and Distant Metastasis

When the mediastinum has metastatic lymph nodes from a primary lung cancer, symptoms often arise from invasion or compression of important structures within the mediastinum, such as the phrenic nerve, the recurrent laryngeal nerve, and the superior vena cava. As a consequence, patients may develop diaphragmatic paralysis (often with accompanying dyspnea), vocal cord paralysis (with hoarseness), or superior vena cava obstruction (with edema of the face and upper extremities resulting from obstruction to venous return), respectively.

Distant metastases, most commonly to brain, bone or bone marrow, liver, and adrenal gland(s), are frequently asymptomatic. In other cases, symptoms depend on the particular organ system involved. As we mentioned in Chapter 20, small cell carcinoma is the cell type most likely to generate distant metastases. Squamous cell carcinoma is least likely, and both adenocarcinoma and large cell carcinoma occupy an intermediate position.

Paraneoplastic Syndromes

Finally, many lung tumors are capable of producing clinical syndromes that are not readily attributable to the space-occupying nature of the tumor or to direct invasion of other structures or organs. These syndromes are sometimes called the "paraneoplastic" manifestations of malignancy and are frequently due to production of a hormone or a hormone-like substance by the tumor. When a detectable hormone is produced by the lung tumor (or, for that matter, by any type of tumor), the patient is said to have "ectopic" hormone production. Sometimes, clinical symptoms result from high circulating levels of the hormone; in other cases, only sensitive techniques of measurement are capable of demonstrating production of the hormone.

Why some tumors are capable of hormone production is not really clear. It has been hypothesized that genetic information coding for the particular hormone is present but not expressed in the normal, well-differentiated nonmalignant cell. In the course of becoming malignant, the cell undergoes a process of de-differentiation, during which it regains the ability to express this normally silent genetic material coding for hormone production.

The cell type most frequently associated with ectopic production of humoral substances is small cell carcinoma, presumably because of its theoretical origin from a cell type (the Kulchitsky cell) with secretory granules and the potential for peptide synthesis. Adrenocorticotropic hormone (ACTH) and antidiuretic hormone (ADH) have been the best described hormones produced by small cell carcinoma, potentially giving rise to the ectopic ACTH syndrome or to the syndrome of inappropriate ADH (SIADH), respectively. Additionally, squamous cell carcinoma is capable of causing hypercalcemia, initially thought to be due to production of a parathyroid hormone-like material but now felt to be due to other humoral substances. Production of other hormones, such as calcitonin and human chorionic gonadotropin (HCG), has also been well described with bronchogenic carcinoma.

Some of the other paraneoplastic syndromes cannot be attributed to a known hormone and their mechanism remains speculative. Examples range from a wide variety of neurologic syndromes to the soft tissue and bony manifestations of clubbing and hypertrophic osteoarthropathy (described in Chapter 3). The nonspecific systemic effects of malignancy, such as anorexia and weight loss, are certainly also potential consequences of lung cancer, and their pathogenesis also remains unknown.

DIAGNOSTIC APPROACH

A wide variety of diagnostic methods are utilized in evaluating the patient with known or suspected lung cancer. Many of the studies that assess the lung on a macroscopic level are used to demonstrate the presence, location, and possibility of spread of a bronchogenic carcinoma. Evaluation on a microscopic level is essential for defining the histologic type of lung cancer, which is an important factor in determining what modalities of therapy are most appropriate. Finally, functional assessment of the patient with lung cancer plays a role primarily in quantitating the severity of underlying lung disease, particularly chronic obstructive lung disease resulting from prior heavy smoking. Knowledge of a patient's functional limitation from lung disease is essential before the clinician can decide whether operative removal of a lung cancer is even feasible without converting the patient into a "respiratory cripple."

Macroscopic Evaluation

Probably the single most valuable test for the detection and macroscopic evaluation of bronchogenic carcinoma is the chest roentgenogram. The presence on chest roentgenogram of a nodule or mass within the lung always raises the question of lung cancer, especially when the patient has a heavy smoking history. As we discussed earlier, the location of the lesion may also give an indirect clue about the histology, since peripheral lesions are more likely to be large cell or adenocarcinoma, whereas central lesions are statistically more likely to be squamous or small cell carcinoma (Figs. 21–1 and 21–2). The chest radiograph is also most useful for determining whether there are additional suspicious lesions, such as a second primary tumor or metastatic spread from the original carcinoma. Involvement of hilar or mediastinal nodes or the pleura (with resulting pleural effusion) may be detected on the chest radiograph and will substantially affect the overall approach to therapy.

The relatively new radiographic technique of computed tomography or CT scanning also helps define the location, extent, and spread of tumor within the chest. Since this is a recent diagnostic technique, its overall usefulness in the evaluation of patients with bronchogenic

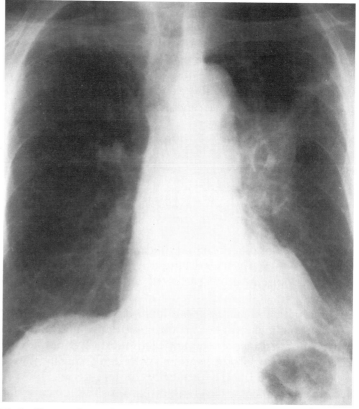

Figure 21–1. Chest radiograph showing a small cell carcinoma of the lung presenting as a left hilar mass.

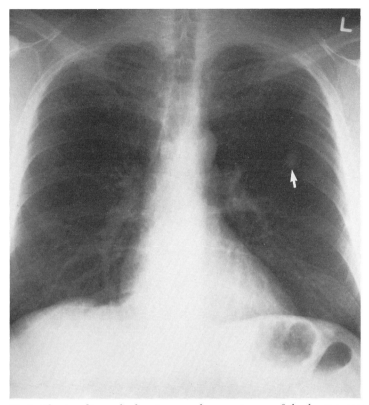

Figure 21–2. Chest radiograph showing an adenocarcinoma of the lung presenting as a solitary pulmonary nodule (arrow).

carcinoma is still being critically examined. However, one important application appears to be the detection of enlarged, potentially malignant lymph nodes within the mediastinum, which are often not seen by conventional radiography.

The best way to examine the airways of a patient with presumed or known bronchogenic carcinoma is via bronchoscopy, either with a rigid or, much more frequently, flexible bronchoscope (see Chapter 3). Not only can the location and intrabronchial extent of many tumors be directly observed, but one can obtain samples from the lesion, either for cytologic or histologic examination. These specimens can be obtained even when the lesion is beyond direct visualization with the bronchoscope. In addition, one can assess whether an intrabronchial carcinoma is impinging significantly on the bronchial lumen and causing either partial or complete airway occlusion.

Staging of Lung Cancer

Once a tumor has been documented, assessment of the extent and spread of the malignancy is often formally done by "staging." In the case of carcinoma of the lung, staging is based on (1) the primary intrathoracic tumor—its size, location, and local complications such as direct extension to adjacent structures or obstruction of the airway lumen; (2) the presence or absence of tumor within mediastinal lymph nodes; and (3) distant spread of tumor beyond the thorax to other tissues or organ systems.

Staging of lung cancer is based on:
1. size, location, and local complications of the primary tumor
2. mediastinal lymph node involvement
3. distant metastasis

The first aspect of staging, taking into account characteristics of the primary tumor itself, is generally done by a combination of chest radiography and bronchoscopy, sometimes with additional information obtained from computed tomographic scanning. The second aspect, based on involvement of mediastinal lymph nodes by tumor, is often initially assessed by CT scanning. Definitive evaluation is done by direct examination (and biopsy) of the nodes by either of two techniques, mediastinoscopy or mediastinotomy. In the procedure called suprasternal mediastinoscopy, the mediastinum is visualized with a scope placed through an incision made just above the sternal notch. The mediastinal nodes can be palpated, and biopsy specimens can be obtained if there is any suspicion that abnormal nodes are present. The other procedure, parasternal mediastinotomy, involves examining the mediastinum through a small incision made adjacent to the sternum. Biopsy of suspicious nodes can also be performed with this technique.

The third component of staging involves determining whether the tumor has disseminated to distant sites. Spread of a lung tumor to other organs is often documented initially with radioisotope scanning methods. For instance, metastatic disease in liver, bone, or brain can be demonstrated well with liver, bone, or brain scans, respectively. Computed tomography is also particularly suitable for detection of brain metastases.

Microscopic Evaluation

Evaluation of lung cancer on a microscopic level is crucial for establishing the specific cell type of the tumor. Some of the techniques used have already been mentioned briefly in Chapter 3. Specimens are obtained either for cytologic examination of abnormal cells shed from the tumor or for histologic examination of a biopsy specimen obtained directly from the lesion. Cytologic examination can be performed on sputum, on washings or brushings obtained through a bronchoscope, or on material aspirated from the tumor with a small gauge needle. Biopsy material can be obtained by passing a biopsy forceps through a bronchoscope, by using a cutting needle passed through the chest wall directly into the tumor, or by directly sampling tissue at the time of a surgical procedure. The staining techniques used for processing these materials are discussed in Chapter 3.

Functional Assessment

Assessment of pulmonary function helps determine whether surgical resection can be tolerated in the functionally compromised patient.

Functional assessment of the patient with lung cancer provides important information for guiding the clinician in the choice of treatment. As we will discuss in the following section on principles of therapy, surgery is usually the procedure of choice if staging techniques have shown that the disease is limited and approachable surgically. However, when surgery is performed, usually a lobe and sometimes even an entire lung may need to be removed. Because these patients are generally smokers, they are at high risk for having significant underlying chronic obstructive pulmonary disease, and they may not tolerate removal of a substantial amount of lung tissue. Useful studies for the clinician in evaluating these patients include pulmonary function tests, measurement of arterial blood gases, and sometimes additional tests to determine the relative amount of function contributed by the area of lung to be removed. Further specification of guidelines precluding surgery is beyond the scope of this discussion but may be found in references listed at the end of the chapter.

PRINCIPLES OF THERAPY

Though many advances have been made over the last two decades in the treatment of a variety of malignancies, patients with lung cancer have unfortunately not seen any significant improvement in their prognosis over the same period of time. The five-year survival of all patients with lung cancer has remained in the range of 8 to 10 percent, certainly a dismal overall outlook.

The three major forms of treatment available for lung cancer are surgery, radiation therapy, and chemotherapy. General guidelines for the clinician suggest when each modality may be most effective, but we still often do not know with certainty what therapy or combination of therapies will prove the most beneficial for a given patient. There appear to be two primary factors determining how a particular tumor should be treated—its staging (i.e., size, location, and extent of spread) and its cell type.

According to current practice for the treatment of bronchogenic carcinoma, surgery is the treatment of choice for localized tumors. When the tumor has extended directly to the pleura or chest wall, the diaphragm, or the mediastinum, it is usually considered unresectable, and alternative therapy is used. Similarly, when mediastinal nodes are involved, the tumor is generally considered unresectable. However, there are exceptions to this latter rule, particularly if the tumor is squamous cell carcinoma and the mediastinal nodes are on the same side as the tumor (i.e., the ipsilateral side). Finally, if there are metastases to distant tissues or organs, then surgery is not an appropriate form of therapy.

The cell type is an important consideration in deciding about management, since small cell carcinoma has a very high likelihood of already having metastasized by the time it is detected. Because of the early spread of small cell carcinoma, surgery is not considered the treatment of choice, unless the particular small cell tumor is a solitary peripheral nodule without any evidence of mediastinal or distant spread. In the more usual presentation of small cell carcinoma as a central mass, unresectable disease is virtually assured, and chemotherapy (with or without radiotherapy) is considered the primary mode of therapy.

When one of the non-small cell tumors is unresectable on the basis of any of the criteria mentioned earlier, then the clinician is faced with a choice of no treatment, radiotherapy, or chemotherapy. The final choice is often a very individual one, depending not only on the particular patient but also on the physician's preferences. In some cases, radiation therapy treatments are instituted early, in an attempt to shrink the tumor and delay local complications. In other circumstances, therapy is withheld until a complication ensues, such as bleeding or airway obstruction. Radiation treatments are then given with the goal of "palliation," or reducing the tumor size for temporary alleviation of the acute problem. Unfortunately, palliation is by definition not curative therapy, and further problems with the tumor are certain to develop.

As we mentioned earlier, the overall 5-year survival in patients with carcinoma of the lung is 10 percent or less. The patients who survive are ones whose disease was localized at presentation and amenable to surgical therapy. However, even among those who have potentially curative surgery, it is a minority who survive five years or more.

Table 21–1 summarizes many of the specific features about lung cancer that we have discussed throughout Chapters 20 and 21. Each of the major cell types is considered separately, with emphasis placed on clinical, radiographic, and therapeutic aspects of each category of tumor.

Table 21–1. LUNG CANCER: COMPARATIVE FEATURES

Cell Type	Frequency*	Location†	Radiographic Appearance‡	Spread	Treatment	Relative Prognosis§	Miscellaneous
Squamous cell	30–35%	Proximal endobronchial	1. Central mass 2. Obstructive atelectasis 3. Postobstructive pneumonia 4. Normal	Contiguous intrathoracic spread; nodal metastasis	Surgery or palliative therapy	Best	Hypercalcemia (occasional)
Small cell (including oat cell)	20%	Proximal, endobronchial (submucosal)	1. Central mass 2. Hilar, mediastinal adenopathy	Hilar, mediastinal nodes; distant metastasis	Chemotherapy (± radiation therapy)	Worst	Ectopic hormone production (ADH, ACTH) relatively common
Adenocarcinoma (including bronchioloalveolar cell)	35%	Peripheral	Solitary peripheral nodule or mass	Contiguous intrathoracic spread; nodal and distant metastasis	Surgery or palliative therapy	Intermediate	
Large cell	15–20	Variable	Variable; often large peripheral mass	Contiguous intrathoracic spread; nodal and distant metastasis	Surgery or palliative therapy	Intermediate	

*Approximate percent of all lung cancers.
†Most common location; for all cell types, variable locations are seen.
‡Common presentations on chest roentgenogram.
§For all cell types, the overall prognosis is generally poor.

BRONCHIAL CARCINOIDS

Bronchial carcinoid tumors have often been called *bronchial adenomas*, because they were thought to represent a benign or ade-nomatous form of neoplasm involving the bronchial tree. In fact, though many of these tumors have an excellent prognosis and are "cured" by surgical removal, it is probably more accurate to view them as low-grade malignancies. Overall, they constitute approximately 5 percent of primary lung tumors.

Bronchial carcinoids arise most commonly in relatively central airways of the tracheobronchial tree (see Fig. 3–8, which is from a patient with a bronchial carcinoid tumor). Though the cell of origin is not known with certainty, it is likely that these tumors arise from the neurosecretory Kulchitsky cells (K cells). It has even been suggested that bronchial carcinoids may represent a more benign variant of small cell carcinoma, which has also been considered by some pathologists to arise from the K cell. In some carcinoid tumors, the histology has "atypical" features more suggestive of frank malignancy; these tumors have a poorer overall prognosis than those without such features.

Two important epidemiologic features distinguish bronchial carci-noids from the other pulmonary neoplasms we have discussed. First, smoking does not appear to be a risk factor. Second, as a group, patients with bronchial carcinoids are younger than those with other pulmonary malignancies; frequently, young adults are the ones affected.

Common features of bronchial carcinoid tumors:
1. often found in young adults
2. hemoptysis
3. pneumonia distal to an obstructing endobronchial mass

Bronchial carcinoids often present with either an abnormal chest radiograph or episodes of hemoptysis or pneumonia distal to an obstructing airway tumor. Ectopic hormone production may also be found, probably relating to the presumed neurosecretory origin of the neoplastic cells.

The treatment of these tumors is surgical resection if at all possible. For many patients, the prognosis is excellent, and recurrent or distant disease is not a problem after surgical removal. However, metastatic disease is commonly found in patients whose tumors have "atypical" histology; the prognosis is certainly worse in this latter group of patients.

MALIGNANT MESOTHELIOMA

Unlike the other tumors discussed, *malignant mesothelioma* pri-marily involves the pleura rather than the airways or the pulmonary parenchyma. Like bronchial carcinoid tumors, it also is not associated with smoking as a risk factor. Although malignant mesothelioma is relatively uncommon, it is important at least partially because we can identify a specific etiologic factor in many of the cases.

The primary risk factor for development of malignant mesothelioma is a prior history of exposure to asbestos, generally in the range of 30 to 40 years earlier. Individuals who have worked in the types of jobs that expose them to asbestos (see Chapter 20) are obviously the ones at highest risk, but a heavy exposure is not necessary for predisposing to malignant mesothelioma. In fact, even wives of asbestos workers

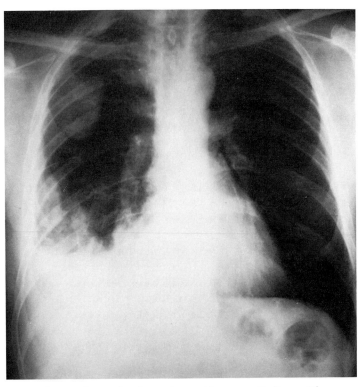

Figure 21–3. Chest radiograph of a patient with a mesothelioma. There are several lobulated, pleura-based masses in the right hemithorax accompanied by a right pleural effusion.

have been noted to develop mesothelioma, presumably because of inhalation of asbestos dust while cleaning their husbands' clothes.

The main symptoms developed by patients with malignant mesothelioma are chest pain and dyspnea; cough may also be present. Chest roentgenogram is usually most notable for the presence of fluid, and there is often irregular or lobulated thickening of the pleura (Fig. 21–3). Diagnosis requires biopsy of the pleura and histologic demonstration of the malignancy. Since the tumor originates in the pleura and does not directly communicate with airways, malignant cells are not shed into the tracheobronchial tree and cannot be found on cytologic examination of sputum.

Mesothelioma is suggested by pleural fluid, irregular or lobulated pleural thickening, and a distant history of asbestos exposure.

Unfortunately, the prognosis for malignant mesothelioma is quite poor. The tumor eventually entraps the lung and spreads to mediastinal structures. Death results, generally from respiratory failure. No clearly effective form of therapy is available, and less than 10 percent of patients survive three years.

THE SOLITARY PULMONARY NODULE

Though the solitary pulmonary nodule on chest radiograph is a common presentation of lung cancer, there is actually a broad differential diagnosis for this radiographic abnormality. The physician is therefore faced with judging the likelihood that a nodule is malignant and choosing the appropriate pathway for diagnosis and management. Since lung cancer presenting as a pulmonary nodule may be curable by surgical resection, it is undesirable to neglect management of such a lesion until it is no longer curable. On the other hand, to subject a patient to thoracotomy, a major surgical procedure, for removal of a benign lesion requiring no therapy is also undesirable.

The diagnostic possibilities for the solitary pulmonary nodule are presented in Table 21–2. Besides primary lung cancer, the major alternative diagnoses are benign pulmonary neoplasms, solitary metastases to the lung from a distant primary carcinoma, and infections (especially healed granulomatous lesions from tuberculosis or fungal disease). Estimating the likelihood of a malignant versus a benign lesion is based on two major factors:

1. Rate of growth. One of the most helpful pieces of information is an old chest radiograph. Comparison of old and new films shows whether a lesion is stable and gives an approximation of the rate of growth. Though it is difficult to say with certainty whether a lesion is benign or malignant based on the rate of growth, the absence of any increase in size over at least a two-year period is an extremely good indication that a lesion is benign.

The likelihood that a solitary pulmonary nodule is malignant can be assessed by: 1. stability or change in size of the lesion 2. presence or absence of calcification

2. Calcification. The presence of calcification within a pulmonary nodule, best demonstrated on either plain tomography or CT scanning, favors the diagnosis of a benign lesion, especially a granuloma or hamartoma. If certain patterns of calcification are found—diffuse speckling, dense calcification, laminated (onion-skin) calcification, or "popcorn" calcification—then the lesion is almost assuredly benign. On the other hand, a speck or an area of calcification at the periphery of a lesion does not rule out malignancy. This appearance is entirely consistent with a scar carcinoma arising in the region of an old, calcified parenchymal scar (such as an old calcified granuloma) and in fact raises the possibility of such a carcinoma.

Additional clinical features may be more suggestive of a benign versus a malignant lesion but are somewhat less reliable. In individuals less than 35 years old, primary lung cancer is an unlikely though certainly not unheard of diagnosis. The presence of a heavy smoking

Table 21–2. DIFFERENTIAL DIAGNOSIS OF THE SOLITARY PULMONARY NODULE

Neoplasms
    Malignant
        Primary lung cancer
        Solitary pulmonary metastasis from distant carcinoma
    ? Low-grade malignant
        Bronchial carcinoid (bronchial adenoma)
    Benign neoplasms
        Hamartoma
        Miscellaneous (fibroma, lipoma, etc.)
Infection
    Tuberculosis ("tuberculoma")
    Histoplasmosis ("histoplasmoma")
    Miscellaneous (e.g., hydatid cyst, dog heartworm)
Vascular abnormality
    Arteriovenous malformation

(and/or asbestos) history indicates a high risk for a malignant lesion; however, the absence of a smoking history does not by any means rule out the diagnosis of lung cancer, particularly a peripheral adenocarcinoma. Finally, the presence of a previously diagnosed distant carcinoma obviously raises the possibility that a lung nodule represents a metastatic focus of tumor.

The practical question of how to evaluate and manage these patients is often a difficult one, and the decision-making process must be individualized for each patient. A simple, non-invasive test such as sputum cytology is most helpful if positive; however, the yield is relatively low, even with peripheral nodules that are eventually proven to be carcinoma. More invasive procedures, such as percutaneous needle aspiration or biopsy and transbronchial biopsy (through a fiberoptic bronchoscope), are available and are frequently used to make a histologic diagnosis. However, in many cases a biopsy negative for malignancy does not obviate the need for surgery, since malignant cells may be missed by the limited sampling of a needle or biopsy forceps. Hence a commonly used approach with a lesion suspicious for carcinoma is to proceed directly with resection, assuming no contraindications to surgery and no clinical evidence that the lesion has spread elsewhere or has metastasized from a distant primary malignancy.

When lung cancer presents as a solitary peripheral nodule, the prognosis is much better than for the general group of patients with lung cancer. As a result of frequently curative surgical resection, approximately 50 percent of patients presenting with a solitary peripheral lung cancer survive 5 years, compared with the less than 10 percent 5-year survival of all lung cancer patients.

REFERENCES

Lung Cancer

Bone, R. C., and Balk, R.: Staging of bronchogenic carcinoma. Chest 82:473–480, 1982.

Cox, J. D., and Yesner, R. A.: Adenocarcinoma of the lung: recent results from the Veterans Administration Lung Group. Am. Rev. Respir. Dis. 120:1025–1029, 1979.

Fontana, R. S.: Early diagnosis of lung cancer. Am. Rev. Respir. Dis. 116:399–402, 1977.

Fontana, R. S.: Lung cancer and asbestos related pulmonary disease. Park Ridge, Ill., American College of Chest Physicians, 1981.

Frank, A. L.: The epidemiology and etiology of lung cancer. Clin. Chest Med. 3:219–228, 1982.

Greco, F. A., and Oldham, R. K.: Small-cell lung cancer. N. Engl. J. Med. 301:355–358, 1979.

Hande, K. R., and Des Prez, R. M.: Current perspectives in small cell lung cancer. Chest 85:669–677, 1984.

Hyde, L., and Hyde, C. I.: Clinical manifestations of lung cancer. Chest 65:299–306, 1974.

Loke, J., Matthay, R. A., and Ikeda, S.: Techniques for diagnosing lung cancer: a critical review. Clin. Chest Med. 3:321–329, 1982.

Merrill, W. W., and Bondy, P. K.: Production of biochemical marker substances by bronchogenic carcinomas. Clin. Chest Med. 3:307–320, 1982.

Mittman, C., and Bruderman, I.: Lung cancer: to operate or not? Am. Rev. Respir. Dis. 116:477–496, 1977.

Mountain, C. F.: Staging of lung cancer. Yale J. Biol. Med. 54:161–172, 1981.

Straus, M. J.: New developments in the treatment of advanced lung cancer. Am. Rev. Respir. Dis. 120:967–971, 1979.

Weiss, R. B.: Small-cell carcinoma of the lung: therapeutic management. Ann. Intern. Med. 88:522–531, 1978.

Woolner, L. B., et al.: Mayo Lung Project: evaluation of lung cancer screening through December 1979. Mayo Clin. Proc. 56:544–555, 1981.

Yesner, R., and Carter, D.: Pathology of carcinoma of the lung: changing patterns. Clin. Chest Med. 3:257–289, 1982.

Bronchial Carcinoids

Lawson, R. M., Ramanathan, L., Hurley, G., Hinson, K. W., and Lennox, S. C.: Bronchial adenoma: review of an 18-year experience at the Brompton Hospital. Thorax 31:245–253, 1976.
Marks, C., and Marks, M.: Bronchial adenoma: a clinicopathologic study. Chest 71:376–380, 1977.

Malignant Mesothelioma

Aisner, J., and Wiernik, P. H.: Malignant mesothelioma: current status and future prospects. Chest 74:438–444, 1978.
Antman, K. H.: Malignant mesothelioma. N. Engl. J. Med. 303:200–202, 1980.
Chahinian, A. P., Pajak, T. F., Holland, J. F., Norton, L., Ambinder, R. M., and Mandel, E. M.: Diffuse malignant mesothelioma. Ann. Intern. Med. 96(Part 1):746–755, 1982.
Legha, S. S., and Muggia, F. M.: Pleural mesothelioma: clinical features and therapeutic implications. Ann. Intern. Med. 87:613–621, 1977.

Solitary Pulmonary Nodule

Cortese, D. A.: Solitary pulmonary nodule: observe, operate, or what? Chest 81:662–664, 1982.
Godwin, J. D.: The solitary pulmonary nodule. Radiol. Clin. North Am. 21:709–721, 1983.
Lillington, G. A.: The solitary pulmonary nodule—1974. Am. Rev. Respir. Dis. 110:699–707, 1974.

22

Lung Defense Mechanisms

In the process of exchanging thousands of liters of air each day for oxygen uptake and carbon dioxide elimination, the lung is exposed to a wide variety of foreign substances transported with the inhaled air. Some of these are potentially injurious; others are relatively harmless. Inhaled air is not the only source of foreign material; secretions from the mouth and pharynx are also frequently aspirated into the tracheobronchial tree, even in normal individuals. This myriad of foreign substances is perhaps best classified into three major categories—small particulate material, noxious gases, and microorganisms. Since the oropharynx is rich with bacteria, aspirated secretions are particularly important as a source of unwanted bacteria entering the airways.

To protect itself against potentially toxic inhaled material, the respiratory system has evolved a complex protective mechanism that can be dissected into a number of different components. Each component appears to have a distinct role, but there is a tremendous degree of interaction and "cooperation" between different components. That the distal lung parenchyma is normally sterile serves as testimony to the effectiveness of the defense system. However, the protective mechanisms can break down, either as a result of certain diseases or frequently as a consequence of treatment, especially medication, that we administer to patients.

Before we discuss infectious disorders of the respiratory system in Chapter 23, it is appropriate to consider first how the lung protects itself against the variety of infectious agents to which it is exposed. Though we will focus on protective mechanisms against infection, we will also mention defenses against noninfectious substances, especially inhaled particulate material. The major categories of defense mechanisms to be discussed include (1) physical or anatomic factors relating to deposition and clearance of inhaled material; (2) phagocytic and inflammatory cells that interact with the inhaled material; and (3) immune responses, which depend upon prior exposure to and recognition of the foreign material. Finally, we will conclude this chapter with a discussion of several ways that the system breaks down, resulting in an inability to handle microorganisms and an increased risk of developing certain types of respiratory tract infection.

PHYSICAL OR ANATOMIC FACTORS

The pathway from the mouth or nose down to the lung parenchyma requires that inhaled air traverse a series of progressively branching airways. Hence, it is possible for inhaled particulate material to be deposited at various points in the airway, never reaching the most distal region of lung, the alveolar spaces. Particle size is an important determinant of deposition along the airway and thus affects the likelihood of a particle's reaching the distal parenchyma. When an inhaled particle is greater than 10 microns in diameter, it is likely to settle high in the upper airway, e.g., in the nose. For particles 5 to 10 microns in diameter, settling tends to occur somewhat lower, in the trachea or the conducting airways but not down to the level of the small airways and alveoli. The particles most likely to reach the distal lung parenchyma range in size from 0.5 to 5 microns. Unfortunately, many bacteria fall within this size range, so that deposition along the airway is not very effective for excluding bacteria from the lower respiratory tract. However, large particles of dust and other inhaled material are effectively excluded from the distal lung parenchyma by virtue of their size.

Factors affecting deposition and physical clearance of particles:
1. particle size
2. cough
3. mucociliary transport

When particles are deposited in the trachea or bronchi, two major processes, cough and mucociliary transport, are responsible for physical removal of these particles from the airways. Cough is certainly an important protective mechanism, often triggered by stimulation of airway irritant receptors that are activated by inhaled or aspirated foreign material. The rapid acceleration and high flow rates of air achieved by a cough are often effective in clearing irritating foreign material from the airways.

The term *mucociliary transport* or *mucociliary clearance* refers to a process of waves of beating cilia moving a blanket of mucus (and any trapped material within the mucus) progressively upward along the tracheobronchial tree. From the trachea down to the respiratory bronchioles, the most superficial layer of epithelial cells lining the airway has cilia projecting into the airway lumen. These cilia have a

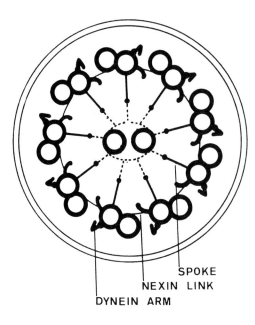

SPOKE
NEXIN LINK
DYNEIN ARM

Figure 22–1. Schematic diagram of the cross-section of a cilium; the two central microtubules and nine pairs of peripheral microtubules are shown. A dynein arm projects from each peripheral doublet, while nexin limbs and radial spokes provide connections within the microtubular structure. (From Eliasson, R., Mossberg, B., Camner, P., and Afzelius, B. A.: N. Engl. J. Med. 297:1–6, 1977. Reproduced with permission.)

structure identical to that of cilia found elsewhere in the body, consisting of longitudinal microtubules arranged in a characteristic way. Specifically, a cross-sectional view of cilia shows two central microtubules, surrounded with 9 pairs of microtubules arranged around the periphery (Fig. 22–1). Small projecting sidearms from each doublet, called dynein arms, are believed to be crucial to the contractile function of the microtubules and hence to the beating of the cilia.

Strikingly, the movement of cilia on a particular cell and the movement between cells are quite coordinated, producing actual "waves" of ciliary motion. How such a pattern of ciliary motion is coordinated from cell to cell or even within the same cell has remained a mystery. What this wavelike motion accomplishes is movement of the overlying mucus layer in a cephalad direction (i.e., from distal to more proximal parts of the tracheobronchial tree), at a speed in the trachea estimated between 6 and 20 mm per minute. If inhaled particles are trapped in the mucous layer, they too are transported upward and eventually either expectorated or swallowed.

There are actually two layers comprising the mucous blanket bathing the epithelial cells. Directly adjacent to the cells is the *sol* layer, within which the cilia are located. Superficial to the sol layer is the more viscous *gel* layer, which is produced by both submucosal mucous glands and goblet cells. In contrast, the origin of the periciliary sol layer is unknown. One can picture the viscous gel layer floating on top of the sol layer and being propelled upward as the cilia are able to beat more freely within the less viscous sol layer.

PHAGOCYTIC AND INFLAMMATORY CELLS

Pulmonary Alveolar Macrophages

Both in the airways and at the level of the alveoli, particles and bacteria can be scavenged by a type of phagocytic cell known as the *pulmonary alveolar macrophage*. This cell is probably the major form of defense against material that has escaped deposition in the upper airway and has reached the lower airway or the alveolar structures. Macrophages also interact and cooperate closely with other parts of the lung's defense system. Their ability to process antigenic material appears to be important for the later immunologic defense provided by lymphocytes. In addition, certain types of antibodies, as we will describe below, are important for enabling macrophages to ingest and kill foreign material.

Alveolar macrophages, which are large cells approximately 15 to 50 microns in diameter, are descendants of circulating monocytes derived from the bone marrow. Their cytoplasm contains a variety of granules of various shapes and sizes, many of which are "packages" of digestive enzymes that can dispose of ingested foreign material.

Phagocytosis

When a macrophage is exposed to inhaled particles or bacteria, attachment of the foreign material to the surface of the macrophage is the first step in the processing sequence. The particles or bacteria are then engulfed within the plasma membrane, which invaginates and pinches off within the cell to form a cytoplasmic phagosome containing the now isolated foreign material. In some circumstances, this sequence of attachment and phagocytosis is facilitated by the presence of *opsonins* coating the foreign material. Opsonins are defined as proteins that bind to extracellular materials and make them more adherent to phagocytic cells and more amenable to engulfment or ingestion. Opsonins can be specific for the particular foreign substance, such as antibodies directed against antigenic material, or they may demonstrate nonspecific binding to a variety of substances. Particularly important specific opsonins are antibodies of the IgG class directed against antigenic foreign material, either bacteria or other antigenic particles. These opsonins greatly promote attachment to and ingestion by macrophages.

Once bacteria or other foreign material is isolated within phagosomes, a process of intracellular digestion takes place within the macrophage. Often the phagosomes combine with lysosomes, forming phagolysosomes, in which proteolytic enzymes supplied by the lysosome digest, detoxify, or destroy the phagosomal contents. In addition to lysosomal enzymes, there are a variety of oxidation products, such as hydrogen peroxide and other intermediate products of oxidative metabolism, that are toxic to bacteria and may play a role in the ability of the macrophage to kill ingested microorganisms.

The macrophage does not always kill or totally eliminate inhaled foreign material to which it is exposed. In some cases, such as with inhaled silica particles, the ingested material is toxic to the macrophage and may eventually kill the cell. In other cases, ingested material is inert but essentially indigestible and may persist indefinitely in the form of an indigestible residue. Finally, in some cases, intracellular processing of antigenic material by macrophages is a crucial preliminary step necessary for further steps in the immune process provided by lymphocytes. Additional discussion of this macrophage-lymphocyte cooperation is beyond the scope of this discussion but can be found in more detailed references listed at the end of this chapter.

Polymorphonuclear Leukocytes (PMN's)

Another important cell type involved in pulmonary defense is the polymorphonuclear leukocyte, or PMN. This cell is a particularly important component of the defense mechanism for an established bacterial infection of the lower respiratory tract. Normally, there are few PMN's that reside in the small airways and alveoli. When bacteria have overwhelmed the initial defense mechanisms that we have already discussed, they may replicate within alveolar spaces, causing a bacterial pneumonia. If we examine the histologic features of a bacterial pneumonitis, we find that a prominent component of the inflammatory response is an outpouring of PMN's into the alveolar spaces. These cells are probably attracted to the lung by a variety of stimuli, particularly products of complement activation and chemotactic factors released by alveolar macrophages. Once PMN's are involved, they play a crucial role in phagocytosis and killing of the population of invading and proliferating bacteria.

IMMUNE RESPONSES

A third major category of defense mechanisms for the respiratory system is the immune response, which involves recognizing and responding to specific antigenic material. Bacteria, viruses, and other microorganisms are perhaps the most important antigens to which the respiratory tract is repetitively exposed. Presumably, immune defense mechanisms are particularly important in protecting the individual against these agents.

We will first briefly describe the two major components of the immune system—the humoral or B-lymphocyte and the cellular or T-lymphocyte related systems. Humoral immunity involves the activation of B-lymphocytes (which do not require the thymus for differentiation) and the production of antibodies by plasma cells (which are derived from B-lymphocytes). In contrast, cellular immunity refers to the activation of T-lymphocytes (which depend upon the thymus for their differentiation) and the execution of certain specific T-lymphocyte functions, including the production of soluble mediators or lymphokines. The two lymphocyte systems are certainly not entirely independent of each other; in particular, T-lymphocytes appear to have an important role in regulating immunoglobulin or antibody synthesis by the humoral immune system.

Both humoral and cellular immunity are important in the protection of the respiratory system against microorganisms. For certain infectious agents, humoral immunity is the primary mode of protection; for other agents, cellular immunity appears to be paramount. In the lung as well as in the blood, T-lymphocytes are more numerous than their B-lymphocyte counterparts, but both systems are essential for effective defense against the wide spectrum of potentially harmful microorganisms.

Lymphocytes can be found in many locations within the respiratory tract, extending from the nasopharynx down to distal regions of the lung parenchyma. True lymph nodes are present around the trachea, the carina, and at the hilum of each lung, in the region of the mainstem bronchi. These lymph nodes receive the lymphatic drainage from most of the airways and lung parenchyma. There is also lymphoid tissue in the nasopharynx, and collections of lymphocytes arranged in nodules are found as well along medium to large bronchi. These latter collections have been termed bronchus-associated lymphoid tissue, or BALT, and may be responsible for intercepting and handling antigens deposited along the conducting airways. Smaller aggregates of lymphocytes can be found in more distal airways and even scattered throughout the pulmonary parenchyma.

Humoral Immune Mechanisms

Humoral immunity in the respiratory tract appears in the form of two major classes of immunoglobulins—IgA and IgG. Antibodies of the IgA class are particularly important in the nasopharynx and upper airways, where they constitute the primary antibody type. The form of IgA present in these areas is secretory IgA, which includes a pair of IgA molecules (joined by a polypeptide) plus an extra glycoprotein component termed the secretory component. Secretory IgA appears to be synthesized locally, and the quantities of IgA are much greater in the respiratory tract than in the serum.

Major components of the immune system operative in the respiratory tract:
1. T-lymphocytes
2. B-lymphocytes
3. IgA
4. IgG

There is evidence to suggest that secretory IgA plays a role as part of the respiratory defense system. In particular, it has been suggested that by virtue of its ability to bind to antigens, IgA may bind to viruses and bacteria, preventing their attachment to epithelial cells. In addition, IgA is efficient in agglutinating microorganisms; the agglutinated microbes might then be more easily cleared by the mucociliary transport system. Finally, IgA appears to have the ability to neutralize a wide variety of respiratory viruses as well as some bacteria.

In contrast to IgA, IgG is particularly abundant within the lower respiratory tract. It is also synthesized locally to a large extent, though a fraction also originates from serum IgG. It has a number of biologic properties—agglutinating particles, neutralizing viruses and bacterial toxins, serving as an opsonin for macrophage handling of bacteria, activating complement, and causing lysis of gram-negative bacteria in the presence of complement.

As best as we can currently tell, the overall role of the humoral immune system in respiratory defenses includes protecting the lung against a variety of bacterial and, to some extent, viral infections. In another section of this chapter, we will discuss the clinical implications of this role and the consequences of impairment in the humoral immune system.

Cellular Immune Mechanisms

Cellular immune mechanisms, those mediated by thymus-dependent or T-lymphocytes, also operate as part of the lung's overall defense system. Sensitized T-lymphocytes produce a variety of soluble, biologically active mediators called lymphokines, some of which have the ability to attract or activate other protective cell types, such as macrophages and PMN's. T-lymphocytes also are capable of interacting with the humoral immune system and modifying antibody production. The place of these actions in overall respiratory defense mechanisms is not really clear. An important but certainly not exclusive role for the cellular immune system is to protect against bacteria that have a pattern of intracellular growth, especially *Mycobacterium tuberculosis* (see the discussion of tuberculosis in Chapter 24).

FAILURE OF RESPIRATORY DEFENSE MECHANISMS

For each of the three major categories of respiratory defense mechanisms, clinically important deficiencies have now been recognized. As a result, respiratory infections may ensue, and analysis of the specific types of infections associated with each type of defect is both extremely informative and useful clinically.

Impairment of Mucociliary Clearance

Impaired mucociliary clearance is caused by
1. immotile cilia syndrome
2. viral respiratory tract infection
3. cigarette smoking
4. high concentrations of O_2 for prolonged periods

Within the category of physical and anatomic factors affecting deposition and clearance of particles, both genetic abnormalities and environmental factors may alter the normal process of particle clearance by the mucociliary transport system. Especially interesting information has been provided by a genetic abnormality termed the *immotile cilia syndrome*. In this disorder, a defect in ciliary structure and function leads to absent or impaired ciliary motility and hence to ineffective mucociliary clearance. Though several different types of defects have now been recognized, the most common is absence of dynein arms on the microtubules. Clinically, the impairment in mucociliary clearance is associated with chronic bronchitis and bronchiectasis. In males, the sperm tail, which has a similar structure to that of cilia, is also abnormal, resulting in poor sperm motility and infertility. As we mentioned in Chapter 7, the disorder called Kartagener's syndrome, consisting of a triad of chronic sinusitis, bronchiectasis, and situs inversus, is a variant of the immotile cilia syndrome, and all of the clinical manifestations are believed to be secondary to the disturbance in ciliary motility.

Viral respiratory tract infections frequently cause temporary structural damage to the tracheobronchial mucosa. Functionally, the alteration of the mucosa is associated with impaired mucociliary clearance, which may retard the transport of invading bacteria out of the tracheobronchial tree. As we will discuss later, this is but one mechanism by which viral respiratory tract infections predispose to complicating bacterial superinfections.

Environmental factors may also cause impairment of mucociliary clearance. Exposure to cigarette smoke is certainly the most important clinically and probably contributes to the predisposition of heavy smokers to develop recurrent respiratory tract infections. Some atmospheric pollutants, such as sulfur dioxide (SO_2), nitrogen dioxide (NO_2), and ozone (O_3), appear to depress mucociliary clearance, but the clinical consequences are not entirely clear. High concentrations of oxygen, such as 90 to 100 percent, inhaled for more than several hours also appear to be associated with impaired mucociliary function; here the consequences are obviously limited to patients with respiratory failure requiring these extremely high concentrations.

Impairment of Phagocytic and Inflammatory Cells

Clinical problems can be seen with deficiencies in number or function of the two major phagocytic and inflammatory cell types that we discussed—alveolar macrophages and polymorphonuclear leukocytes. One of the more important ways that macrophage function can be impaired is by viral respiratory tract infections. These infections may paralyze the ability of the macrophage to kill bacteria, an additional reason why patients with viral infections are more susceptible to getting superimposed bacterial bronchitis or pneumonia.

Problems with macrophage function result from
1. viral respiratory tract infections
2. cigarette smoking
3. alcoholism
4. starvation
5. cold exposure
6. hypoxia
7. corticosteroid therapy

Cigarette smoking also depresses the ability of alveolar macrophages to take up and kill bacteria. Hypoxia, starvation, alcoholism, and cold exposure similarly appear to be conditions in which impaired bacterial killing is at least partly due to depressed macrophage function. Treatment with corticosteroids, given for a myriad of diseases, seems to alter migration and function of macrophages, which may compound additional adverse effects of steroids on lymphocytes and the immune system.

Polymorphonuclear leukocytes are depressed in number in several clinical circumstances, generally as a result of an underlying disease of the bone marrow, such as leukemia, or as a result of treatment we administer. Chemotherapeutic agents used to treat malignancy commonly destroy rapidly proliferating cells of the bone marrow, resulting in a temporary loss of PMN precursors and a marked depression in the number of circulating PMN's. When PMN's are present at less than 1000 per mm^3 of blood, the risk of bacterial infection begins to rise, becoming particularly marked when the count drops below 500 per mm^3.

Causes of decreased numbers of polymorphonuclear leukocytes:
1. bone marrow replacement by tumor
2. cancer chemotherapeutic agents

Defects in Immune System

Finally, the immune system is subject to defects in function affecting both its humoral and cellular arms. Deficiencies in the humoral immune system, such as decreased or absent immunoglobulin production (i.e., hypo- or agammaglobulinemia), are associated with recurrent bacterial respiratory infections, often leading to bronchiectasis. Cellular immunity is disturbed perhaps most frequently by treatment with corticosteroids or cytotoxic drugs and in some well-defined disease states, such as Hodgkin's disease and the acquired immunodeficiency syndrome (AIDS). Unlike most other deficits in respiratory defenses, problems with cell-mediated immunity may lead to infection with a special group of microorganisms—intracellular bacteria (especially *Mycobacterium tuberculosis*), fungi, and certain types of protozoa—that rarely affect individuals with normal cellular immunity.

Causes of immune deficiency:
1. humoral—decreased or absent immunoglobulins
2. cellular—corticosteroids, cytotoxic drugs, Hodgkin's disease, AIDS

In summary, the defense mechanisms available to protect the respiratory tract from invading microorganisms are varied and complex. Unfortunately, we as individuals are capable of thwarting these defenses by exposing ourselves to such damaging influences as cigarette smoke and ethanol. Just as importantly, we as physicians often treat our patients with agents that disrupt the defense mechanisms, making it incumbent upon us to beware of potential infectious complications of our therapy.

In the clinical setting, deficiencies in immunoglobulins and in PMN's are strongly associated with an increased risk of bacterial infections. Though problems with mucociliary clearance and with macrophage function are somewhat less well defined in terms of the specific infectious risk, bacterial infections also appear to be prominent in these settings. In contrast, disturbances in cellular immunity are characterized by an increased risk of a different subset of infections— especially tuberculosis and infections due to certain fungi and protozoans.

Because of the frequency and serious nature of respiratory infections in immunosuppressed patients, we will conclude this chapter with a brief consideration of the problems posed by the immunocompromised patient with pulmonary infiltrates. More detailed discussions can be found in several excellent review articles listed in the references at the end of this chapter.

THE IMMUNOSUPPRESSED PATIENT WITH PULMONARY INFILTRATES

Over the past 10 to 15 years, physicians have been faced with increasing numbers of patients who have impaired host defense mechanisms, particularly granulocytopenia (decreased PMN's) and depressed cellular immunity; these occur frequently as a result of chemotherapy given for malignancy. Within the past few years, an entirely new population of individuals at risk for opportunistic infections has emerged. These patients have the *acquired immunodeficiency syndrome (AIDS)*, with its devastating consequences on the cellular immune system.

Immunocompromised patients are extremely susceptible to development of respiratory tract infections with a variety of organisms, some of which rarely cause disease in the immunocompetent host. When the immunosuppressed patient presents with fever and new pulmonary infiltrates, the possibility of an "opportunistic" infection comes to mind immediately. However, patients with malignancy are also susceptible to noninfectious complications of their tumor or its treatment; such complications must also be seriously considered in the differential diagnosis.

The wide spectrum of infectious and noninfectious etiologies of pulmonary infiltrates in the immunosuppressed host is shown in Table 22–1. Even though we commonly think of fungi and protozoa as the major causes of infiltrates in patients receiving treatment for malignancy, bacterial pneumonia is actually the most frequent problem in this setting. Granulocytopenia is the primary predisposing factor for bacterial pneumonias, which are frequently due to gram-negative rods or to *Staphylococcus*.

Other bacteria, namely mycobacteria (*Mycobacterium tuberculosis* or atypical mycobacteria) and *Nocardia* cause problems mainly in the

Table 22–1. CAUSES OF PULMONARY INFILTRATES IN THE IMMUNOCOMPROMISED HOST

Infections
    Bacteria
        Gram-positive cocci, especially *Staphylococcus*
        Gram-negative bacilli
        Mycobacterium tuberculosis
        Atypical mycobacteria
        Nocardia
    Viruses
        Cytomegalovirus (CMV)
        Herpes virus
    Fungi
        Aspergillus
        Cryptococcus
        Candida
        Mucor
    Protozoa
        Pneumocystis carinii
        Toxoplasma gondii
Pulmonary effects of therapy
    Chemotherapeutic agents
    Radiation therapy
Pulmonary hemorrhage
Congestive heart failure
Disseminated malignancy
Nonspecific interstitial pneumonitis (no defined etiology)

patient with impaired cellular immunity. Defective cellular immunity also predisposes to infections with certain protozoa (especially *Pneumocystis carinii*), fungi, and viruses. The fungus *Aspergillus*, which causes an invasive pneumonia in the immunosuppressed patient, seems to be most commonly found in the patient who is neutropenic (and also has impaired cellular immunity) from cytotoxic chemotherapy.

Common noninfectious diagnoses are interstitial lung disease complicating radiation therapy or a variety of chemotherapeutic agents (see Chapter 10). However, congestive heart failure (often secondary to cardiac toxicity from chemotherapeutic agents), pulmonary dissemination of the underlying malignancy, and hemorrhage into the pulmonary parenchyma are also additional causes of infiltrates that can closely mimic infectious etiologies. In many circumstances, an interstitial inflammatory process can be proved histologically, but no definite etiology can be identified. These cases are often diagnosed as nonspecific interstitial pneumonitis, with the realization that neither the pathology nor the clinical history provides clues to an etiologic diagnosis.

The approach to the immunocompromised patient with pulmonary infiltrates revolves around trying to identify an infectious agent by examination of sputum or bronchial washings or brushings obtained by bronchoscopy. Frequently, a diagnosis is made by histologic examination of lung tissue obtained by transbronchial or open lung biopsy. The particular procedure chosen is based on specific clinical features relevant to each patient, such as the nature of the underlying disease, the suspected cause of the pulmonary infiltrate, the presence or absence of other predisposing factors, and the potential risks of a diagnostic procedure. Alternatively, it is common for patients to be treated empirically, particularly when they are at high risk for invasive procedures or when a specific diagnosis appears to be fairly certain.

Acquired Immunodeficiency Syndrome

Before concluding this brief discussion of the immunocompromised host, we will consider a few aspects of the acquired immunodeficiency syndrome (AIDS), since it has emerged as such an important public health problem over the past few years. This recently recognized syndrome has been best described in homosexual men, but it has also been seen in a few other selected groups of individuals, such as intravenous drug users and patients with hemophilia (receiving frequent blood products). Identifying the cause of this syndrome is currently under active and intense investigation; recent evidence suggests a form of retrovirus known as HTLV-III (human T-cell lymphotropic virus type III). Clinically, patients with AIDS have a form of impairment of their cell-mediated immune system, characterized by decreased numbers of circulating T-lymphocytes and an abnormal distribution of subsets of T-lymphocytes. Specifically, such patients exhibit a deficiency in "helper" T-cells and thus a decrease in the proportion of "helper" relative to "suppressor" T-cells.

In AIDS, a deficiency of helper T-lymphocytes and a decrease in the helper:suppressor T-cell ratio is most likely due to a retrovirus.

The most common opportunistic pathogen in these patients has been the protozoan *Pneumocystis carinii*, but they also can develop a number of other unusual infections. A relatively unusual form of malignancy, Kaposi's sarcoma, has also been well described in these patients.

Major complications of AIDS include infection and Kaposi's sarcoma.

So far, the prognosis for patients with this syndrome has been dismal, with almost all patients dying from either opportunistic infection or malignancy within two years. However, because of the amount of interest and active investigation that this syndrome has generated, there is optimism that prevention and/or management may be feasible within the next decade.

AUGMENTATION OF RESPIRATORY DEFENSE MECHANISMS

Rather than leave this chapter with the negative side of what physicians and disease can do to impair normal lung defense mechanisms, we should keep in mind that progress has also been made in augmenting defense mechanisms and protecting against some forms of respiratory tract infection. Immunization against certain respiratory pathogens has induced production of antibodies against the organisms and has conferred either relative or complete protection against infection by these microbes. Perhaps the most notable examples are immunization against the bacteria causing pertussis (whooping cough) and more recently immunization against influenza virus and many subtypes of the common bacterium *Streptococcus pneumoniae* (pneumococcus). We look to the future for additional vaccines that will enhance immunity against other respiratory pathogens and allow us to approach these infections more from a preventive standpoint.

REFERENCES

Lung Defense Mechanisms

Green, G. M., Jakab, G. J., Low, R. B., and Davis, G. S.: Defense mechanisms of the respiratory membrane. Am. Rev. Respir. Dis. 115:479–514, 1977.

Hocking, W. G., and Golde, D. W.: The pulmonary-alveolar macrophage. N. Engl. J. Med. 301:580–587; 639–645, 1979.

Kaltreider, H. B.: Expression of immune mechanisms in the lung. Am. Rev. Respir. Dis. 113:347–379, 1976.

Lauweryns, J. M., and Baert, J. H.: Alveolar clearance and the role of the pulmonary lymphatics. Am. Rev. Respir. Dis. 115:625–683, 1977.

Newhouse, M., Sanchis, J., and Bienenstock, J.: Lung defense mechanisms. N. Engl. J. Med. 295:990–998; 1045–1052, 1976.

Pulmonary Disease Associated With Impaired Defense Mechanisms

Dukes, R. J., Rosenow, E. C., III, and Hermans, P. E.: Pulmonary manifestations of hypogammaglobulinemia. Thorax 33:603–607, 1978.

Eliasson, R., Mossberg, B., Camner, P., and Afzelius, B. A.: The immotile cilia syndrome. N. Engl. J. Med. 297:1–6, 1977.

Fanta, C. H., and Pennington, J. E.: Fever and new lung infiltrates in the immunocompromised host. Clin. Chest Med. 2:19–39, 1981.

Murray, J. F., et al.: Pulmonary complications of the acquired immunodeficiency syndrome. N. Engl. J. Med. 310:1682–1688, 1984.

Williams, D. M., Krick, J. A., and Remington, J. S.: Pulmonary infection in the compromised host. Am. Rev. Respir. Dis. 114:359–394; 593–627, 1976.

23

Pneumonia

By any of several criteria, pneumonia, or infection of the pulmonary parenchyma, must be considered one of the most important categories of disease affecting the respiratory system. First of all, it is extraordinarily common, accounting for nearly 10 percent of admissions to many large general hospitals. Overall, it has been estimated that more than a million cases of bacterial pneumonia alone occur in the United States each year. Secondly, it is an important cause of death; more precisely, over 50,000 Americans die of bacterial pneumonia each year, making it the fifth most common cause of death in the nation. It is no wonder that Sir William Osler referred to pneumonia as "the captain of the men of death," particularly when speaking before the era of effective antibiotic therapy. Finally, for many types of pneumonia, medical therapy with antibiotics (along with supportive care) has an extraordinary impact on the duration and outcome of the illness. Because of the effect of treatment, the diseases discussed in this chapter (as well as tuberculosis, which is discussed in the next chapter) are particularly gratifying to treat for all involved medical personnel.

Though we will certainly consider many of the specific agents causing pneumonia, this chapter will be organized primarily as a general discussion of the problem of pneumonia. When appropriate, we will focus on individual etiologic agents in order to outline some of the characteristic features of each that are particularly useful to the physician.

ETIOLOGY AND PATHOGENESIS

As we discussed in Chapter 22, the host defenses of the lung are constantly challenged by a variety of organisms, both viruses and bacteria. Viruses in particular are likely to avoid or overwhelm some of the defenses of the upper respiratory tract, causing a transient, relatively mild clinical illness with symptoms limited to the upper respiratory tract. When host defense mechanisms of the upper and lower respiratory tracts are overwhelmed, microorganisms may establish residence, proliferate, and cause a frank infectious process within the pulmonary parenchyma. With particularly virulent organisms, there need not be any major impairment of host defense mechanisms, and pneumonia may be seen even in essentially normal individuals. At the other extreme, if host defense mechanisms are quite impaired, microorganisms that are not particularly virulent, i.e., ones that are unlikely to cause disease in a normal host, may produce a life-threatening pneumonia.

In practice, there are several factors that frequently cause enough impairment of host defenses to contribute to the development of pneumonia, even though we do not usually consider individuals with such impairment to be "immunosuppressed." Viral upper respiratory tract infections, ethanol abuse, cigarette smoking, and pre-existing chronic obstructive pulmonary disease are just a few of these contributing factors. More severe impairment of host defenses is caused by various underlying malignancies, particularly leukemia and lymphoma, and by the use of corticosteroids and cytotoxic drugs. In these cases, individuals are susceptible both to bacterial and to more unusual nonbacterial infections, which will be covered in subsequent chapters.

Contributing factors for pneumonia in the immunocompetent host:
1. viral upper respiratory tract infection
2. ethanol abuse
3. cigarette smoking
4. chronic obstructive pulmonary disease

There are two major ways that microorganisms, especially bacteria, find their way to the lower respiratory tract. The first is inhalation, whereby organisms are usually carried in small droplet particles that are inhaled into the tracheobronchial tree. The other mechanism is aspiration, by which secretions from the oropharynx pass through the larynx and into the tracheobronchial tree. We usually think of aspiration as a process occurring in individuals unable to protect their airway from secretions by glottic closure and coughing. Although it is true that clinically significant aspiration is more likely in individuals unable to protect their airway, it is also true that all of us are subject to aspirating small amounts of oropharyngeal secretions, particularly while sleeping. Fortunately, our defense mechanisms seem able to cope with this nightly onslaught of bacteria, and we do not experience frequent bouts of aspiration pneumonia.

Less commonly, bacteria may reach the pulmonary parenchyma through the bloodstream rather than the airways. This route is an important one for the spread of certain organisms, particularly *Staphylococcus*. With such spread, i.e., bacteremia, the implication is either that a distant, primary source of bacterial infection is present or that bacteria were introduced directly into the bloodstream, e.g., as a consequence of intravenous drug abuse.

Many individual infectious agents are associated with the development of pneumonia. The frequency with which individual agents are responsible for pneumonia is quite difficult to assess and depends to a large extent on the specific population studied. The largest single category of such agents is probably bacteria; the other two major categories are viruses and mycoplasma. Of the bacteria, the organism most frequently associated with pneumonia is *Streptococcus pneumoniae*, in common parlance often called the pneumococcus. It has been estimated that more than half of all pneumonias in the adult serious enough to require hospitalization are pneumococcal in origin.

Streptococcus pneumoniae (pneumococcus) is the most common cause of bacterial pneumonia; the polysaccharide capsule is an important factor in its virulence.

Bacteria

Streptococcus pneumoniae, a normal inhabitant of the oropharynx in a large proportion of adults, is a gram-positive coccus seen in pairs or diplococci. Pneumococcal pneumonia is commonly acquired in the community, i.e., in nonhospitalized patients, and frequently occurs after a viral upper respiratory tract infection. The organism has a polysaccharide capsule, which protects the bacteria from phagocytosis and is therefore an important factor in its virulence. There are many antigenic types of capsular polysaccharide; in order for host defense cells to phagocytize the organism, antibody against the particular capsular type must be present. As discussed in Chapter 22, antibodies contributing in this way to the phagocytic process are called opsonins.

Staphylococcus aureus is another gram-positive coccus, usually appearing in clusters when examined microscopically. There are three major settings in which this organism is seen as a cause of pneumonia: (1) as a secondary complication of respiratory tract infection with the influenza virus; (2) in the hospitalized patient, who often has some impairment of host defense mechanisms, and whose oropharynx has been colonized by *Staphylococcus*; and (3) as a complication of widespread dissemination of staphylococcal organisms through the bloodstream.

A wide variety of gram-negative organisms, normally considered inhabitants of the gastrointestinal tract, are potential causes of pneumonia. In the normal nonhospitalized individual, these organisms are not an important cause of pneumonia. In hospitalized patients with a variety of underlying diseases or in those who have received antibiotics, however, these organisms may take up residence in the oropharynx. From this point they have access to the lower respiratory tract, presumably when secretions are aspirated, and can be responsible for initiating pneumonia.

**Factors predisposing to oropharyngeal colonization and pneumonia with gram-negative organisms:
1. hospitalization
2. underlying disease and compromised host defenses
3. recent antibiotic therapy**

The bacterial flora normally present in the mouth are also potential etiologic agents in the development of pneumonia. A multitude of organisms (both gram-positive and gram-negative) that favor or require anaerobic conditions for growth are the major organisms comprising mouth flora. The most common predisposing factor for anaerobic pneumonia is aspiration of secretions from the oropharynx into the tracheobronchial tree. Patients with impaired consciousness, e.g., as a result of coma, alcohol ingestion, or seizures, and those with difficulty swallowing, e.g., as a result of diseases causing muscle weakness, are prone to aspirate and are at risk for developing pneumonia due to anaerobic mouth organisms.

Anaerobes normally found in the oropharynx are the usual cause of aspiration pneumonia.

In some settings, such as prolonged hospitalization or recent use of antibiotics, the type of bacteria residing in the oropharynx may change. Specifically, aerobic gram-negative bacilli and *Staphylococcus aureus* are then more likely to colonize the oropharynx, and any subsequent pneumonia due to aspiration of oropharyngeal contents may include these aerobic organisms as part of the process.

The final type of bacteria we will mention is a newcomer to the list of etiologic agents. This organism, called *Legionella pneumophila*, was first identified as the cause of a mysterious outbreak of pneumonia in 1976 affecting American Legion members at a convention in Phila-delphia. Since then it has been recognized as an important cause of pneumonia occurring in epidemics as well as in isolated, sporadic cases. Additionally, it seems to affect both previously normal individuals and those with prior impairment of respiratory defense mechanisms. In retrospect, several prior outbreaks of unexplained pneumonia have now been shown to be due to this organism. Though the organism is a gram-negative bacillus, it stains very poorly and is generally not seen by conventional staining methods.

Many other types of bacteria can certainly cause pneumonia. We cannot cover all of them in this chapter, and the interested reader should consult some of the more detailed references listed at the end of this chapter.

Viruses

Though viruses are extremely common causes of upper respiratory tract infections, they are diagnosed relatively infrequently as a cause of frank pneumonia except in children. In adults, influenza virus is the most commonly diagnosed agent; outbreaks of pneumonia due to adenovirus are also well recognized, particularly in military recruits.

Mycoplasma

Mycoplasma appears to be a class of organisms intermediate between viruses and bacteria. Unlike bacteria, they have no rigid cell wall; unlike viruses, they do not require the intracellular machinery of a host cell in order to replicate and are capable of free-living growth. Similar in size to a large virus, mycoplasmas are the smallest free-living organisms that have yet been identified. These organisms are now recognized as a very common cause of pneumonia, perhaps responsible for a minimum of 10 to 20 percent of all cases of pneumonia. Though mycoplasmal pneumonia occurs most frequently in young adults, it is certainly not limited to this age group. The pneumonia is generally acquired in the community, i.e., in previously normal, nonhospitalized individuals, and may occur either in isolated cases or in localized outbreaks.

Mycoplasma, the smallest known free-living organism, is a frequent cause of pneumonia in young adults.

PATHOLOGY

The pathologic process common to all pneumonias is infection and inflammation of the distal pulmonary parenchyma. An influx of poly-morphonuclear leukocytes, edema fluid, erythrocytes, mononuclear cells, and fibrin is seen to a variable extent in all cases. The bacterial pneumonias in particular are characterized by an exuberant outpouring of PMN's into alveolar spaces as they attempt to limit proliferation of the invading bacteria.

The individual types of pneumonia may differ in the exact location and mode of spread of the infection. In the past, a distinction was often made between those pneumonias that follow a "lobar" distribution, those that behave more like a "bronchopneumonia," and those with the pattern of an "interstitial pneumonia." However, these distinctions are often difficult to make, as individual cases of pneumonia frequently do not adhere to any one particular pattern but have mixtures of the three in varying proportions. Given this limitation, we will briefly mention the three major types.

Lobar Pneumonia. Lobar pneumonia has classically been described as a process not limited to segmental boundaries but rather tending to spread throughout an entire lobe of the lung. Spread of the infection is believed to occur from alveolus to alveolus and from acinus to acinus through interalveolar pores, known as the pores of Kohn. The classic example of a lobar pneumonia is that due to *Streptococcus pneumoniae*, though many cases of pneumonia now recognized as being due to pneumococcus do not necessarily follow this typical pattern.

Bronchopneumonia. In bronchopneumonia, distal airway inflammation is prominent along with alveolar disease, and spread of the infection and the inflammatory process tends to occur through airways rather than through adjacent alveoli and acini. Whereas lobar pneumonias appear as dense consolidations involving part or all of a lobe, bronchopneumonias are more patchy in distribution, depending upon where spread by airways has occurred. Many of the other bacteria, such as staphylococci and gram-negative bacilli, may produce the latter pattern.

Interstitial Pneumonia. Interstitial pneumonias are characterized by an inflammatory process within the interstitial walls rather than the alveolar spaces. Though viral pneumonias classically start as interstitial pneumonias, severe cases generally show extension of the inflammatory process to alveolar spaces as well.

In some cases of pneumonia, the organisms are not very destructive to lung tissue, even though an exuberant inflammatory process may be seen. Pneumococcal pneumonia classically (though certainly not always) behaves in this way, and the healing process is associated with restoration of relatively normal parenchymal architecture. In other cases, when the organisms are more destructive, tissue necrosis can occur, with resulting abscess formation or scarring of the parenchyma. Many cases of staphylococcal and anaerobic pneumonias follow this more destructive course.

PATHOPHYSIOLOGY

Infections of the pulmonary parenchyma produce their clinical sequelae not only by altering the normal functioning of the lung parenchyma, but also by inducing a more generalized, systemic response to the invading microorganisms. The major pathophysiologic consequence of inflammation and infection involving the distal airspaces is a decrease in ventilation to the affected areas. If perfusion is relatively maintained, as it often is, ventilation-perfusion mismatch results, with low ventilation-perfusion ratios in the diseased regions. When alveoli are totally filled with inflammatory exudate, there may be no ventilation to these regions, and an extreme of ventilation-perfusion inequality (i.e., shunt) results.

If we then translate this ventilation-perfusion inequality into effects on gas exchange, we find that patients with pneumonia generally are hypoxemic. Though frank shunting may explain part of the hypoxemia, ventilation-perfusion mismatch with areas of low ventilation-perfusion ratio is usually a more important factor. Carbon dioxide retention is not a feature of pneumonia unless the patients already have an extremely limited reserve, especially from underlying chronic obstructive lung disease. In fact, patients with pneumonia frequently hyperventilate and have a P_{CO_2} that is less than 40 torr.

Pneumonia commonly results in ventilation-perfusion mismatch (with or without shunting) and hypoxemia.

The systemic response to pneumonia is certainly not unique but rather a reflection of the body's response to serious infection. Perhaps the most apparent aspects of this response are fever, an outpouring of PMN's into the circulation (particularly with bacterial pneumonia), and often a "toxic" appearance to the patient. These indirect systemic responses can be clues that an infectious process is the etiology of a new pulmonary infiltrate.

CLINICAL FEATURES

In many ways, the clinical manifestations of pneumonia are similar, even when different infectious agents are involved; in other ways, the presentations and manifestations are quite different. Though recognition of subtle clinical differences sometimes allows the astute clinician to suggest an etiologic diagnosis, methods for identifying a specific infectious agent play an equally if not more important role in the final diagnosis.

Perhaps the most important constellation of symptoms in almost any type of pneumonia includes fever, cough, and often shortness of breath. The cough is nonproductive in some cases, particularly in those pneumonias due to viruses or mycoplasma; in others, especially bacterial pneumonias, sputum production is a prominent feature. When the inflammatory process in the pulmonary parenchyma extends out to the pleural surface, the patient often complains of pleuritic chest pain. If the fever is high and "spiking," patients frequently experience shaking chills associated with the rapid rise in body temperature.

Frequent clinical features in patients with pneumonia:
1. fever (± chills)
2. cough (± sputum)
3. dyspnea
4. pleuritic chest pain
5. crackles overlying affected region
6. dullness and bronchial breath sounds with frank consolidation
7. polymorphonuclear leukocytosis

Physical examination reflects the systemic response to infection as well as the ongoing inflammatory process in the lung. Patients often have tachycardia, tachypnea, and fever. Examination of the chest typically reveals crackles or rales overlying the region of the pneumonia. If there is dense consolidation and the bronchus supplying the area is patent, then sound transmission is greatly increased through the consolidated, pneumonic area. As a result, breath sounds may be bronchial in quality, fremitus is increased, and egophony is present. The consolidated area is also characteristically dull to percussion of the overlying chest wall. Examination of the peripheral blood generally shows an increase in the white blood count (leukocytosis). Especially in patients with bacterial pneumonia, the leukocytosis is composed primarily of PMN's, and there may be a shift towards immature, younger neutrophils, i.e., bands.

In pneumococcal pneumonia, the onset of the clinical illness is often relatively abrupt, with shaking chills and high fever. Cough may be productive of yellow, green, or blood-tinged (rusty-colored) sputum. Prior to the development of pneumonia, the patients have often experienced a viral upper respiratory tract infection, which presumably was an important predisposing feature.

Mycoplasmal pneumonia, in contrast to pneumococcal pneumonia, characteristically has a somewhat slower, more insidious onset. Cough is a particularly prominent symptom, but it is often non-productive. Fever is not as high, and shaking chills are uncommon. Young adults are the individuals most likely to have mycoplasmal pneumonia, though the disease is certainly not limited to this age group.

Patients with either staphylococcal or gram-negative bacillary pneumonias are often quite ill. Frequently, they are patients with complex underlying medical problems who have already been hospitalized, and many have impaired defense mechanisms or have recently received antibiotics. As we mentioned earlier, staphylococcal pneumonia may also be seen as a secondary complication of influenza infection or as a result of dissemination of the organism through the bloodstream.

Pneumonia with anaerobic organisms generally occurs in patients with impaired consciousness or difficulty swallowing, who cannot adequately protect the airway from aspiration of oropharyngeal secretions. Dentition is often poor, and patients frequently have gingivitis or periodontal abscesses. Clinical onset of the pneumonia tends to be gradual, and sputum may have a foul odor, suggesting anaerobic infection. Since the organisms are likely to cause substantial tissue destruction, necrosis of affected tissue and abscess formation are relatively common sequelae.

As we mentioned earlier, pneumonia due to *Legionella pneumophila*, commonly called Legionnaires' disease, can be seen as isolated cases or in the form of localized outbreaks. Otherwise normal hosts may be affected, but patients with impaired respiratory defense mechanisms also appear to be predisposed. Patients are often extremely ill, not only with respiratory compromise and even respiratory failure, but also with nonrespiratory manifestations. Specifically, gastrointestinal, central nervous system, hepatic, and renal abnormalities may accompany the pneumonia.

DIAGNOSTIC APPROACH

As with other disorders affecting the pulmonary parenchyma, the single most useful tool for assessing pneumonia at a macroscopic level is the chest radiograph. The radiograph not only confirms the presence of a pneumonia; it also shows the distribution and extent of disease and sometimes gives clues about the nature of the etiologic agent. The classic pattern for *Streptococcus pneumoniae*, the pneumococcus, is a lobar pneumonia (Fig. 23–1). Staphylococcal and gram-negative pneu-

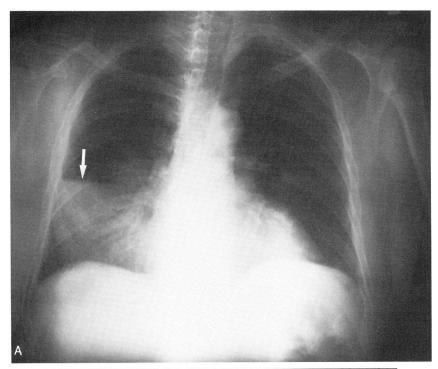

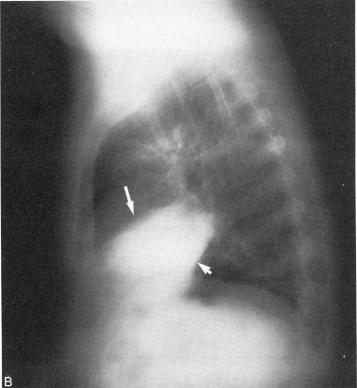

Figure 23–1. Posteroanterior (A) and lateral (B) chest radiographs demonstrating a lobar pneumonia (probably due to *Streptococcus pneumoniae*) affecting the right middle lobe. In *A*, the arrow points to the minor fissure, which defines the upper border of the middle lobe. In *B*, the long arrow points to the minor fissure; the short arrow, to the major fissure. (Courtesy of Dr. Christopher Fanta.)

monias may be localized or extensive and often follow a patchy distribution (Fig. 23–2). Mycoplasma can produce a variety of roentgenographic presentations, classically described as being more impressive than the clinical picture would suggest. Pneumonias due to aspiration of oropharyngeal secretions characteristically involve the dependent regions of lung—the lower lobe in the upright patient, or the posterior segment of the upper lobe or superior segment of the lower lobe in the supine patient (Fig. 23–3).

The chest radiograph is also useful for demonstrating pleural fluid, which frequently accompanies pneumonia, particularly of bacterial origin. As we discuss later in the chapter, the pleural fluid can be either thin and serous or thick and purulent; in the latter case the term empyema is used.

Microscopic examination of the sputum plays a particularly important role in the evaluation of patients with pneumonia. In a good sputum specimen, i.e., one that contains few squamous epithelial cells picked up in transit through the upper respiratory tract, inflammatory cells and bacteria can be seen. In most bacterial pneumonias, large numbers of PMN's are seen in the sputum; mycoplasma and viral pneumonias, in contrast, have fewer PMN's and more mononuclear inflammatory cells. Pneumococcal, staphylococcal, and gram-negative bacillary pneumonias commonly demonstrate a relatively homogeneous population of the infecting bacteria. Anaerobic aspiration pneumonias, since they are caused by a mixture of organisms from the oropharynx,

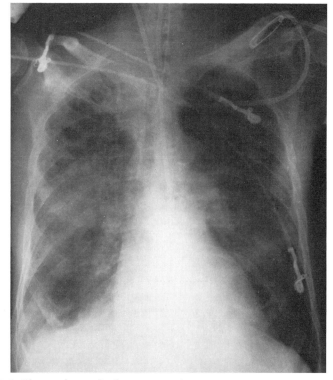

Figure 23–2. Chest radiograph of a patient with an extensive gram-negative pneumonia. There are patchy infiltrates throughout both lungs, more prominent on the right.

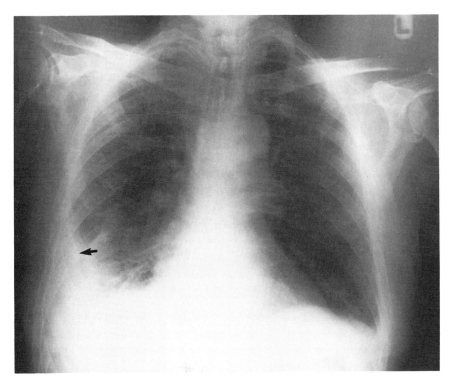

Figure 23–3. Chest radiograph of a right lower lobe aspiration pneumonia. In addition to the infiltrate at the right base, there is a loculated pleural effusion, which represents an empyema complicating the pneumonia. Arrow points to the edge of the loculated effusion. (Courtesy of Dr. T. Scott Johnson.)

show a mixed population of bacteria of many different morphologies. In Legionnaires' disease, the bacterium does not stain well with the usual gram stain reagent and is therefore not seen with conventional staining techniques. In mycoplasmal and viral pneumonia, the infecting agent is not visualized at all, and one can see only the predominantly mononuclear cell inflammatory response.

In conjunction with the initial gram stain and microscopic examination of sputum, the specimen is also cultured for bacteria. However, it is well recognized that some bacteria are relatively difficult to grow, and in many if not most cases the initial gram stain is just as important in making the etiologic diagnosis.

When sputum is not spontaneously expectorated by the patient, other methods for obtaining respiratory secretions (or even material directly from the lung parenchyma) may be necessary. The techniques that have been used, including transtracheal aspiration, fiberoptic bronchoscopy, needle aspiration of the lung, and occasionally even open lung biopsy, have all been described in more detail in Chapter 3.

The functional assessment of patients with acute infectious pneumonia is usually limited to evaluation of gas exchange. Arterial blood gases characteristically demonstrate hypoxemia, accompanied by a normal or decreased P_{CO_2}. Pulmonary function tests have little usefulness in this setting except in the patient with previously compromised lung function, for whom it may be important to assess the extent of further acute compromise.

GENERAL PRINCIPLES OF THE THERAPEUTIC APPROACH

The cornerstone of treatment of bacterial pneumonia is antibiotic therapy directed at the infecting organism. In the case of pneumococcal pneumonia, penicillin is generally the most appropriate agent, assuming the patient is not allergic to penicillin. Staphylococci that are now identified generally produce penicillinase, which requires that a penicillinase-resistant form of penicillin, such as oxacillin or nafcillin, be used. Gram-negative bacillary pneumonias often display resistance to a variety of antibiotics. Aminoglycosides such as gentamicin or tobramycin may be used initially while sensitivity testing against various antibiotics is performed for the bacteria isolated from sputum. Erythromycin is now the antibiotic of choice for pneumonias due either to Legionella or to Mycoplasma. Finally, viral pneumonias do not yet have specific forms of therapy, though rapid advances in this field may lead to development of clinically useful therapeutic agents.

Frequently used antibiotics for common pneumonias:
1. Strep. pneumoniae (penicillin)
2. Staphylococcus (oxacillin, nafcillin)
3. Gram-negative rods (gentamycin, tobramycin)
4. Mycoplasma (erythromycin)
5. Legionella (erythromycin)

Other modalities of therapy are mainly supportive. Chest physical therapy and other measures to assist clearance of respiratory secretions are useful in many patients with pneumonia. If patients have inadequate gas exchange, as demonstrated by significant hypoxemia, administration of supplemental oxygen is beneficial. Occasionally, patients develop frank respiratory failure, in which case the therapeutic measures discussed in Chapter 28 are called into action. Before concluding this chapter, we will also briefly mention two specific intrathoracic complications of pneumonia—lung abscess and empyema—since they represent relatively common clinical problems.

INTRATHORACIC COMPLICATIONS OF PNEUMONIA

Lung Abscess

A *lung abscess*, like an abscess elsewhere, represents a localized collection of pus. In the lung, abscesses generally result from tissue destruction complicating a pneumonia. The abscess contents are primarily PMN's, often with collections of bacterial organisms. When antibiotics have already been administered, organisms may no longer be obtainable from the abscess cavity.

Etiologic agents associated with formation of a lung abscess are generally those bacteria causing significant tissue necrosis. Most commonly, anaerobic organisms are responsible, suggesting that aspiration of oropharyngeal contents is the predisposing event. However, aerobic organisms, such as *Staphylococcus* or enteric gram-negative rods, can also cause significant tissue destruction, with excavation of a region of lung parenchyma and abscess formation.

Anaerobic bacteria are the agents most frequently responsible for lung abscesses.

Treatment of a lung abscess revolves around appropriate antibiotic therapy, often given for a more prolonged duration than for an uncomplicated pneumonia. Though abscesses elsewhere in the body are drained by surgical incision, lung abscesses generally drain through the tracheobronchial tree, and surgical intervention is only rarely needed.

Empyema

When a pneumonia extends to the pleural surface, the inflammatory process may eventually lead to another intrathoracic complication of pneumonia—*empyema*. The term empyema refers to pus in the pleural space; in its most florid form, an empyema represents thick, creamy, or yellow fluid within the pleural space. The fluid contains enormous numbers of leukocytes, primarily PMN's, often accompanied by bacterial organisms. With a frank empyema, or often even with other grossly inflammatory pleural effusions accompanying pneumonia (parapneumonic effusions), the pleural inflammation can result in (1) formation of localized pockets of fluid or (2) substantial scarring and limitation of mobility of the underlying lung.

Several different bacterial organisms can be associated with development of an empyema. Anaerobes are particularly common, but staphylococci and other aerobic organisms are also potential causes. Once an empyema has been demonstrated, usually by thoracentesis and sampling of pleural fluid, drainage of the fluid is required. Most commonly, a relatively large tube is inserted into the pleural space for adequate drainage. Alternative techniques are used in some specific clinical situations, but these are beyond the scope of this chapter.

Adequate drainage of pleural fluid is important in the management of empyema.

REFERENCES

General Reviews

Pennington, J. E. (ed.): Respiratory Infections: Diagnosis and Management. New York, Raven Press, 1983.

Bacterial Pneumonia

Bartlett, J. G.: Anaerobic bacterial pneumonitis. Am. Rev. Respir. Dis. 119:19–23, 1979.
Bartlett, J. G., and Finegold, S. M.: Anaerobic infections of the lung and pleural space. Am. Rev. Respir. Dis. 110:56–77, 1974.
Edelstein, P. H., and Meyer, R. D.: Legionnaires' disease: a review. Chest 85:114–120, 1984.
Finland, M.: Pneumonia and pneumococcal infections, with special reference to pneumococcal pneumonia. Am. Rev. Respir. Dis. 120:481–502, 1979.
George, W. L., and Finegold, S. M.: Bacterial infections of the lung. Chest 81:502–507, 1982.
Jakab, G. J.: Mechanisms of virus-induced bacterial superinfections of the lungs. Clin. Chest Med. 2:59–66, 1981.
LaForce, F. M.: Hospital-acquired gram-negative rod pneumonias: an overview. Am. J. Med. 70:664–669, 1981.
Mufson, M. A.: Pneumococcal infections. JAMA 246:1942–1948, 1981.
Pierce, A. K., and Sanford, J. P.: Aerobic gram-negative bacillary pneumonias. Am. Rev. Respir. Dis. 110:647–658, 1974.
Sanford, J. P.: Legionnaires' disease—the first thousand days. N. Engl. J. Med. 300:654–656, 1979.
Schwartz, J. S.: Pneumococcal vaccine: clinical efficacy and effectiveness. Ann. Intern. Med. 96:208–220, 1982.

Viral Pneumonia

Anderson, L. J., Patriarca, P. A., Hierholzer, J. C., and Noble, G. R.: Viral respiratory illness. Med. Clin. North Am. 67:1009–1030, 1983.
Reichman, R. C., and Dolin, R.: Viral pneumonias. Med. Clin. North Am. 64:491–506, 1980.

Mycoplasmal Pneumonia

Cassell, G. H., and Cole, B. C.: Mycoplasmas as agents of human disease. N. Engl. J. Med. 304:80–89, 1981.
Murray, H. W., Masur, H., Senterfit, L. B., and Roberts, R. B.: The protean manifestations of Mycoplasma pneumoniae infection in adults. Am. J. Med. 58:229–242, 1975.

24

Tuberculosis

Etiology and Pathogenesis
Pathology
Pathophysiology
Clinical Manifestations
Diagnostic Approach
Principles of Therapy

Over the span of centuries, few diseases have claimed so many lives, caused so much morbidity, and been so dreaded as tuberculosis. At the turn of this century, tuberculosis was the single most common cause of death in the United States; over 80 percent of the population was infected before the age of 20. However, since that time few diseases have seen so great a decline in the frequency of cases and the mortality of the disease as tuberculosis. Two main factors have been responsible—an overall improvement in living conditions and the development of effective chemotherapy, which has now made tuberculosis a curable disease.

However, as we now enter the second century since the identification of the tubercle bacillus by Robert Koch in 1882, it is important that we not become complacent about this disease. There are still numerous cases discovered each year, and in conditions of poverty and crowding tuberculosis remains a major public health problem.

ETIOLOGY AND PATHOGENESIS

The etiologic agent causing tuberculosis, *Mycobacterium tuberculosis*, is an aerobic rod-shaped bacterium. As we discuss later, an important property of the tubercle bacillus is its ability to retain certain stains even after exposure to acid; hence mycobacteria are said to be *acid-fast*.

Transmission of the disease occurs by means of small aerosol droplets, generally from 1 to 5 microns in size, that contain the microorganism. The source of these droplets is an individual with tuberculosis who harbors the organism, often excreting tubercle bacilli in the sputum or in small droplets produced during such commonplace activities as speaking, coughing, singing, or laughing. Most commonly, transmission occurs with relatively close contact, often between related individuals or others living in the same household. The disease is not transmitted by fomites, i.e., articles of clothing, eating utensils, or the like; direct inhalation of droplets aerosolized by another individual is almost exclusively the mode of spread.

When droplets containing mycobacteria are inhaled and reach the distal pulmonary parenchyma, a small focus of *primary* infection develops, consisting of the organisms and an inflammatory process mounted by the host. At this time, organisms frequently spread via lymphatics to draining lymph nodes as well as via the bloodstream to distant organs and to other regions of lung, particularly the apices. In the vast majority of cases, even though lymphatic and hematogenous spread may occur, the body's defense mechanisms (in the lung and elsewhere) are capable of controlling and limiting the primary infection. An important component of the body's defense appears to be the development of cell-mediated immunity, i.e., delayed hypersensitivity, against the mycobacterial organisms. This sensitization and development of a cell-mediated immune response generally occur within several weeks of initial exposure.

The patient is usually unaware of the primary infection, and the only tracks left by the organism are those related to the host's response to the bacillus—either the local tissue response or evidence that the host has become sensitized to the tubercle bacillus, i.e., a positive skin test. In a few patients, probably 10 percent or less, the defense mechanisms are unable to control the primary infection, and clinically apparent primary tuberculosis results.

Even when the primary infection has been apparently controlled, the tubercle bacillus may not be completely eliminated from the host. Rather, a small number of organisms often appear to remain in a dormant state, not actually killed but also not proliferating or causing any apparent active disease. The majority of such patients will never have any further difficulty with development of clinically active tuberculosis. In some patients, though, the delicate balance between the organism and host defense mechanisms eventually breaks down, often after many years, and a dormant focus of infection becomes active. These patients with active disease occurring at a time distant from the primary infection are said to have *reactivation* tuberculosis.

Overall, the large majority of cases of active tuberculosis are of the reactivation variety, occurring many years after the initial or primary infection. For both primary and reactivation disease, the lungs are certainly the most commonly affected site. However, with either variety of disease, distant organ systems may be involved as a result of hematogenous spread during the primary phase of the infection. Additionally, there may be disseminated disease, known as miliary tuberculosis, again resulting from hematogenous dissemination of the organisms.

Before we proceed with a discussion of the pathology of tuberculosis, a few other terms are worth defining since they are used relatively frequently. The term *progressive primary tuberculosis* reflects primary disease that has not been controlled by host defense mechanisms and

Transmission of tuberculosis is by inhalation of small aerosol droplets containing the organism.

The majority of active tuberculosis cases involve reactivation of a previously dormant focus within the lungs.

has continued to be active beyond the point at which delayed hypersensitivity has developed. As a general rule, cellular immunity develops between 2 and 10 weeks after the initial infection, and continuing active disease beyond this point has many of the features of reactivation tuberculosis. The term *postprimary tuberculosis* refers to disease beyond the initial, primary infection. Though this term usually refers to reactivation disease, it also includes cases of progressive primary tuberculosis. Finally, the term *reinfection tuberculosis* refers to disease in a previously infected person that results not from reactivation of dormant tubercle bacilli but rather from new exposure to another source of organisms. This type of infection is quite uncommon, since it is believed that individuals with prior exposure to tuberculosis, who manifest delayed hypersensitivity to the organism, are relatively resistant to exogenous reinfection from another source. The risk for these individuals is from reactivation of their own latent disease, not from a new exposure.

PATHOLOGY

Following development of delayed hypersensitivity, the pathologic hallmarks of tuberculosis are granulomas and caseous necrosis, often with cavity formation.

The pathologic features of pulmonary tuberculosis vary according to the stage of infection. The primary infection in the lung consists of organisms along with a relatively nonspecific inflammatory response in the involved region of parenchyma. Regional lymph nodes often become involved by local spread of the organism, and the combination of the primary area in the lung and involved lymph nodes is termed the primary or Ghon complex.

When delayed hypersensitivity is present, either weeks after the primary infection or during a period of reactivation disease, a different pathologic pattern emerges. The hallmarks at this time are the presence of (1) granulomas, i.e., collections of phagocytic cells termed epithelioid histiocytes, and (2) caseous necrosis, i.e., foci of necrosis and softening at the center of a granuloma. Within the region of caseous necrosis, the contents can liquefy and slough, leaving behind a cavity, another hallmark of tuberculosis. Other features of the granulomas include multinucleated giant cells and often the presence of tubercle bacilli themselves.

A process of healing also tends to occur at the sites of disease. Fibrosis or scarring ensues, often associated with contraction of the affected area and deposition of calcium. With full-blown tuberculosis, there is extensive destruction of lung tissue, resulting from large areas of inflammation, granuloma formation, caseous necrosis, and cavitation, along with fibrosis, contraction, and foci of calcification.

As we mentioned earlier, tuberculosis is capable of spread, and in fact spread of organisms through the bloodstream at the time of primary infection is probably the rule rather than the exception. When defense mechanisms break down, disease can become apparent at other sites as well, e.g., liver, kidney, adrenal glands, bones, or central nervous system. Spread also occurs to other regions of lung, either as a result of hematogenous seeding during the primary infection or as a result of spilling of infected secretions or caseous material into the bronchi and into other regions of lung.

Within the lung, characteristic locations for reactivation tuberculosis are the apical regions of the upper lobes and, to a lesser extent, the superior segment of the lower lobes. It is believed that these are not the sites of the primary infection but rather the favored location for organisms to implant after hematogenous spread. These regions have a very high Po_2 and are thus particularly suitable for survival of the aerobic tubercle bacilli.

PATHOPHYSIOLOGY

Most of the clinical features of pulmonary tuberculosis can be attributed to either of two aspects of the disease—the presence of a poorly controlled chronic infection or the presence of a chronic destructive process within the lung parenchyma. A variety of other manifestations result from extrapulmonary spread of tuberculosis, but we will not consider these consequences in any detail.

Why the chronic infection within the lung produces systemic manifestations is not entirely clear. However, as implied by the term "consumption," used so frequently in the past, tuberculosis is a disease in which systemic manifestations such as weight loss, wasting, and loss of appetite have been prominent features. These and other systemic effects of tuberculosis will be discussed in more detail when we consider clinical aspects of the disease.

The chronic destructive process involving the pulmonary parenchyma entails progressive scarring and loss of lung tissue. However, it is of interest that respiratory function is generally preserved more than one would expect, perhaps because the disease is often limited to the apical and posterior regions of the upper lobes as well as to the superior segment of the lower lobes. Oxygenation also tends to be surprisingly preserved, presumably because ventilation and perfusion are destroyed simultaneously in the affected lung. Consequently, ventilation-perfusion mismatch is not nearly so great as in many other parenchymal and airway diseases.

CLINICAL MANIFESTATIONS

For the purposes of discussion in this and subsequent sections of this chapter, it is important to make a distinction between tuberculous infection and the disease tuberculosis. Tuberculous infection is the consequence of primary exposure, by which the bacilli have become established in the patient, but in this case the host defense mechanisms have prevented any clinically apparent disease. Specific immunity to the tubercle bacillus can be demonstrated by a positive skin test for delayed hypersensitivity; otherwise, there is no evidence for proliferation of bacteria or for tissue involvement by disease. On the other hand, the disease tuberculosis is associated with proliferation of organisms, accompanied by a tissue response and generally (though not always) clinical problems of which the patient is aware.

Patients with pulmonary tuberculosis can present with (1) systemic symptoms, (2) symptoms referable to the respiratory tract, or (3) an abnormal chest radiograph but no clinical symptoms. When symptoms occur, they are generally insidious rather than acute in onset.

The systemic symptoms are often relatively nonspecific, e.g., weight loss, anorexia, fatigue, low-grade fever, and night sweats. The most common symptoms resulting from pulmonary involvement are cough, sputum production, and hemoptysis; chest pain is also occasionally present. Many patients have neither systemic nor pulmonary symptoms and come to the attention of a physician because of an abnormal chest radiograph, often performed for an unrelated reason.

Patients with extrapulmonary involvement frequently have pulmonary tuberculosis as well, but occasional cases are limited to an extrapulmonary site. Pericardium, pleura, kidney, peritoneum, adrenal glands, and central nervous system may each be involved, with symptoms resulting from the particular organ or region that is affected. With miliary tuberculosis, the disease is disseminated, and the patients are usually systemically quite ill.

Physical examination of the patient with pulmonary tuberculosis may show the ravages of a chronic infection, with evidence of wasting and weight loss. However, though this was a common appearance in the past, it is now seen in a minority of patients. Chest examination also tends to be relatively unremarkable, though there is sometimes evidence of crackles or rales over affected areas. If a tuberculous pleural effusion is present, the physical findings characteristic of an effusion may be found.

DIAGNOSTIC APPROACH

One of the most commonly used diagnostic tests, the tuberculin skin test, is actually a test to document tuberculous infection rather than the disease tuberculosis. In this test, a small amount of protein derived from the tubercle bacillus (PPD, or purified protein derivative) is injected intradermally. Individuals who have been exposed to *Mycobacterium tuberculosis* and have acquired cellular immunity to the organism demonstrate a positive test, i.e., induration or swelling at the site of injection after 48 to 72 hours. The test does not at all distinguish between individuals who have active tuberculosis and those who merely have acquired delayed hypersensitivity from previous exposure. However, since most cases of active tuberculosis are of the reactivation variety, occurring in patients with previous exposure and tuberculous infection, a positive skin test does identify individuals at higher risk for subsequent development of active disease.

As is true of most diagnostic tests, false negative results can be seen with the tuberculin skin test. Faulty administration, an inactive batch of skin testing material, and underlying diseases that depress cellular immunity are but a few of the causes of a falsely negative skin test. On the other hand, not all patients who react to tuberculoprotein have been exposed to *Mycobacterium tuberculosis*. Exposure to, or disease resulting from, nontuberculous mycobacteria, often called atypical mycobacteria, is also sometimes associated with a positive or a borderline positive skin test.

In order to diagnose tuberculosis, i.e., actual tuberculous disease, the most important initial diagnostic technique is the chest radiograph. In primary disease, the chest radiograph may simply show a nonspecific infiltrate, often but certainly not exclusively in the lower lobes (contrast this with the upper lobe predominance of reactivation disease). There may be hilar (and sometimes paratracheal) lymph node enlargement, reflecting involvement of the draining node by the organism and by the primary infection. Pleural involvement may also be seen, with development of a pleural effusion.

Common features of the chest radiograph in primary tuberculosis:
1. nonspecific infiltrate (often lower lobe)
2. hilar (and paratracheal) node enlargement
3. pleural effusion

When the primary disease heals, the chest roentgenogram frequently shows some residua of the healing process. Most common are small calcified lesions within the pulmonary parenchyma, reflecting calcified granulomas. There may also be calcification within hilar or paratracheal lymph nodes.

With reactivation tuberculosis, the most common sites of disease are the apical and posterior segments of the upper lobes, and to a lesser extent the superior segment of the lower lobes. A variety of patterns can be seen—infiltrates, cavities, nodules, and scarring and contraction (Fig. 24–1). The presence of chest radiographic abnormalities, however, does not necessarily indicate active disease. The disease may be old, stable, and currently inactive; and it is quite difficult if not impossible to gauge activity on the basis of the radiographic appearance.

Radiographic location of reactivation tuberculosis: most commonly apical and posterior segments of upper lobe(s), superior segment of lower lobe(s).

Definitive diagnosis of tuberculosis rests upon culturing the organism, either from secretions (e.g., sputum) or from tissue. However, the organisms are slow growing, and six weeks may be required for growth and final identification of the organism.

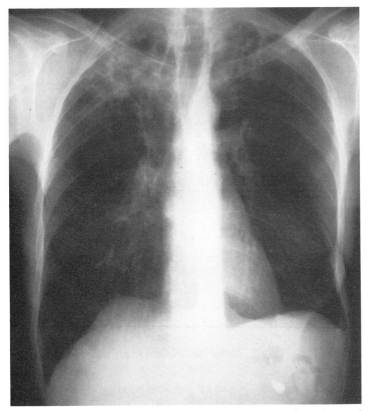

Figure 24–1. Chest radiograph of a patient with reactivation tuberculosis. There are infiltrates with cavitation at both apices, more prominent on the right.

Another extremely useful procedure, for which results are available almost immediately, is staining of material obtained from the tracheobronchial tree, primarily sputum. As we mentioned earlier, a hallmark of mycobacterial organisms is their ability to retain certain dyes even after exposure to acid. This property of being "acid-fast" is generally demonstrated with either Ziehl-Neelsen or Kinyoun stains, or with a fluorescent stain that utilizes auramine-rhodamine. Even the finding of only one acid-fast bacillus from sputum or from tracheobronchial washings is clinically significant in the large majority of cases. One qualification is that nontuberculous mycobacteria, which either cause disease or are sometimes present as colonizing organisms or contaminants, also have the same staining properties. It is only by certain growth characteristics on culture that these organisms can be distinguished from *Mycobacterium tuberculosis*.

In order for even one tubercle bacillus to be seen on smear, large numbers of organisms must be present in the lung. Therefore, if fewer organisms are present, even if they are causing disease, the smear may be negative, whereas culture will often be positive in this setting. In general, the infectiousness of a patient with tuberculosis correlates both with the number of organisms he or she is harboring and with the presence of organisms on smear. Patients who have a positive smear tend to be much more infectious than those who are culture positive but smear negative.

If the patient is not producing sputum even after attempts at induction, material can easily be obtained from the tracheobronchial tree by fiberoptic bronchoscopy. Other techniques are also available for obtaining specimens, but since they have less clinical utility, they will not be discussed further.

Functional assessment of the patient with tuberculosis, as we mentioned earlier, often shows surprisingly little impairment of pulmonary function. Such testing is useful primarily for the patient who already has compromised pulmonary function, when there is concern about how much of the patient's reserve has been lost. Similarly, arterial blood gases are often relatively preserved, with Po_2 being either normal or decreased, depending on the amount of ventilation-perfusion mismatch that has resulted.

PRINCIPLES OF THERAPY

Treatment for most cases of pulmonary tuberculosis is currently INH and rifampin given for 9 months.

Fortunately, effective chemotherapy is now available for tuberculosis. Whereas treatment for tuberculosis used to be essentially ineffective, involving prolonged hospitalization (usually in a sanatorium) or a variety of surgical procedures, the large majority of cases are now curable with appropriate drug therapy. Patients are treated for a prolonged period, generally with two effective antituberculous agents. Until recently, two drugs were continued for a period of 18 to 24 months. Now, therapy for nine months with two very effective antituberculous agents, isoniazid (INH) and rifampin, is commonly used in cases of pulmonary tuberculosis, with excellent results. Treatment can be administered in an outpatient setting, unless the patient is sufficiently ill to require hospitalization. After approximately two weeks of chemotherapy, patients are no longer considered infectious, including even those whose sputum smears were initially positive for acid-fast bacilli.

In addition to two-drug therapy administered for active tuberculosis, therapy with isoniazid alone (for one year) is generally given for household members of patients with recently diagnosed tuberculosis or for newly infected persons (documented by recent conversion to a positive skin test). Such therapy substantially decreases the chances of developing active tuberculosis in these individuals, who are at particularly high risk.

Certain other patients with previous tuberculous infection, documented by a positive tuberculin skin test, are also felt to be candidates for one year of treatment with isoniazid alone. Specifically, this category includes patients satisfying additional criteria (besides a positive PPD) that put them at high risk for developing reactivation of a dormant infection. Examples include the presence of stable radiographic findings of old tuberculosis but no prior therapy, or the presence of underlying diseases or treatment that impair host defense mechanisms. Though this form of single-drug therapy is often called "prophylactic," it is actually treatment aimed at eradicating a small number of dormant but viable organisms. In any case, it has been shown to be quite effective in achieving its goal, namely to decrease substantially the eventual risk of developing reactivation tuberculosis.

Isoniazid alone for one year is frequently given to patients without currently active tuberculosis who are at high risk for developing active disease.

REFERENCES

General Reviews

Glassroth, J., Robins, A. G., and Snider, D. E., Jr.: Tuberculosis in the 1980's. N. Engl. J. Med. 302:1441–1450, 1980.
Green, G. M., Daniel, T. M., and Ball, W. C., Jr. (ed.): Koch Centennial Supplement: 100th Anniversary of the Announcement of the Discovery of the Tubercle Bacillus by Robert Koch, March 24, 1882. Am. Rev. Respir. Dis. 125 (part 2):1–132, 1982.
Stead, W. W., and Dutt, A. K. (ed.): Tuberculosis. Clin. Chest Med. 1:167–284, 1980.

Clinical Manifestations and Diagnostic Approach

Alvarez, S., and McCabe, W. R.: Extrapulmonary tuberculosis revisited: a review of experience at Boston City and other hospitals. Medicine 63:25–55, 1984.
American Thoracic Society: Diagnostic standards and classification of tuberculosis and other mycobacterial diseases (14th edition). Am. Rev. Respir. Dis. 123:343–358, 1981.
Berger, H. W., and Mejia, E.: Tuberculous pleurisy. Chest 63:88–92, 1973.
Khan, M. A., Kovnat, D. M., Bachus, B., Whitcomb, M. E., Brody, J. S., and Snider, G. L.: Clinical and roentgenographic spectrum of pulmonary tuberculosis in the adult. Am. J. Med. 62:31–38, 1977.
Sahn, S. A., and Neff, T. A.: Miliary tuberculosis. Am. J. Med. 56:495–505, 1974.

Treatment

American Thoracic Society: Guidelines for short-course tuberculosis chemotherapy. Am. Rev. Respir. Dis. 121:611–614, 1980.
American Thoracic Society: Preventive therapy of tuberculous infection. Am. Rev. Respir. Dis. 110:371–374, 1974.
American Thoracic Society: Treatment of tuberculosis and other mycobacterial diseases. Am. Rev. Respir. Dis. 127:790–796, 1983.
Dutt, A. K., and Stead, W. W.: Short-course treatment regimens for patients with tuberculosis. Arch. Intern. Med. 140:827–829, 1980.
Van Scoy, R. E., aand Wilkowske, C. J.: Antituberculous agents. Mayo Clin. Proc. 58:233–240, 1983.

25

Miscellaneous Infections—Fungal and Protozoan

Fungal Infections
   Histoplasmosis
      Types of Infection
   Coccidioidomycosis
   Aspergillosis
      Allergic Bronchopulmonary Aspergillosis
      Aspergilloma
      Invasive Aspergillosis
   Other Fungi
Protozoan Infections
   Pneumocystis
   Other Protozoa

In this chapter, we will complete our discussion of infectious diseases involving the lungs by considering miscellaneous infections due to fungi and to protozoa. Since this is a relatively broad topic with many organisms potentially causing disease, we will limit ourselves to the most common organisms in each category. In addition, given the varied types of clinical presentation seen with even a single organism, we will try to offer an overview of the major clinical problems posed by these organisms, rather than an exhaustive review.

For some of the organisms we will discuss, infection is clearly a potential problem for the relatively normal host, i.e., the individual with intact host defense mechanisms. Histoplasmosis and coccidioidomycosis are the two fungal infections falling within this category; but even for these two diseases impairment of normal defense mechanisms may substantially alter the presentation, clinical consequences, and natural history of the illness.

For many other fungi and protozoa, the normal host is essentially protected from the organism, and disease occurs almost exclusively as a consequence of an underlying illness or a breakdown of normal defense mechanisms. *Aspergillus* is perhaps the most important fungus of this sort and will be the main one considered in this chapter. Of the protozoan infections, pulmonary involvement by *Pneumocystis* is the most important and is also seen almost exclusively in the setting of impaired host defenses. The less common fungi (e.g., *Cryptococcus*, *Mucor*, and *Candida*) and protozoa (e.g., *Toxoplasma*) affecting the immunosuppressed host will not be considered in detail, but further information can be obtained from references listed at the end of this chapter.

FUNGAL INFECTIONS

Histoplasmosis

Histoplasmosis is caused by the fungus *Histoplasma capsulatum*, found primarily in the soil of river valleys in temperate zones of the world. The central United States, e.g., the Mississippi and Ohio River valleys, is a particularly notable endemic region for the organism. *Histoplasma* is a dimorphic fungus, meaning that it exhibits two types of morphology, depending on the conditions for growth. In the soil, the organism takes the form of branching hyphae; in the body at 37° C, it appears as a round or oval yeast.

Features of Histoplasma capsulatum:
1. *common in river valleys of central U.S.*
2. *found in soil contaminated by bird droppings*
3. *present in yeast form in tissue*
4. *elicits granulomatous response in tissue*

Histoplasma flourishes best in soil that has been contaminated by bird droppings. When the soil becomes dry, the infectious spores become airborne and are inhaled by man, eventually reaching the distal regions of the lung. Contact with chicken houses, bat caves, and starling, blackbird, and pigeon roosts often provides exposure for individuals or groups working in the contaminated area.

After an individual has been exposed and *Histoplasma capsulatum* has entered the lung, the organism (at body temperature) undergoes conversion to the yeast phase. An inflammatory response ensues in the lung parenchyma, with recruitment of phagocytic cells (macrophages). Commonly, there is also spread of the organism to regional lymph nodes. Within three weeks, patients have generally developed delayed hypersensitivity against *Histoplasma*, and the pathologic response becomes granulomatous in nature. Central areas of caseation necrosis are often seen within the granulomas, making the pathologic response similar to that of tuberculosis.

When the initial or primary lesions heal, residua either are absent or take the form of small, fibrotic pulmonary nodules, which may contain areas of calcification. However, there are alternatives to this quite benign pathologic course following exposure. In some cases, particularly in the immunosuppressed host or in the infant or young child, the organism becomes disseminated to many organs, and the patient is said to have disseminated histoplasmosis. In other cases, particularly in patients with significant underlying airways disease or emphysema, progressive parenchymal inflammation, destruction, and cavity formation occur, often called progressive or chronic pulmonary histoplasmosis.

Types of Infection

Three main clinical syndromes are associated with histoplasmosis, corresponding to the three types of pathologic response we just mentioned. The normal, immunocompetent host generally develops a benign, self-limited infection called *acute* or *primary histoplasmosis*, with relatively few if any clinical sequelae. Often the patients are asymptomatic during the acute infection. Other individuals have a variety of nonspecific symptoms, ranging from cough, fever, chills, and chest pain to headache, malaise, myalgias, and weight loss. The chest radiograph can present with several types of patterns, commonly a pulmonary infiltrate, with or without either hilar adenopathy or pleural effusion. The clinical syndrome resolves within a few weeks, even without therapy. The only clues remaining from the acute infection are often one or several pulmonary nodules (which can be calcified) seen on chest roentgenogram. Immunologic testing, using skin tests or serologic studies, may also indicate prior exposure to the organism.

The syndrome of *disseminated histoplasmosis* usually occurs in immunocompromised hosts or in infants or young children. What these patients appear to have in common that predisposes them to disseminated histoplasmosis is impairment of cell-mediated immunity. In this potentially life-threatening illness, there is often widespread pulmonary involvement, accompanied by prominent systemic symptoms and infection of other organ systems.

Finally, *chronic pulmonary histoplasmosis* is generally seen in individuals with pre-existing structural abnormalities of the lung, primarily chronic obstructive lung disease with emphysema. The clinical and roentgenographic patterns often resemble those of tuberculosis. Patients may have cough, sputum production, fever, fatigue, and weight loss. The chest radiograph also shows disease localized mainly to the upper lobes, with parenchymal infiltrates, often streaky in appearance, and cavity formation.

Diagnosis of histoplasmosis depends upon the type of infection, i.e., acute, disseminated, or chronic. The options available to the clinician are culture of the organism, identification in tissue, or documentation of an immunologic response by serologic studies. In order to identify the organism microscopically, special stains, such as methenamine silver, are required. The specific usefulness and limitations of each of these methods are beyond the scope of this discussion but can be found in references listed at the end of this chapter.

Treatment of pulmonary histoplasmosis also depends on the particular type of infection. Acute histoplasmosis generally requires no therapy and is a self-limited illness. Disseminated histoplasmosis requires treatment with the antifungal agent amphotericin B. Chronic pulmonary histoplasmosis is generally also treated with amphotericin B; surgery to remove localized disease is occasionally performed but clearly has a very limited role.

Coccidioidomycosis

Like histoplasmosis, *coccidioidomycosis* also affects normal hosts but may have its clinical consequences altered in special categories of patients, especially those with impairment of host defense mechanisms. The causative organism, *Coccidioides immitis*, is also a dimorphic fungus, with mycelia present in soil but the yeast form of the organism growing in tissues.

However, unlike *Histoplasma*, *Coccidioides* is limited to the Western hemisphere, particularly to the San Joaquin Valley region of California. Other areas in which the organism is endemic include parts of New Mexico, Nevada, Texas, and Arizona, as well as regions in Mexico and South America.

After inhalation of the infectious spore, the host develops primary disease. Pathologically, the inflammatory response to the organism is also a granulomatous one, once delayed hypersensitivity to *Coccidioides* has developed. The normal host generally has a relatively self-limited illness resulting from the primary infection. When dissemination occurs, it is usually in specific groups of predisposed individuals—immunosuppressed patients, pregnant women, and for unclear reasons, certain ethnic groups, particularly Filipinos and blacks. Chronic pulmonary coccidioidomycosis is found in some patients as a sequel to primary disease, perhaps related either to underlying lung disease or to immune impairment.

Clinically, primary infection with *Coccidioides immitis* may be subclinical and unassociated with symptoms, or it may produce respiratory tract symptoms or manifestations of hypersensitivity to the organism. When symptoms occur, they often include fever, cough, headache, and chest pain. Skin manifestations, presumably representing a form of hypersensitivity, are also common. One of these, erythema nodosum, consists of tender, red nodules on the anterior surface of the lower legs. Chest radiograph during the primary infection frequently shows a pulmonary infiltrate, often with associated hilar adenopathy and sometimes a pleural effusion.

The primary infection is usually self-limited, resolving within a few weeks. Residual findings on chest roentgenogram may be absent or may consist of one or more pulmonary nodules (with or without calcification) or thin-walled cavities.

Disseminated disease, resulting from hematogenous spread of the organism, is often associated with an ominous prognosis. As mentioned earlier, certain ethnic groups are at high risk for this complication, as are immunosuppressed patients and pregnant women.

Clinical syndromes with coccidioidomycosis:
1. acute (primary) coccidioidomycosis
2. disseminated coccidioidomycosis
3. chronic pulmonary coccidioidomycosis

Chronic pulmonary involvement by coccidioidomycosis can take several forms, including one or more chronic cavities, or upper lobe disease with streaky infiltrates and/or nodules resembling tuberculosis. Patients often have fever, cough (sometimes with hemoptysis), malaise, and weight loss and may appear subacutely or chronically ill.

As with histoplasmosis, diagnosis of coccidioidomycosis depends on the type of clinical presentation and rests upon culture, demonstration in tissue (e.g., with methenamine silver staining), and evidence of an immune response to the organism. The specific uses and interpretation of skin testing and serologic techniques for diagnosis are beyond the scope of this chapter and are discussed in the more detailed references to this chapter.

Treatment considerations are similar to those for histoplasmosis. Primary infections generally do not require therapy, whereas disseminated disease is treated with amphotericin B. Chronic pulmonary disease frequently requires therapy with amphotericin B, but occasionally surgery plays a role in specific clinical settings.

Aspergillosis

Of all the fungi, *Aspergillus* is particularly notable for the variety of clinical presentations seen and the types of individuals predisposed. Unlike *Histoplasma* and *Coccidioides*, *Aspergillus* species are widespread throughout nature and are not limited to particular geographic areas. Also unlike these other two types of fungi, *Aspergillus* species are not dimorphic in appearance but always occur as mycelia, i.e., branching hyphal forms. Since virtually everyone is exposed to the organism, it is clear that disease must be associated with certain predisposing factors, which are now quite well-defined.

We will consider three major clinical forms of disease due to *Aspergillus*, and the three settings in which these diseases occur. The first of these, *allergic bronchopulmonary aspergillosis*, is a hypersensitivity reaction to airway colonization with *Aspergillus*, seen almost exclusively in patients with underlying asthma. The second, *aspergilloma*, is a saprophytic colonization of a pre-existing cavity in the lung by a "fungus ball" composed of a mass of *Aspergillus* hyphae. The third form, *invasive aspergillosis*, involves tissue invasion by the organism and is seen in patients who have significant impairment of their immune defense mechanisms.

Features of Aspergillus:
1. widespread distribution
2. present as branching hyphae in tissue

Clinical syndromes with aspergillosis:
1. allergic bronchopulmonary aspergillosis
2. aspergilloma
3. invasive aspergillosis

Allergic Bronchopulmonary Aspergillosis

The presence of underlying reactive airways disease, i.e., asthma, appears to be the important predisposing factor for development of allergic bronchopulmonary aspergillosis. In this condition, the organism resides in the patient's airways, where it appears to be important as an antigen rather than as an infectious, invasive fungus. Patients develop both Type I (immediate, IgE-mediated) and Type III (immune complex, IgG-mediated) immune reactions to the organism.

Clinically, patients with allergic bronchopulmonary aspergillosis not only have manifestations of asthma, such as wheezing, dyspnea, and cough, but they also may have low-grade fever and production of characteristic brownish plugs of sputum. *Aspergillus* can frequently be cultured from these plugs of sputum. The chest radiograph may show transient pulmonary infiltrates, which can be a consequence of bronchial obstruction by the plugs or a result of eosinophilic infiltration of lung tissue. In addition, bronchiectasis of proximal airways can be present, and these dilated airways may also be filled with mucous plugs.

Diagnosis is made in the proper clinical setting of underlying asthma, and it is based on culturing the organism and/or demonstrating the host's immune response to the fungus. For example, skin tests against *Aspergillus* antigen show a positive immediate reaction (reflecting Type I immunity) and a delayed (Arthus) reaction after several hours (reflecting Type III immunity). Precipitins in the blood can also frequently be identified.

Treatment of allergic bronchopulmonary aspergillosis is not aimed at the fungus but rather at the host's immunologic response to the organism. Therefore, corticosteroids are the treatment for this syndrome, not the antifungal agent amphotericin B.

Aspergilloma

The second type of clinical problem resulting from *Aspergillus* is the aspergilloma, or fungus ball. The major predisposing feature for this entity is the presence of a pre-existing cavity within the pulmonary parenchyma. Tuberculosis, sarcoidosis, and other fungal infections are a few examples of diseases in which cavities may be seen and therefore in which an aspergilloma may be a complicating problem. In these cases, the organism is essentially a saprophyte or colonizer of the cavity, with little tissue invasion. The fungus ball itself is just a mass of fungal mycelia lying within the cavity proper.

Clinically, patients with an aspergilloma present either with hemoptysis or with no symptoms but suggestive findings on chest radiograph. Classically, the radiograph demonstrates an apparent mass surrounded by a lucent rim, representing air in the cavity around the fungus ball (Fig. 25–1). When the patient changes position, the fungus ball often can be shown to change position within the cavity, according to the effects of gravity.

Diagnosis of an aspergilloma is generally suggested by the char-

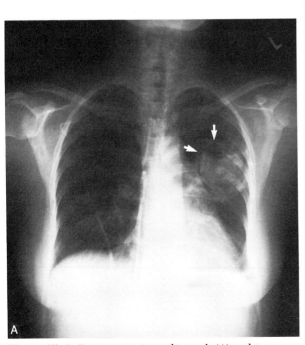
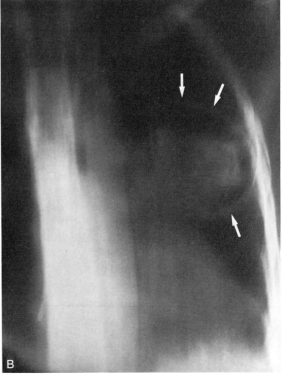

Figure 25–1. Posteroanterior radiograph (A) and tomogram (B) demonstrating an aspergilloma in the left lung. The fungus ball appears as a mass sitting within a radiolucent, thin-walled cavity. Arrows outline the wall of the cavity. (Courtesy of Dr. Ferris·Hall.)

acteristic roentgenographic appearance and is confirmed by culturing the organism or by demonstrating the presence of precipitins against *Aspergillus*. Treatment is often unnecessary, as the clinical sequelae are frequently inconsequential. In some cases, particularly those with significant amounts of hemoptysis, surgery is performed to remove the diseased area containing the fungus ball. Amphotericin B is not effective in treatment of this syndrome.

Invasive Aspergillosis

The final clinical presentation of *Aspergillus* infection in the lung is invasive aspergillosis. This is certainly the most life-threatening manifestation of *Aspergillus* infection, occurring almost exclusively in patients with marked impairment of host immune defense mechanisms. Characteristically, patients are neutropenic, i.e., have insufficient numbers of polymorphonuclear leukocytes, and often have impairment of cellular immunity as a consequence of treatment with steroids or immunosuppressive agents.

Pathologically, the organism invades and spreads through lung tissue, but it also tends to invade blood vessels within the lung. As a result of vascular involvement by the fungus, vessels can become occluded, and patients can develop areas of pulmonary infarction.

Clinically, patients are extremely ill, demonstrating fever, cough, dyspnea, and often pleuritic chest pain. The chest radiograph may show localized or diffuse pulmonary infiltrates, reflecting either tissue invasion and a fungal pneumonia or pulmonary infarction secondary to vascular occlusion.

Diagnosis of invasive aspergillosis generally requires demonstrating the organism, e.g., by methenamine silver staining, on a biopsy specimen of lung tissue. Treatment consists of amphotericin B, but even with appropriate use of this agent the mortality is extremely high.

Other Fungi

The fungi we have not discussed occur less frequently. Blastomycosis, due to the organism *Blastomyces dermatitidis*, is seen in normal hosts and is associated with pulmonary disease as well as potential problems with other organ systems. *Candida albicans*, though an extraordinarily common contaminant of sputum (particularly in the patient treated with antibiotics), is an uncommon cause of pneumonia, even in immunosuppressed patients. *Cryptococcus neoformans* is found primarily in immunosuppressed patients, in whom it causes lung disease as well as meningitis. Finally, *Mucor* is an opportunistic fungus that may cause pulmonary infection in the immunocompromised host.

PROTOZOAN INFECTIONS

Pneumocystis

The main protozoan causing lung disease is the organism *Pneumocystis carinii*. Though the natural habitat of this organism is not

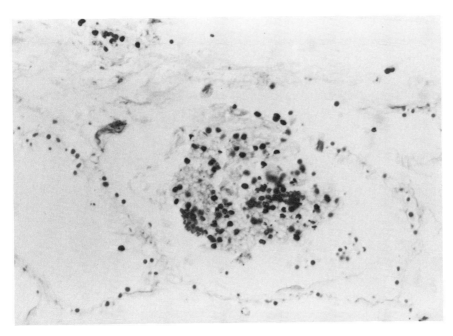

Figure 25–2. High-power photomicrograph of many Pneumocystis cysts, as seen with methenamine silver staining. The darkly staining cysts are within the alveolar lumen. There is also a foamy exudate in the alveolar lumen. (Courtesy of Dr. Earl Kasdon.)

known with certainty, it is probably widely distributed in nature. However, pulmonary infection with the organism is not seen in normal individuals and is clearly related to abnormal host defense mechanisms. A major setting for *Pneumocystis* infection is the patient with malignancy treated with steroids or other immunosuppressive agents. Recently, however, several new populations of individuals have been recognized to be at risk—homosexuals, intravenous drug abusers, and others who manifest the newly described syndrome of acquired immunodeficiency (see Chapter 22 for a discussion of AIDS).

Pneumocystis cysts, which are seen in the lung tissue of infected patients, appear on light microscopy as round or cup-shaped structures. They do not stain well with the routine hematoxylin-eosin stain and require instead special stains such as methenamine silver (Fig. 25–2). The tissue response to the organism, seen on microscopic examination of lung tissue, includes infiltration of mononuclear cells within the pulmonary interstitium and exudation of foamy fluid into alveolar spaces.

Clinically, *Pneumocystis* pneumonia usually presents in the immunocompromised patient with dyspnea and fever. The chest radiograph commonly shows diffuse infiltrates, frequently taking the appearance of a bilateral alveolar filling pattern (Fig. 25–3). Hypoxemia is often a particularly prominent clinical feature in these patients. Though the disease is sometimes insidious in onset, it usually presents as an acute pneumonia and, if untreated, may progress to respiratory failure and death within days.

Since the organism is extremely difficult to cultivate in the laboratory setting, diagnosis depends on demonstrating the organism on stains of tissue sections or respiratory "secretions" (e.g., washings obtained by fiberoptic bronchoscopy). No serologic or skin testing methods are available for diagnosis. The current treatment of choice for *Pneumocystis* infection is a combination of trimethoprim and sulfa-

Features of **Pneumocystis carinii:**
1. ubiquitous distribution
2. diagnosis by methenamine silver stain
3. tissue response is primarily exudation of foamy fluid into alveoli

Clinical features of **Pneumocystis** *pneumonia:*
1. symptoms—dyspnea, fever
2. chest radiograph—frequently diffuse alveolar infiltrates
3. hypoxemia

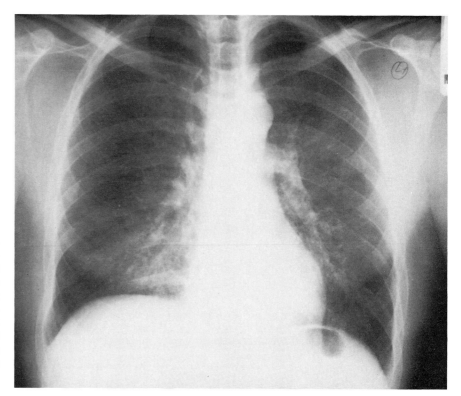

Figure 25–3. Chest radiograph of a patient with acquired immunodeficiency syndrome (AIDS) and pneumonia due to *Pneumocystis carinii*. Infiltrates representing alveolar filling are most prominent at the right base, but they are also seen in the left mid-lung field as a diffuse haziness.

methoxazole, which is effective in approximately 80 percent of patients. In high-risk patients, low doses of the same agents have often been used prophylactically to prevent the infection.

Other Protozoa

The only other protozoan we will mention is *Toxoplasma gondii*. It is associated with a variety of clinical syndromes, one of which is pulmonary infection in the immunocompromised host. However, it is quite uncommon even in this setting, occurring much less frequently than *Pneumocystis carinii*.

REFERENCES

General

Fanta, C. H., and Pennington, J. E.: Fever and new lung infiltrates in the immunocompromised host. Clin. Chest Med. 2:19–39, 1981.
Williams, D. M., Krick, J. A., and Remington, J. S.: Pulmonary infection in the compromised host. Am. Rev. Respir. Dis. 114:359–394; 593–627, 1976.

Fungal Infections (General References)

American Thoracic Society: Treatment of fungal diseases. Am. Rev. Respir. Dis. 120:1393–1397, 1979.
Gold, J. W. M.: Opportunistic fungal infections in patients with neoplastic disease. Am. J. Med. 76:458–463, 1984.
Sarosi, G. A.: Management of fungal diseases. Am. Rev. Respir. Dis. 127:250–253, 1983.
Stamm, A. M., and Dismukes, W. E.: Current therapy of pulmonary and disseminated fungal diseases. Chest 83:911–917, 1983.

Histoplasmosis

Goodwin, R. A., Loyd, J. E., and Des Prez, R. M.: Histoplasmosis in normal hosts. Medicine 60:231–266, 1981.
Goodwin, R. A., Jr. and Des Prez, R. M.: Histoplasmosis. Am. Rev. Respir. Dis. 117:929–956, 1978.

Coccidioidomycosis

Bayer, A. S.: Fungal pneumonias: pulmonary coccidioidal syndromes. Chest. 79:575–583; 686–691, 1981.
Drutz, D. J., and Catanzaro, A.: Coccidioidomycosis. Am. Rev. Respir. Dis. 117:559–595; 727–771, 1978.

Aspergillosis

Glimp, R. A., and Bayer, A. S.: Fungal pneumonias. Part 3. Allergic bronchopulmonary aspergillosis. Chest 80:85–94, 1981.
Glimp, R. A., and Bayer, A. S.: Pulmonary aspergilloma: diagnostic and therapeutic considerations. Arch. Intern. Med. 143:303–308, 1983.
Herbert, P. A., and Bayer, A. S.: Fungal pneumonia (Part 4): invasive pulmonary aspergillosis. Chest 80:220–225, 1981.
Rosenberg, M., Patterson, R., Mintzer, R., Cooper, B. J., Roberts, M., and Harris, K. E.: Clinical and immunologic criteria for the diagnosis of allergic bronchopulmonary aspergillosis. Ann. Intern. Med. 86:405–414, 1977.

Protozoa—Pneumocystis

Follansbee, S. E., et al.: An outbreak of *Pneumocystis carinii* pneumonia in homosexual men. Ann. Intern. Med. 96(Part 1):705–713, 1982.
Haverkos, H. W.: Assessment of therapy for *Pneumocystis carinii* pneumonia. Am. J. Med. 76:501–508, 1984.
Hughes, W. T.: *Pneumocystis carinii* pneumonia. N. Engl. J. Med. 297:1381–1383, 1977.
Hughes, W. T.: *Pneumocystis carinii* pneumonitis. Chest 85:810–813, 1984.

26

Classification and Pathophysiologic Aspects of Respiratory Failure

By the time the reader has reached this point in the book, it should be obvious that many different types of respiratory disease have the capability of impairing the lung's normal function as a gas-exchanging organ. In some cases, the degree of impairment is mild, and the patient suffers relatively few consequences. In other cases, dysfunction is marked, and the patient experiences disabling or life-threatening clinical sequelae. When the respiratory system can no longer function to keep gas exchange at an acceptable level, the patient is said to be in *respiratory failure*, irrespective of the underlying cause.

The tempo for development of respiratory failure varies depending on the nature of the underlying problem. Many of the diseases we have discussed so far, such as chronic obstructive lung disease and interstitial lung disease, are characterized by a chronic clinical course, accompanied by relatively slow deterioration of pulmonary function and gas exchange. However, because of their limited pulmonary reserve, patients with pre-existing pulmonary disease are also susceptible to episodes of acute respiratory failure, either from an intercurrent illness or from transient worsening of their underlying disease. On the other hand, individuals without pre-existing lung disease may also develop respiratory failure, generally acute or subacute in onset. The initiating problem in the latter patient is often a primary respiratory illness or a disorder of another organ system, complicated by major respiratory problems.

The goal of this chapter is to present an overview of the problem of respiratory failure and to discuss the different pathophysiologic types and consequences of respiratory insufficiency. In the following chapter, we will discuss a specific form of acute respiratory failure known as the adult respiratory distress syndrome, which does not require the presence of pre-existing lung disease. And finally, the last chapter of this book will consider some principles of management of respiratory failure as well as specific modalities of therapy currently available to us.

DEFINITION OF RESPIRATORY FAILURE

Respiratory failure is probably best defined as inability of the respiratory system to maintain adequate gas exchange. Exactly where we draw the line for adequate gas exchange is somewhat arbitrary, but in the previously normal individual an arterial PO_2 lower than 60 torr or a PCO_2 greater than 50 torr can be considered evidence for acute respiratory failure. In the individual with pre-existing lung disease, the situation is even more complicated, since the patient chronically has impaired gas exchange and abnormal blood gases.

Arterial blood gas criteria for respiratory failure: $PO_2 < 60$ torr or $PCO_2 > 50$ torr.

For example, it would not be unusual for a patient with significant chronic bronchitis to undergo his usual daily activities with a PO_2 of perhaps 60 torr and a PCO_2 of 50 to 55 torr. By the blood gas criteria we have set, this patient is always in respiratory failure, but this is obviously chronic, not acute. When we look at the patient's pH, we find that his kidneys have compensated for the CO_2 retention and that his pH is not far from the normal value of 7.40.

When do we say that this patient has gone into acute respiratory failure? Certainly, if he develops an acute respiratory illness such as an acute pneumonia, his gas exchange becomes even worse. The PO_2 falls further, while the PCO_2 may rise even higher. In this case, we are forced to define acute respiratory failure as a significant change from the patient's baseline gas exchange status. If we know the patient's usual arterial blood gases, our task is easier. If we do not, examination of the patient's pH can at least give us a clue about whether his CO_2 retention is acute or chronic. When a patient presents with a PCO_2 of 70 torr, the implications are quite different if the accompanying pH is 7.15 as opposed to 7.36.

CLASSIFICATION OF ACUTE RESPIRATORY FAILURE

Hypoxemic Type

In practice, it is most convenient to classify acute respiratory failure into two major categories, based on the pattern of gas exchange abnormalities. In the first category, hypoxemia is the major problem, and the patient's PCO_2 is normal or even low. For our purposes, we

Categories of acute respiratory failure:
1. hypoxemic (with normal or low PCO_2)
2. hypercapnic/hypoxemic

will call this the hypoxemic variety of acute respiratory failure. As an example, localized diseases of the pulmonary parenchyma, such as pneumonia, can result in this type of respiratory failure, if the disease is sufficiently severe. However, an even broader group of etiologic factors causes hypoxemic respiratory failure via a generalized increase in fluid within the alveolar spaces, often as a result of leakage of fluid from pulmonary capillaries. The latter problem is frequently called the *adult respiratory distress syndrome (ARDS)* and can be the consequence of a wide variety of disorders that cause an increase in pulmonary capillary permeability. Because of the importance of this syndrome as a major form of acute respiratory failure, we have reserved the following chapter entirely for discussion of this problem.

Examples of hypoxemic respiratory failure:
1. severe pneumonia
2. ARDS

Hypercapnic/Hypoxemic Type

In the second category, hypercapnia is present; for the respiratory failure to be considered acute, the pH must show that there is absent or incomplete metabolic compensation for the respiratory acidosis. If we recall the discussion of alveolar gas composition and the alveolar gas equation in Chapter 1, it is apparent that hypercapnia is associated with a decreased arterial oxygen tension by virtue of an altered alveolar P_{O_2}. Therefore, even if ventilation and perfusion are relatively well-matched and the fraction of blood shunted across the pulmonary vasculature is not increased, the arterial P_{O_2} falls in the presence of hypercapnia. In fact, many cases of hypercapnic respiratory failure have marked ventilation-perfusion mismatch occurring as well, which further accentuates the hypoxemia. With these concepts in mind, it is clear that the hypercapnic form of respiratory failure generally involves not just hypercapnia but rather may be more appropriately considered as the hypercapnic/hypoxemic form of respiratory failure.

A number of types of respiratory disease are potentially associated with this second form of respiratory failure. In a subsequent section of this chapter, we will discuss exactly how the various disorders result in hypercapnic/hypoxemic respiratory failure. These disorders primarily include (1) depression of the neurologic system responsible for respiratory control; (2) disease of the respiratory bellows, either the chest wall or the neuromuscular apparatus responsible for thoracic expansion; and (3) chronic obstructive lung disease. It is also quite common for more than one of these three factors to be present, thus compounding the potential for respiratory insufficiency.

Causes of hypercapnic/hypoxemic respiratory failure:
1. depression of central nervous system ventilatory control
2. disease of the respiratory bellows
3. chronic obstructive lung disease

In the hypercapnic/hypoxemic form of respiratory failure, the patients generally have pre-existing disease that is responsible either for chronic respiratory insufficiency or for limitations in respiratory reserve sufficient to make them much more susceptible to "going over the brink" with an acute superimposed problem. In common parlance, this form of respiratory failure is frequently called *acute on chronic respiratory failure*, obviously reflecting the prior problems or limitations with respiratory reserve. This expression has especially been used to describe the patient with chronic obstructive pulmonary disease who develops acute respiratory failure at the time of an infection or another acute respiratory insult.

PRESENTATION OF GAS EXCHANGE FAILURE

When patients develop acute respiratory failure, their symptom complex generally includes the manifestations of hypoxemia and/or hypercapnia, accompanied by the specific symptoms related to the precipitating disorder. Dyspnea is also present in the majority of cases and is the symptom that often suggests to the physician the possibility of respiratory failure.

Impairment of mental abilities is also a frequent result of either hypoxemia or hypercapnia. Patients may become disoriented, confused, and unable to conduct their normal level of activity. With profound hypercapnia, patients may become stuporous and eventually lapse into a frank coma. Headache is commonly found in patients with hypercapnia. Dilation of cerebral blood vessels as a consequence of increased P_{CO_2} is probably important in the pathogenesis of the headache.

Physical findings associated with abnormal gas exchange are relatively few. Patients may be tachypneic, tachycardic, and restless, findings that are relatively nonspecific. Examination of the optic fundus may show papilledema (an elevation of the optic disk) resulting from hypercapnia, cerebral vasodilation, and an increase in pressure at the back of the eye. Findings in the lung are related to the specific form of disease that is present, e.g., wheezing and/or rhonchi in chronic obstructive lung disease, crackles as a result of fluid in the small airways and alveolar spaces. When hypoxia is severe, patients may become cyanotic, which is apparent as a dusky or bluish hue to the nailbeds and the lips.

Clinical presentation with respiratory failure:
1. dyspnea
2. impaired mental status
3. headache
4. tachycardia
5. papilledema (with $\uparrow P_{CO_2}$)
6. variable lung exam
7. cyanosis (with severe hypoxemia)

PATHOGENESIS OF GAS EXCHANGE ABNORMALITIES

Since we discussed the basic principles of abnormal gas exchange in Chapter 1, we will now focus on applications of these principles to the patient with respiratory failure. We will first consider hypoxemic respiratory failure and then proceed with a discussion of hypercapnic/hypoxemic failure.

Hypoxemic Respiratory Failure

In the patient with hypoxemic respiratory failure, two major pathophysiologic factors contribute to the lowering of arterial P_{O_2}—ventilation-perfusion mismatch and shunting. As we discussed earlier, in the patient with significant ventilation-perfusion mismatch, regions having a low ratio of ventilation to perfusion contribute relatively desaturated blood to the systemic circulation. What sorts of problems cause ventilation to be decreased relative to perfusion in a particular region of lung? If an alveolus or group of alveoli is partially filled with fluid, then a limited amount of ventilation reaches that particular area, whereas perfusion to the region may remain relatively preserved. Similarly, if an airway supplying a region of lung is diseased, either by pathology of the airway wall or by secretions occupying the lumen, then ventilation is again limited.

When these problems become most extreme, ventilation to a region of lung may be totally absent, so that a true shunt exists. For example, alveoli may be completely filled with fluid or an airway may be completely obstructed, preventing any ventilation to the involved area. Though the response of the pulmonary vasculature is to constrict and thereby limit perfusion to an under- or nonventilated portion of the lung, this protective mechanism is often unable to compensate fully for the loss of ventilation, and hypoxemia results.

As we will discuss in Chapter 27, alveolar filling with fluid as well as collapse of small airways and alveoli seem to be the main pathogenetic features leading to $\dot{V}/\dot{Q}$ mismatch and shunting in the adult respiratory distress syndrome. When we considered the ability of supplemental oxygen to raise the PO_2 under conditions of $\dot{V}/\dot{Q}$ mismatch versus shunt, we mentioned that oxygen is unable to improve the PO_2 significantly for truly shunted blood (see Chapter 1). Therefore, when the shunt fraction of the cardiac output is quite high, oxygenation may be helped surprisingly little by the administration of supplemental oxygen.

Despite the marked derangement in oxygenation in ARDS, CO_2 elimination remains adequate, as the patients are able to maintain alveolar ventilation at an acceptable level. In fact, even when there are regions of lung that have a high ventilation-perfusion ratio and thus effectively act as dead space, the patients are generally able to compensate by increasing their overall minute ventilation.

Hypercapnic/Hypoxemic Respiratory Failure

In the hypercapnic form of respiratory failure, patients are unable to maintain a level of alveolar ventilation sufficient to eliminate CO_2 and keep arterial PCO_2 within the normal range. Since ventilation is determined by a sequence of events ranging from the generation of impulses by the respiratory controller to the movement of air through the airways, there are several stages at which problems can adversely affect total minute ventilation. This sequence is shown in Figure 26-1, which also lists some of the disorders that can interfere at each level. Not only is the total ventilation per minute important, but the "effectiveness" of the ventilation for CO_2 excretion, i.e., the relative amount of alveolar versus dead space ventilation, is also important to assure proper utilization of inspired gas. If the proportion of each breath going to dead space (i.e., V_D/V_T ratio) increases substantially, then alveolar ventilation may fall to a level sufficient to cause an elevated PCO_2, even if total minute ventilation is preserved.

In the hypercapnic form of respiratory failure, hypoventilation also leads to a decrease in alveolar PO_2. Thus arterial PO_2 may fall even if ventilation-perfusion matching and gas exchange at the alveolar level are well maintained. In practice, however, many of the diseases associated with alveolar hypoventilation, ranging from neuromuscular and chest wall disease to chronic airflow obstruction, are accompanied by significant ventilation-perfusion mismatch. Therefore, these patients generally have two major reasons for hypoxemia—hypoventilation and $\dot{V}/\dot{Q}$ mismatch. Interestingly, true shunts usually play a very

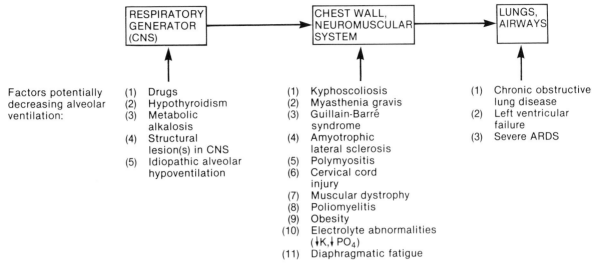

Figure 26–1. Levels at which there may be interference with normal ventilation, giving rise to alveolar hypoventilation. Factors contributing to decreased ventilation are listed under each level.

limited role in causing hypoxemia in these disorders, unlike the situation in ARDS.

Given the causes of hypoxemia in the hypercapnic/hypoxemic form of respiratory failure, it is not surprising that patients frequently respond to supplemental oxygen with a substantial rise in arterial Po_2. However, most of these patients have at least mild chronic CO_2 retention, with their acute respiratory failure due to some precipitating insult or to worsening of their underlying disease. As we mentioned in Chapter 18, for a number of reasons that are not yet entirely clear, administration of supplemental oxygen to these chronically hypercapnic patients may lead to a further increase in arterial Pco_2. Fortunately, with judicious use of supplemental oxygen, substantial additional elevation of arterial Pco_2 can usually be avoided.

We will proceed now with an elaboration of further features of the hypercapnic/hypoxemic form of respiratory failure. Discussion of ARDS, the major form of hypoxemic respiratory failure, will be reserved for Chapter 27.

CLINICAL AND THERAPEUTIC ASPECTS OF HYPERCAPNIC/HYPOXEMIC RESPIRATORY FAILURE

Whether the underlying disease is chest wall disease, such as kyphoscoliosis, or chronic obstructive lung disease, patients who go into this type of respiratory failure often have chronic respiratory insufficiency as their starting point. This is not true of all cases, however, since there are certain neurologic problems, such as Guillain-Barré syndrome, in which hypercapnic respiratory failure occurs in a previously normal individual.

When the patient has chronic disease upon which acute respiratory failure is superimposed, the phrase "acute on chronic respiratory failure" is frequently used, as mentioned earlier. In such cases, there is often a specific additional problem that precipitates the acute deterioration, and it is important to identify the problem if at all possible.

Frequent precipitants for acute on chronic respiratory failure:
1. respiratory tract infection
2. drugs, e.g., sedatives, narcotics
3. congestive heart failure
4. less common—pulmonary emboli, exposure to environmental pollutants

What are some of the intercurrent problems or factors that precipitate acute respiratory failure in these patients? Perhaps the most common is an acute respiratory tract infection, such as bronchitis, usually but not always due to a virus. Bacterial etiologies must always be investigated, however, since they are often amenable to specific therapy. Use of drugs that suppress the respiratory center, such as sedatives or narcotics, may also precipitate hypercapnic respiratory failure by virtue of depressing central respiratory drive in a previously marginal individual. Other intercurrent problems include congestive heart failure, pulmonary emboli, and exposure to environmental pollutants, each of which may be sufficient to push the borderline compensated patient "over the brink" with regard to CO_2 retention.

The general therapeutic approach to these patients involves several main areas: (1) support of gas exchange; (2) treatment of the acute precipitating event; and (3) treatment of the underlying pulmonary disease. Support of gas exchange involves maintaining adequate oxygenation and elimination of CO_2; we will discuss these problems in more detail in Chapter 28. Briefly, supplemental oxygen, generally in a concentration not much higher than that found in ambient air, is administered to raise the Po_2 to an acceptable level, i.e., greater than 60 torr. If CO_2 elimination deteriorates much beyond the usual level of Pco_2, then the patient develops an acute respiratory acidosis superimposed upon his or her usual acid-base status. If the patient becomes quite acidemic or if his or her mental status changes significantly as a result of CO_2 retention, then intubation and mechanical ventilation may be required.

Treating the precipitating factor for acute respiratory failure is most successful when bacterial infection or congestive heart failure is responsible for the acute deterioration. Antibiotics for suspected bacterial infection and diuretics and a digitalis glycoside for congestive heart failure are appropriate forms of therapy in these circumstances. For patients in whom respiratory secretions seem to be playing a role either chronically or in an acute exacerbation of their disease, attempts to assist in clearance of secretions may be beneficial. In particular, chest physical therapy, in which percussion and vibration of the chest are given, followed by appropriate positioning to allow gravity assistance in drainage of secretions, may be beneficial.

How effective treatment of the underlying pulmonary disease is obviously depends on the nature of the disease. For patients with obstructive lung disease, intensive therapy with bronchodilators and sometimes corticosteroids may be helpful in reversing whatever component of bronchoconstriction is present. If neuromuscular or chest wall disease is the underlying problem, then therapy is sometimes available, as is the case with myasthenia gravis. Unfortunately, for most neuromuscular or chest wall diseases no specific form of therapy exists, and support of gas exchange and treatment of any precipitating factors are the major modes of therapy.

When patients with irreversible chest wall or neuromuscular disease are in frank respiratory failure, they may require some form of ventilatory assistance on a chronic basis. Though consideration of the alternative modalities for chronic ventilatory support is beyond the scope of this discussion, it is important to realize that the primary decision is whether chronic ventilatory support should be given to a patient with this type of irreversible disease. In many cases, the joint decision of the patient, the family, and the physician is that life should not be prolonged with chronic ventilator support, given the projected quality of life and the irreversible nature of the process.

REFERENCES

General

Bone, R. C. (ed.): Symposium on Respiratory Failure. Med. Clin. North Am. 67:551–746, 1983.
Zwillich, C., Kryger, M., and Weil, J.: Hypoventilation: consequences and management. Adv. Intern. Med. 23:287–306, 1978.

Respiratory Failure in Obstructive Lung Disease

Aubier, M., et al.: Effects of the administration of O_2 on ventilation and blood gases in patients with chronic obstructive pulmonary disease during acute respiratory failure. Am. Rev. Respir. Dis. 122:747–754, 1980.
Bone, R. C., Pierce, A. K., and Johnson, R. L., Jr.: Controlled oxygen administration in acute respiratory failure in chronic obstructive pulmonary disease. Am. J. Med. 65:896–902, 1978.
Burk, R. H., and George, R. B.: Acute respiratory failure in chronic obstructive pulmonary disease. Arch. Intern. Med. 132:865–868, 1973.

Respiratory Failure in Neuromuscular and Chest Wall Disease

Bergofsky, E. H.: Respiratory failure in disorders of the thoracic cage. Am. Rev. Respir. Dis. 119:643–669, 1979.
Gracey, D. R., Divertie, M. B., and Howard, F. M., Jr.: Mechanical ventilation for respiratory failure in myasthenia gravis. Mayo Clin. Proc. 58:597–602, 1983.
Gracey, D. R., McMichan, J. C., Divertie, M. B., and Howard, F. M., Jr.: Respiratory failure in Guillain-Barré syndrome. Mayo Clin. Proc. 57:742–746, 1982.

27

Adult Respiratory Distress Syndrome

Physiology of Fluid Movement in the Alveolar Interstitium
    Two Mechanisms of Fluid Accumulation
Etiology
    Inhaled Injurious Agents
    Injury Via the Pulmonary Circulation
Pathogenesis
Pathology
Pathophysiology
    Effects on Gas Exchange
    Changes in the Pulmonary Vasculature
    Effects on the Mechanical Properties of the Lungs
Clinical Features
Diagnostic Approach
Treatment

As a continuation of our discussion of respiratory failure, we will proceed with more detailed consideration of one important type of acute respiratory failure—the *adult respiratory distress syndrome* or *ARDS*. This syndrome represents a major form of hypoxemic respiratory failure; its clinical and pathophysiologic features differ considerably from those we discussed for acute on chronic respiratory failure.

Rather than a specific disease, adult respiratory distress syndrome is truly a syndrome, resulting from any of a number of etiologic factors. It is perhaps easiest to consider this syndrome as the nonspecific result of acute injury to the lung, characterized by breakdown of the normal barrier preventing leakage of fluid out of the pulmonary capillaries and into the interstitium and alveolar spaces. A number of other names have also been used to describe ARDS, including noncardiogenic pulmonary edema, shock lung, and post-traumatic pulmonary insufficiency, just to name a few.

In this chapter, we will first consider the dynamics of fluid transfer between the pulmonary vessels and the alveolar interstitium, since an alteration in this process is so important in the pathogenesis of ARDS.

We will then outline the many types of injury that can result in ARDS and present some of the theories proposed to explain how such a diverse group of disorders can produce this syndrome. A discussion of the pathologic, pathophysiologic, and clinical consequences will follow. Finally, a general approach to treatment will conclude the chapter, but more specific details about support of gas exchange will be presented in Chapter 28.

PHYSIOLOGY OF FLUID MOVEMENT IN THE ALVEOLAR INTERSTITIUM

Despite the diverse group of disorders that can cause ARDS, the net result of this syndrome is the same—a disturbance in the normal barrier limiting leakage of fluid out of the pulmonary capillaries and into the pulmonary parenchyma. Before we discuss some of the theories explaining how this barrier is damaged, we will briefly consider the determinants of fluid transport between the pulmonary vessels, the interstital space, and the alveolar lumen. For this purpose, we can view the pulmonary parenchyma as shown in Figure 27–1, consisting

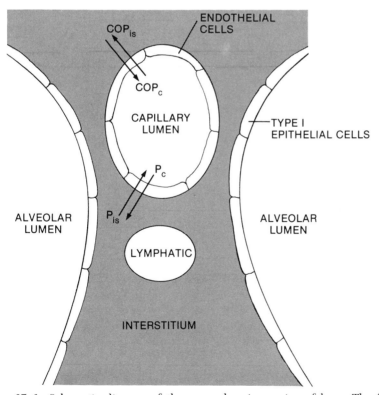

Figure 27–1. Schematic diagram of the gas-exchanging region of lung. The forces governing fluid movement between the pulmonary capillary lumen and the alveolar interstitium are shown. P_c = pulmonary capillary hydrostatic pressure; P_{is} = interstitial space hydrostatic pressure; COP_c = pulmonary capillary colloid osmotic pressure; COP_{is} = interstitial space colloid osmotic pressure. Arrows show the direction of fluid movement favored by each of the important forces.

of (1) small vessels coursing through the alveolar walls, which for simplicity's sake we will refer to as the pulmonary capillaries; (2) the pulmonary capillary endothelium, the lining cells that normally limit but do not completely prevent fluid movement out of the capillaries; (3) the pulmonary interstitium, which for our purposes here refers to the alveolar wall exclusive of vessels and the epithelial cells lining the alveolar lumen; (4) lymphatic channels, which are found largely in perivascular connective tissue in the lung; (5) alveolar epithelial cells, lining the surface of the alveolar lumen; and (6) the alveolar lumen or alveolar space.

Movement of fluid out of the pulmonary capillaries and into the interstitial space is determined by a number of factors, including the hydrostatic pressures in the vessels and in the pulmonary interstitium, the colloid osmotic pressures in these same two compartments, and the permeability of the endothelium. The effect of these factors in determining fluid transport is summarized in the Starling equation, which we examined earlier in Chapter 15 with regard to fluid transport across the pleural space. This equation is reproduced again as Equation 27–1:

$$F = K[(P_c - P_{is}) - \sigma (COP_c - COP_{is})] \qquad (27\text{--}1)$$

where F = fluid movement; P_c and P_{is} = pulmonary capillary and interstitial hydrostatic pressures; COP_c and COP_{is} = pulmonary capillary and the interstitial colloid osmotic (oncotic) pressures; K = the filtration coefficient; and σ the reflection coefficient (a measure of the permeability of the endothelium for protein).

Fluid normally moves from the pulmonary capillaries to the interstitial space; resorption by lymphatics prevents accumulation.

If we substitute an estimate of the actual numbers for normal hydrostatic and oncotic pressures in Equation 27–1, we find that F is a positive number, indicating that fluid normally moves out of the pulmonary capillaries and into the interstitial space. Even though the rate of fluid movement out of the pulmonary capillaries is estimated to be approximately 20 ml per hr, this fluid does not accumulate; the lymphatics are quite effective in absorbing both protein and fluid that have left the vasculature and entered the interstitial space. However, if fluid movement into the interstitium increases substantially or if lymphatic drainage is impeded, then fluid accumulates within the interstitial space, resulting in interstitial edema. When sufficient fluid accumulates or when the alveolar epithelium is damaged, fluid also moves across the epithelial cell barrier and into the alveolar spaces, resulting in alveolar edema.

Two Mechanisms of Fluid Accumulation

In practice, the forces described in the Starling equation become imbalanced in two main ways, producing interstitial and often alveolar edema (Table 27–1). The first occurs when hydrostatic pressure within the pulmonary capillaries (P_c) is increased, generally as a consequence of elevated left ventricular or left atrial pressures (e.g., in left ventricular failure or mitral stenosis). The resulting pulmonary edema is called *cardiogenic* or *hydrostatic* pulmonary edema, and the cause is essen-

Table 27–1. CATEGORIES OF PULMONARY EDEMA

Feature	Cardiogenic	Noncardiogenic
Major etiologies	Left ventricular failure, mitral stenosis	ARDS
Pulmonary capillary pressure	Increased	Normal
Pulmonary capillary permeability	Normal	Increased
Protein content of edema fluid	Low	High

tially an imbalance between the hydrostatic and oncotic forces governing fluid movement. In this form of edema, the permeability barrier that limits movement of protein out of the intravascular space is intact, and the fluid that leaks out has a very low protein content.

In the second mechanism by which fluid accumulates, hydrostatic pressures are normal, but the permeability of the capillary endothelial and alveolar epithelial barriers is increased as a result of damage to one or both of these cell populations. Movement of proteins out of the intravascular space now occurs as a consequence of the increase in permeability. The fluid that leaks out has a relatively high protein content, often close to that found in plasma. This second mechanism is the one operative in ARDS. Since an elevation in pulmonary capillary pressure from cardiac disease is not involved, this form of edema is called *noncardiogenic* pulmonary edema.

In subsequent parts of this chapter, we will not concern ourselves with cardiogenic or hydrostatic pulmonary edema but rather will focus our discussion on noncardiogenic edema, i.e., adult respiratory distress syndrome. However, it is important to remember that even patients with a permeability defect of their pulmonary capillary bed can simultaneously have high pulmonary capillary pressure as a result of coincidental left ventricular failure. In these cases, both a permeability defect and the elevated hydrostatic pressure contribute to leakage of fluid out of the pulmonary vasculature. Not only is the fluid leak compounded, but when both factors are involved it is often quite difficult to sort out the relative importance of each.

ETIOLOGY

As can be seen from Table 27–2, numerous and varied disorders have now been associated with the potential to produce ARDS. What these diverse etiologies of ARDS have in common is their ability to cause diffuse injury to the pulmonary parenchyma. Beyond that, it is hard with our present knowledge to define other features linking the underlying causes. Even the route of injury varies. Some etiologies involve inhaled injurious agents; others appear to be brought to the lung via the circulation rather than the airway.

Inhaled Injurious Agents

Numerous injurious agents that reach the pulmonary parenchyma through the airway have now been identified. In some cases, a liquid

Table 27–2. CAUSES OF ADULT RESPIRATORY DISTRESS SYNDROME (ARDS)

Aspiration	Trauma
Gastric contents	
Salt/frsh water near drowning)	Disseminated intravascular coagulation
Hydrocarbons	
	Embolism
Gas inhalation	Fat embolism
Oxygen toxicity	Amniotic fluid embolism
Nitrogen dioxide (NO_2)	
Smoke	Drugs
Ammonia	Narcotics
Phosgene	Sedatives
	Aspirin (rare)
Diffuse pneumonia	Thiazides (rare)
Viral	
Bacterial	Pancreatitis
Pneumocystis carinii	
	Neurogenic
Sepsis	Head trauma
	Intracranial hemorrhage
Shock	Seizures

is responsible; examples include gastric contents, salt or fresh water, or hydrocarbons. With acid gastric contents, especially when the pH is lower than 2.5, patients sustain a "chemical burn" to the pulmonary parenchyma, resulting in damage to the alveolar epithelium. In the case of near drowning, in either fresh or salt water, not only does the inhaled water fill alveolar spaces, but secondary damage to the alveolar-capillary barrier also causes fluid to leak out of the pulmonary vasculature. Since salt water is hypertonic to plasma, it is capable of drawing fluid from the circulation as a result of an osmotic pressure gradient. Fresh water, on the other hand, is hypotonic to plasma and to cellular contents and thus may enter pulmonary parenchymal cells with resulting cellular edema. In addition, fresh water appears to' inactivate surfactant, a complicating factor that we will shortly discuss in more detail. Finally, aspirated hydrocarbons can be quite toxic to the distal parenchyma, perhaps also in part because they inactivate surfactant and cause significant changes in surface tension.

Of the inhaled, potentially toxic gases perhaps the most important one is oxygen, which causes injury when inhaled at high concentrations for a prolonged period of time. It is ironic that oxygen can itself be a causative factor for ARDS, since it is so important in the supportive treatment of this syndrome. In patients requiring high concentrations of supplemental oxygen to maintain an adequate Po_2, the therapy itself may certainly compound the problem by furthering cellular damage and increasing alveolar-capillary permeability. The mechanism of oxygen toxicity is believed to be generation of free radicals and superoxide anions, by-products of oxidative metabolism that are toxic to pulmonary epithelial and endothelial cells.

Several other inhaled gases have been identified as potential acute toxins and precipitants of ARDS. Nitrogen dioxide is one example, as are some chemical products of combustion inhaled in smoke.

Infectious agents may also produce injury via airway access to the pulmonary parenchyma. Perhaps the most important example is viral pneumonia, which has the capability of damaging parenchymal cells and altering alveolar-capillary permeability. With the recent appearance of the acquired immunodeficiency syndrome, pneumonia due to *Pneumocystis carinii* has become another important, relatively common example.

Injury Via the Pulmonary Circulation

For those etiologies of ARDS that do not involve inhaled agents or toxins, it has been presumed that the pulmonary circulation in some way initiates the injury. However, in most cases a specific circulating factor has not been identified with certainty, even though several possibilities have been proposed. One of the most common precipitants for ARDS is sepsis, in which microorganisms or their products (especially endotoxin) circulating through the bloodstream can initiate a sequence of events resulting in toxicity to parenchymal cells.

Though the term *shock lung* has been used in the past for ARDS, the presence of hypotensive shock alone is probably not sufficient for the development of ARDS. Patients who develop ARDS seemingly as a result of hypotension usually have complicating potential etiologies (e.g., trauma, sepsis) or have received therapy (e.g., blood transfusions) also capable of cellular damage.

Patients who have developed a coagulation disorder known as disseminated intravascular coagulation (DIC) also appear to have the potential to develop ARDS. In DIC, patients have ongoing activation of both the clotting mechanism and the protective fibrinolytic system that prevents clot formation and propagation. Like ARDS, DIC is also a syndrome and can occur for a variety of primary or underlying reasons. However, it is not entirely clear how ARDS and DIC are related. Though there is frequently an association between these two problems, whether and exactly how one causes the other remains uncertain.

When fat or amniotic fluid enters the circulation, the material is transported to the lung, resulting in the clinical problems of fat embolism and amniotic fluid embolism, respectively. Presumably, these materials are directly toxic to endothelial cells of the pulmonary capillaries, and they certainly have been associated with the development of ARDS.

A variety of drugs, many of which fall into the class of narcotics, are potential causes of ARDS. In most cases, an overdose of the drug has been taken, though this is not always the situation. One of the agents most frequently recognized has been heroin, and the name "heroin pulmonary edema" has sometimes been used. In addition to heroin and other narcotics, several other drugs have been described as occasionally causing ARDS, including even aspirin and thiazide diuretics. Though the problem of drug-induced pulmonary edema has been well-described, the mechanism by which it occurs is not at all certain.

Some patients with acute pancreatitis develop a clinical picture consistent with noncardiogenic pulmonary edema. In this situation, it has been proposed that enzymes released into the circulation from the damaged pancreas may directly injure pulmonary parenchymal cells or initiate other indirect pathways resulting in injury.

Finally, certain disorders of the central nervous system, particularly trauma or intracerebral bleeding associated with increased intracranial pressure, are known to be associated with development of ARDS. Similarly, ARDS occasionally occurs after generalized seizures. Though there has been speculation about the cause of this so-called "neurogenic pulmonary edema," the mechanism is currently unknown.

PATHOGENESIS

The initial injury in ARDS affects alveolar epithelial (type I) and/or capillary endothelial cells.

How do these diverse clinical problems all result in the syndrome of increased pulmonary capillary permeability that we call ARDS? It appears that one important factor is the ability to produce injury to pulmonary capillary endothelial and alveolar epithelial cells (primarily type I epithelial cells, whose cytoplasmic processes provide most of the surface area lining the alveolar walls). Given the wide variety of insults that can damage these cell types, it seems unlikely that a single common mechanism is operative for all kinds of injury.

When we discussed some of the specific etiologies of ARDS, we also briefly mentioned a few of the theories of pathogenesis for individual disorders. However, it is worthwhile now to consider some of the more generalized theories proposed to explain how epithelial and endothelial cells become damaged, particularly during the course of sepsis. The two main theories that have enjoyed some popularity revolve around toxic products of neutrophils and disturbances in coagulation resulting in microemboli. We will consider these in turn.

Theories of pathogenesis of ARDS induced by sepsis: 1. neutrophil-derived injury— via superoxide radicals, proteolytic enzymes 2. coagulation-derived injury—via products from disseminated intravascular coagulation, microemboli

In the neutrophil theory an important role is played by the complement pathway. When complement is activated by sepsis, C5a is released and is responsible for aggregation of neutrophils within the pulmonary vasculature. These neutrophils may then release a variety of substances potentially toxic to cellular and noncellular components of the alveolar wall. Superoxide radicals, other by-products of oxidative metabolism, and various proteolytic enzymes can all be released by neutrophils and may be important pathogenetically in producing structural and functional injury to the alveolar wall.

The possibility that the coagulation system is important in the pathogenesis of ARDS is suggested by the frequent finding of small thrombi or microemboli in the lungs of patients dying with ARDS. In many cases, there is frank evidence of widespread disturbance of the coagulation system in the form of disseminated intravascular coagulation (DIC). Products of this process do circulate in the blood and also have the potential for being toxic to alveolar constituents. Finally, it has also been suggested that prostaglandins may play a role in the pathogenesis of ARDS, particularly in terms of mediating the pulmonary artery hypertension so frequently observed.

How the complement cascade, neutrophil aggregation (with release of oxygen radicals and proteolytic enzymes), coagulation pathway, and prostaglandins interact in the various forms of ARDS is not at all clear. Suffice it to say these are now important areas of research, from which we may see major advances during the next decade.

PATHOLOGY

Despite the number of etiologies of ARDS, the pathologic findings are relatively similar, no matter what the underlying cause. In most cases, injury to the type I alveolar epithelial cell and the pulmonary capillary endothelial cell appears to be primary in the pathogenesis. However, damage to these cells is relatively difficult, if not impossible, to recognize by light microscopy. What we actually observe are some of the secondary consequences that follow later in the sequence of events.

Early in the course of ARDS, fluid can be seen in the interstitial space of the alveolar septum as well as in the alveolar lumen. One may sometimes see scattered bleeding as well as regions of alveolar collapse, which are at least partly related to a surfactant abnormality that is thought to be a secondary phenomenon rather than a primary initiator of ARDS.

The lung parenchyma also demonstrates an influx of inflammatory cells, both in the interstitial space and often in the alveolar lumen as well. The cellular response is relatively non-specific, consisting of neutrophils and macrophages. Additionally, one may see fibrin and cellular debris located in or around alveoli. As part of the reparative process, alveolar type II epithelial cells generally replicate, in an attempt to replace the damaged type I epithelial cells. Therefore, hyperplastic type II epithelial cells often figure quite prominently in the pathologic picture of ARDS.

Another characteristic finding often seen in the pathology of ARDS is the presence of hyaline membranes. These membranes are actually believed to represent a combination of fibrin, cellular debris, and plasma proteins that are deposited or formed on the alveolar surface. Though they are nonspecific, their presence suggests that alveolar injury and a permeability problem, rather than elevated hydrostatic pressures, are the cause of pulmonary edema.

In severe cases, the damaged lung parenchyma is not repaired, but goes on to develop significant scar tissue, i.e., fibrosis. Exactly what determines which patients heal the damage and which develop fibrosis is not at all clear. However, it has been postulated that maintenance of the integrity of the basement membrane adjacent to alveolar epithelial cells is quite important. When the basement membrane is spared, the alveolar wall can regenerate reasonably normal structure; the type II cells become hyperplastic and eventually differentiate into a new population of type I lining cells. In contrast, when the primary injury has destroyed the basement membrane, a scaffolding for regrowth of alveolar epithelial cells is lost, and restoration of normal architecture does not occur.

Pathologic features of ARDS:
1. interstitial and alveolar fluid
2. areas of alveolar collapse
3. inflammatory cell infiltrate
4. hyperplasia of alveolar type II epithelial cells
5. hyaline membranes
6. fibrosis

PATHOPHYSIOLOGY

Effects on Gas Exchange

Most of the clinical consequences of ARDS follow in reasonably logical fashion from the presence of interstitial and alveolar edema.

Pathophysiologic features of ARDS:
1. shunting and $\dot{V}/\dot{Q}$ mismatch
2. secondary alterations in function of surfactant
3. increased pulmonary vascular resistance
4. decreased pulmonary compliance
5. decreased FRC

shunt - due to filling of alveoli w/ fluid

= hypoxemia blood doesn't get O_2

also areas of V/Q mismatch uneven distrib? of ds across lng
- changes in airflow not followed by Δ's in blood flow ∴ V/Q mismatch

if lots of fluid surfactant is inactive ; alveoli collapse

hypoxemia due to V/Q & shunting

w/ shunt 100% O_2 will ↑ oxygenat? but not nearly to (N)

100 O_2 ineffective in true shunt

pt incr total ventilat? w/ pts no diffic w/ CO_2 retention

The most striking problem is alveolar flooding, which effectively prevents ventilation of affected alveoli even though perfusion may be relatively preserved. These alveoli, perfused but not ventilated, act as regions in which blood is shunted from the pulmonary arterial to pulmonary venous circulation without ever being oxygenated. As we mentioned in Chapter 1, shunting is one of the mechanisms of hypoxemia, and there is perhaps no better example of shunting than the adult respiratory distress syndrome.

Not only are there regions of true shunting in ARDS, but there are also regions of ventilation-perfusion mismatch. To some extent, this phenomenon results from an uneven distribution of the pathologic process within the lungs. In areas where the interstitium is more edematous or where there is more fluid in alveoli, ventilation is more impaired (even though some ventilation remains) than in areas that have been relatively spared. Changes in blood flow do not necessarily follow the same distribution as changes in ventilation, and ventilation-perfusion mismatch results.

In addition to the direct effects of interstitial and alveolar fluid on oxygenation, other changes also appear to be secondary to alterations in the effectiveness of surfactant. We mentioned in Chapter 8 that surfactant is a phospholipid responsible for decreasing surface tension and maintaining alveolar patency. When surfactant is absent, as is seen in the respiratory distress syndrome of neonates, there is extensive collapse of alveoli. In the adult respiratory distress syndrome, no primary deficiencies or abnormalities appear to affect surfactant. However, evidence suggests that as a result of extensive fluid within the alveoli surfactant is inactivated and therefore ineffective in preventing alveolar collapse.

In terms of oxygenation, both ventilation-perfusion mismatch (with regions of low $\dot{V}/\dot{Q}$ ratio) and true shunting ($\dot{V}/\dot{Q} = 0$) are responsible for hypoxemia. Insofar as shunting is responsible for the drop in P_{O_2}, supplemental oxygen alone may not be capable of restoring oxygenation to normal. In practice, the P_{O_2} does rise somewhat with administration of 100 percent oxygen but not nearly to the level expected after such high concentrations of oxygen. Considering the nature of the problem of ARDS, this response to supplemental oxygen should not strike us as surprising. Oxygen improves whatever component of hypoxemia is due to ventilation-perfusion mismatch, but it is ineffective for true shunting.

On the other hand, the absolute level of ventilation in the patient with ARDS remains intact or even increases. As a result, patients do not have difficulty with CO_2 retention, except in terminal stages of the disease or if another underlying pulmonary process is present. Even though substantial amounts of what is effectively dead space may be present (as part of the overall ventilation-perfusion mismatch), the patient is able to increase total ventilation to compensate for the regions of maldistribution.

Changes in the Pulmonary Vasculature

The pulmonary vasculature is also subject to changes resulting from the overall pathologic process. Pulmonary vascular resistance increases, probably for a variety of reasons. Hypoxemia certainly produces vasoconstriction within the pulmonary arterial system, while fluid in the interstitium may increase interstitial pressure, resulting in a decrease in size and an increase in resistance of the small pulmonary vessels. In those cases with evidence of disseminated intravascular coagulation, small thrombi may be widespread throughout the pulmonary vasculature and may contribute to increased pulmonary vascular resistance.

One consequence of the pulmonary vascular changes is an alteration in the normal distribution of pulmonary blood flow. Naturally, blood flows preferentially to areas with lower resistance, which do not necessarily correspond to those regions receiving the most ventilation. Hence, ventilation-perfusion mismatch again results, with some areas having high and other areas low ventilation-perfusion ratios.

Effects on the Mechanical Properties of the Lungs

The pathologic processes seen in ARDS have an important effect not only on gas exchange but also on the mechanical properties of the lungs. The combination of fluid within the pulmonary interstitium as well as in the alveoli and alveolar collapse contributes to a "stiffening" of the lung parenchyma. In other words, the compliance of the lung is decreased, so that less expansion occurs for any given level of distending or inflating pressure. One effect of the decrease in compliance is an increase in the work of breathing, which is associated with decreased tidal volume and an increase in respiratory frequency.

Additionally, as a result of fluid occupying alveolar spaces and collapse of small airways and alveoli, the volume of gas within the lungs is significantly decreased. Specifically, lung volume at the end of expiration is much lower than normal, i.e., FRC is decreased. Therefore, as a consequence of the fluid accumulation and collapse that are so integral to the pathophysiology of ARDS, patients breathe at a much lower lung volume than normal, and their respiratory pattern consists of rapid but shallow breaths. This type of breathing is inefficient, demanding increased energy expenditure by the patient, and probably contributes to the dyspnea that is so characteristic of patients with ARDS.

CLINICAL FEATURES

Since ARDS is a clinical syndrome with many different etiologies, the clinical picture reflects not only the presence of noncardiogenic pulmonary edema but also the presence of the underlying disease. We are concerned here with the respiratory consequences of ARDS, irrespective of the etiology, and we will therefore focus on the clinical effects of the syndrome itself and not on those of the underlying disorder.

After the initial insult, whatever it may be, there generally is a lag of several hours to a day or more before respiratory consequences ensue. In most cases, the first symptom experienced by the patient is

Clinical features of ARDS:
1. *dyspnea, tachypnea*
2. *rales*
3. *↓ P_{O_2}, normal or ↓ P_{CO_2}, ↑ AaD_{O_2}*
4. *radiography—interstitial and alveolar edema*

dyspnea. At this time, examination often shows the patient to be tachypneic, though the chest radiograph may still be relatively unremarkable. However, arterial blood gases reflect a disturbance of oxygenation, often with an increase in the alveolar-arterial oxygen difference (AaD_{O_2}). Alveolar ventilation is either normal or more frequently increased, so that P_{CO_2} is generally low.

As fluid and protein continue to leak from the vasculature into the interstitial and alveolar spaces, the clinical findings become even more florid. Patients may become extremely dyspneic and tachypneic, and chest examination may now show the presence of rales. The chest radiograph becomes grossly abnormal, revealing interstitial and alveolar edema that can be quite extensive. The roentgenographic aspects of ARDS will be discussed further in the following section on Diagnostic Approach.

The course of ARDS is certainly variable from patient to patient, though many patients succumb, either as a result of the ARDS itself or from the underlying disorder that precipitated it. Overall, the mortality for patients with ARDS is greater than 50 percent, indicating how gravely ill these patients are. Prior to the development of ARDS, the patients often have entirely normal lungs. Yet they may progress to life-threatening respiratory failure within a matter of days.

However, in those patients who are fortunate enough to recover, there may be surprisingly few permanent sequelae. Pulmonary function may return essentially to normal, though sophisticated assessment often shows some relatively subtle abnormalities.

DIAGNOSTIC APPROACH

The diagnosis of ARDS is generally based on a combination of clinical and radiographic information (assessment at a macroscopic level) and arterial blood gases (assessment at a functional level). Though some clinicians and investigators have advocated lung biopsies in patients with presumed ARDS, these have been done primarily for research purposes and have not yet achieved general clinical acceptance.

As we mentioned above, the chest radiograph in patients with ARDS is not necessarily abnormal at the onset of the clinical presentation. However, within a short period of time the patient generally develops evidence of interstitial and alveolar edema, the latter being the most prominent finding on the radiograph. The edema is diffuse, affecting both lungs relatively symmetrically. As an indication that the fluid is filling alveolar spaces, air bronchograms are often seen within the diffuse infiltrates. Unless the patient has prior heart disease and cardiac enlargement that is unrelated to the present problem, the heart size remains normal. A characteristic example of a chest radiograph in a patient with severe ARDS is shown in Figure 3–7.

Arterial blood gases show hypoxemia and hypocapnia (respiratory alkalosis). If one calculates the alveolar-arterial difference in oxygen tension (AaD_{O_2}), it is clear that gas exchange is actually worse than it appears at first glance, since the alveolar P_{O_2} is elevated as a result of hyperventilation. As the amount of interstitial and alveolar edema increases, oxygenation becomes progressively more abnormal, and severe hypoxemia results. Because true shunting of blood across nonventilated alveoli is important in the pathogenesis of hypoxemia, the Po_2 may be relatively unresponsive to the administration of supplemental oxygen.

In many cases of ARDS, it has proved useful to obtain a direct measurement of pressures within the pulmonary circulation. This has been facilitated by use of a catheter inserted into a systemic vein and then passed through the right atrium and right ventricle into the pulmonary artery. The relatively easy passage of this catheter (commonly known as a Swan-Ganz catheter) results from a balloon at the tip, which can be inflated with air and then carried along with blood flow through the tricuspid and pulmonic valves into the pulmonary artery. The catheter is then positioned at a point in the pulmonary artery where inflation of the balloon occludes the lumen and prevents forward flow. Consequently, if pressure is measured at the tip of the catheter when forward flow has been prevented, the measured pressure is theoretically a reflection of pressure in the pulmonary capillaries. The pressure measured with the balloon inflated is commonly called the *pulmonary capillary wedge (PCW)* or *pulmonary artery occlusion pressure*.

Using measurement of pressure within the pulmonary capillary system, we can distinguish whether the observed pulmonary edema is cardiogenic or noncardiogenic in origin. In cardiogenic pulmonary edema, the hydrostatic pressure within the pulmonary capillaries is high as a result of "back-pressure" from the pulmonary veins and left atrium. On the other hand, in non-cardiogenic pulmonary edema or ARDS, the pressure within the pulmonary capillary system, measured as the PCW pressure, is normal, indicating that the interstitial and alveolar fluid results from increased permeability of the pulmonary capillaries, not from high intravascular pressure.

Though use of these catheters in measurement of intravascular pressures is not essential to the diagnosis of ARDS, the information obtained is often useful for determining whether high intravascular pressures are contributing to the observed pulmonary edema. Additionally, the catheters often provide helpful information during the course of the complicated management of these patients.

A pulmonary artery (Swan-Ganz) catheter can measure pulmonary vascular pressures and cardiac output.

TREATMENT

Management of patients with ARDS centers on three main issues: treatment of the precipitating disorder, control of the permeability defect causing leakage of fluid and protein, and support of gas exchange until the pulmonary process improves. Though treatment of the precipitating disorder is not always possible or successful, the principle is relatively simple—as long as the underlying problem persists, the pulmonary capillary leak may remain. In the case of a disorder like sepsis, management of the infection with appropriate antibiotics (and drainage, if necessary) is crucial in allowing the pulmonary vasculature to regain the normal permeability barrier for protein and fluid.

At the present time, there is no proven way to control or reverse the capillary permeability defect allowing fluid and protein to leak into

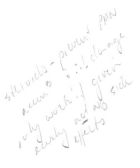

the interstitium and alveolar spaces. Corticosteroids have been used with this goal in mind, as experimental evidence suggests that steroids inhibit aggregation of neutrophils induced by activated complement. Consequently, it has been proposed that steroids might prevent damage to capillary endothelial cells resulting from complement activation. However, clinical results have been equivocal, and there are potentially harmful effects from using high doses of corticosteroids. If steroids are effective, it is probably only if they are given relatively early in the course of the syndrome.

Finally, supportive management of the patient with ARDS, particularly with regard to maintaining adequate gas exchange, is essential if these patients are to survive the acute illness. Considering the importance of supportive measures, we are devoting Chapter 28 to a discussion of modalities for supporting gas exchange.

REFERENCES

Divertie, M. B.: The adult respiratory distress syndrome. Mayo Clin. Proc. 57:371–378, 1982.

Hopewell, P. C., and Murray, J. F.: The adult respiratory distress syndrome. Ann. Rev. Med. 27:343–356, 1976.

Moser, K. M., and Spragg, R. G.: Use of the balloon–tipped pulmonary artery catheter in pulmonary disease. Ann. Intern. Med. 98:53–58, 1983.

Overland, E. S., and Severinghaus, J. W.: Noncardiac pulmonary edema. Adv. Intern. Med. 23:307–326, 1978.

Petty, T. L., and Fowler, A. A., III: Another look at ARDS. Chest 82:98–104, 1982.

Pontoppidan, H., Geffin, B., and Lowenstein, E.: Acute respiratory failure in the adult. N. Engl. J. Med. 287:690–698; 743–752; 799–806, 1972.

Rinaldo, J. E., and Rogers, R. M.: Adult respiratory–distress syndrome: changing concepts of lung injury and repair. N. Engl. J. Med. 306:900–909, 1982.

Robin, E. D., Cross, C. E., and Zelis, R.: Pulmonary edema. N. Engl. J. Med. 288: 239–246; 292–304, 1973.

Staub, N. C.: Pulmonary edema due to increased microvascular permeability. Ann. Rev. Med. 32:291–312, 1981.

Staub, N. C.: "State of the art" review. Pathogenesis of pulmonary edema. Am. Rev. Respir. Dis. 109:358–372, 1974.

Tate, R. M., and Repine, J. E.: State of the art: Neutrophils and the adult respiratory distress syndrome. Am. Rev. Respir. Dis. 128:552–559, 1983.

28

Principles and Methods of Supporting Gas Exchange in Respiratory Failure

In many ways, survival of patients with acute respiratory failure depends upon their ability to maintain adequate gas exchange with the aid of supportive forms of therapy. We have already discussed a few aspects of managing acute on chronic respiratory failure and ARDS. However, in this chapter, we will specifically focus on the way in which adequate gas exchange can be maintained during the course of respiratory failure. Since the principles for supportive management differ considerably in the two main categories of respiratory failure, we will emphasize these differences in the course of our discussion. First, however, we will briefly consider the goals of supportive therapy.

GOALS OF SUPPORTIVE THERAPY FOR GAS EXCHANGE

Adequate uptake of oxygen by the blood, delivery of oxygen to the tissues, and elimination of CO_2 are all parts of normal gas exchange. In terms of oxygen uptake by the blood, we must remember that almost all the oxygen carried by blood is bound to hemoglobin and that only a small portion is dissolved in plasma. It is apparent from the oxyhemoglobin dissociation curve that elevating the Po_2 beyond the point at which hemoglobin is almost completely saturated does not significantly increase the oxygen content of blood. On the average, assuming that the dissociation curve is not shifted, hemoglobin is approximately 90 percent saturated at a Po_2 of 60 torr. Increasing the

Goals for optimizing oxygen transport to tissues:
1. arterial oxygen saturation >90% (i.e., Po_2 >60 torr)
2. acceptable hemoglobin level (e.g., >10 gm/dl, corresponding to a hematocrit >30%)
3. normal or near normal cardiac output

311

Po_2 to this level is important, but a Po_2 much beyond this level does not provide any particular benefit. In practice, patients with respiratory failure are often kept at a Po_2 slightly higher than 60 torr to allow a "margin of safety" for fluctuations in Po_2.

Oxygen delivery to the tissues, however, depends not only on the arterial Po_2, but also on the hemoglobin level and the cardiac output. In patients who are anemic, oxygen content and hence oxygen transport can be compromised as much by the low hemoglobin level as by hypoxemia (see Equation 1–3). In selected circumstances, blood transfusion may be useful in raising the hemoglobin and the oxygen content to a more desirable level.

Similarly, when cardiac output is impaired, tissue oxygen delivery also decreases, and measures to augment cardiac output may improve overall oxygen transport. Unfortunately, some of the measures we use to improve arterial Po_2 may have a detrimental effect on cardiac output. As a result, tissue oxygen delivery may not improve (and may even worsen) despite an increase in Po_2. The use of positive pressure ventilation, particularly with positive end-expiratory pressure, is most important in this regard. We will discuss this technique shortly.

CO$_2$ is eliminated to maintain an acceptable pH rather than a "normal" Pco$_2$.

Elimination of carbon dioxide by the lungs is important for maintaining adequate acid-base homeostasis. However, achieving acceptable pH, not a "normal" Pco_2, is actually the primary goal in managing patients with respiratory failure and impaired elimination of CO_2. In patients with chronic hypercapnia (and metabolic compensation), abruptly restoring the Pco_2 to normal (40 torr) may cause a significant alkalosis and risk precipitating either arrhythmias or seizures.

MAINTENANCE OF CO$_2$ ELIMINATION

As we have mentioned, there are several types of patients for whom CO_2 retention is an important aspect of respiratory failure. Most frequently, these patients have some degree of chronic CO_2 retention, and their acute problem is appropriately termed "acute on chronic" respiratory failure. Patients with chronic obstructive lung disease, chest wall disease, and neuromuscular disease are all subject to developing hypercapnia. There is also a group of patients in whom hypercapnia may be acute—for example, individuals who have suppressed their respiratory drive with drugs ingested in a suicide attempt, or occasional patients with severe asthma and status asthmaticus.

Mechanical ventilation is often indicated when arterial Pco$_2$ has risen sufficiently to:
1. lower pH to 7.25–7.30 or below
2. impair the patient's mental status

If the degree of CO_2 retention is sufficiently great to cause a marked decrease in the patient's pH (less than 7.25 to 7.30), then ventilatory assistance with a mechanical ventilator is often necessary.* Similarly, if marked CO_2 retention has resulted in impairment of the patient's mental status, then ventilatory assistance is again indicated. For the patient in whom there is a good chance of rapid reversal of CO_2 retention with therapy (assuming the level of CO_2 retention is not life-threatening), this therapy is often attempted first with the hope of avoiding mechanical ventilation.

---

*To initiate ventilatory support, the patient is intubated (i.e., a tube is placed through the nose or mouth, through the vocal cords, and into the trachea), and a mechanical ventilator is connected to the endotracheal tube.

There are also measurements reflecting muscle strength and pulmonary function that are useful for the patient with acute or impending respiratory failure. These measurements serve as an indirect guide to the patient's ability to maintain adequate CO_2 elimination. Hence they are also often used as criteria for instituting ventilatory assistance or, conversely, for deciding when a patient aided by a mechanical ventilator might be weaned from ventilatory support. Perhaps the most commonly used measurements (along with the criteria for mechanical ventilation) are

1. vital capacity: less than 10 ml/kg body weight, and
2. inspiratory force: less than 25 cm H_2O negative pressure.

This latter test is performed by having the patient inspire as deeply as possible through tubing connected to a pressure gauge, which quantitates the negative pressure that the patient can generate.

Though these and other specific measurements are frequently used to determine when a patient requires ventilatory assistance for eliminating CO_2, it is important to realize that none of the guidelines are absolute. Some of the many additional factors that enter into such decisions include the nature of the underlying disease, the tempo and direction of change of the patient's illness, and the presence of additional medical problems.

MAINTENANCE OF OXYGENATION

Though hypoxemia is a feature of virtually all patients with respiratory failure when breathing air (21 percent oxygen), the ease of supporting the patient and restoring an adequate Po_2 depends to a great degree on the type of respiratory failure. In most cases of acute on chronic respiratory failure, ventilation-perfusion mismatch and hypoventilation are responsible for hypoxemia. For these mechanisms of hypoxemia, administration of supplemental oxygen is quite effective at improving the Po_2, and particularly high concentrations of inspired oxygen are not necessary. Frequently, oxygen can be administered by face mask or by nasal prongs to give inhaled concentrations of oxygen not exceeding 40 percent, with which patients are able to achieve a Po_2 greater than 60 torr.

However, as we discussed in Chapter 18, patients with chronic hypercapnia are subject to further increases in their Pco_2 when they receive supplemental oxygen. If the Pco_2 rises to an unacceptably high range, then the patient may require intubation and assisted ventilation with a mechanical ventilator in order to maintain an acceptable Pco_2.

In the patient with hypoxemic respiratory failure, e.g., ARDS, ventilation-perfusion mismatch and shunting are responsible for hypoxemia. When a large fraction of the cardiac output is being shunted and does not achieve oxygenation during passage through the lungs, supplemental oxygen is relatively ineffective at raising the Po_2 to an acceptable level. In these cases, patients may require inspired oxygen concentrations in the range of 60 to 100 percent, and even then they may have difficulty in maintaining a Po_2 greater than 60 torr.

Such patients with ARDS also require ventilatory assistance but generally for a different reason than the patient with acute on chronic respiratory failure. In the latter patient, an unacceptable degree of CO_2 retention is generally the indication for intubation and mechanical ventilation. In the patient with ARDS, CO_2 retention is rarely a problem, whereas oxygenation is extremely difficult to support.

For patients with hypoxemic respiratory failure regardless of etiology, inability to achieve a Po_2 of 60 torr or greater on supplemental oxygen readily administered by face mask (40 percent or less) is often considered reason for intubation and mechanical ventilation. Another way of quantifying the difficulty with oxygenation is by calculation of the alveolar-arterial oxygen difference ($AaDo_2$) with the patient breathing 100 percent O_2. An $AaDo_2$ greater than 350 torr is often considered a criterion for intubation and mechanical ventilation. Again, we stress that such decisions for ventilatory support are not based just on one number but generally also take many other factors into account.

In the setting of ARDS, intubation and mechanical ventilation serve several useful purposes. First, high concentrations of oxygen can be administered much more reliably through a tube inserted into the trachea than through a mask placed over the face. Second, administration of positive pressure by a ventilator allows the patient to receive much larger tidal volumes than he or she would spontaneously take, particularly since the poorly compliant lungs of ARDS promote shallow breathing and low tidal volumes. Finally, when a tube is in place in the trachea, positive pressure can be maintained in the airway throughout the respiratory cycle, not just during the inspiratory phase. In common usage, positive airway pressure maintained at the end of expiration in a mechanically ventilated patient is termed *positive end-expiratory pressure*, or *PEEP*. This particular modality will be discussed more in the final section of this chapter.

Why is positive pressure throughout the respiratory cycle beneficial in patients with ARDS? As we mentioned earlier, patients with ARDS often have a great deal of microatelectasis, most likely because of fluid occupying alveolar spaces, low tidal volumes, and probably inactivation of surfactant. The resting end-expiratory volume of the lung, i.e., FRC, is quite low in these patients but can be increased substantially by the administration of PEEP. At the higher FRC, many small airways and alveoli that were formerly closed and therefore received no ventilation are opened and capable of gas exchange. Therefore, blood supplying these regions no longer courses through unventilated alveoli and can now be oxygenated. Indeed, measurement of the "shunt fraction" shows that PEEP is quite effective at decreasing the amount of blood that would otherwise not be oxygenated during passage through the lungs.

When the shunt fraction is decreased by PEEP, supplemental oxygen is much more effective at elevating the patient's Po_2 to an acceptable level. The concentration of inspired oxygen can then be lowered, and the patient is less likely to experience oxygen toxicity from extremely high concentrations of oxygen.

MECHANICAL VENTILATION

Mechanical ventilators, which have gained widespread use over the past 20 to 30 years, are critical to the effective management of

Mechanical ventilation is often indicated when Po_2 ≥ 60 torr cannot be achieved with inspired O_2 concentration ≤ 40%.

Beneficial effects of ventilatory assistance in ARDS:
1. more reliable administration of high concentrations of inspired O_2
2. use of higher tidal volumes than achieved spontaneously by the patient
3. use of PEEP

PEEP is effective in ARDS by increasing FRC and preventing closure of small airways and alveoli.

patients in respiratory failure. By supporting gas exchange for as long a period as necessary, mechanical ventilators can keep a patient alive while the acute process precipitating respiratory failure is treated or allowed to resolve spontaneously. We will briefly describe the operation of mechanical ventilators, the available modes of ventilation, and the complications that can ensue from their use.

Ventilators currently used for the management of acute respiratory failure are positive pressure devices—that is, they deliver gas under positive pressure to the patient during inspiration. Most of these ventilators are *volume-cycled*, meaning that each inspiration is terminated (and passive expiration allowed to occur) after a specified volume has been delivered by the machine. In contrast, with *pressure-cycled* ventilators, which are used infrequently, inspiration ends when a specified airway pressure has been reached. Volume-cycled ventilators are much more reliable in delivering constant, specifiable tidal volumes than are pressure-cycled ventilators. With the latter, changes in either lung compliance or airway resistance alter the volume of gas delivered before the specified pressure limit has been reached.

Several ventilatory patterns or modes are available with most mechanical ventilators (Fig. 28–1). *Controlled ventilation* provides for ventilation to be supplied entirely by the ventilator at a respiratory rate, tidal volume, and inspired oxygen concentration chosen by the physician. If the patient tries to take a spontaneous breath between the machine-delivered breaths, he or she does not receive any inspired gas. This type of ventilation is quite uncomfortable to the awake patient capable of initiating inspiration and is generally reserved for patients who are comatose, anesthetized, or unable to make any inspiratory effort.

In the *assist-control* mode of ventilation, the ventilator is able to "sense" when the patient initiates inspiration, at which point the machine assists by delivering a specified tidal volume to the patient. Though the tidal volume is set by the machine, the respiratory rate is determined by the number of spontaneous inspiratory efforts made by the patient. However, should the patient's spontaneous respiratory rate fall below a specified level, the machine provides a back-up by delivering at least this minimum number of breaths. For example, if the back-up rate set on the machine is 10 breaths per minute, the ventilator will automatically deliver a breath if and when 6 seconds have elapsed from the previous breath. Since the respiratory rate with this mode of ventilation is determined by the patient (once the rate is higher than the specified minimum level), wide swings in minute ventilation can occur if the patient's respiratory rate changes significantly.

Finally, a very commonly used ventilatory mode is known as *intermittent mandatory ventilation*, or *IMV*. With IMV, the machine delivers a preset number of breaths per minute at a specified tidal volume and inspired oxygen concentration. In between the machine-delivered breaths, the patient is able to breathe spontaneously from a gas source providing the same inspired oxygen concentration given during the machine-delivered breaths. However, the machine does not assist these spontaneous breaths, and the tidal volume for these breaths is therefore determined by the patient. In a variant of IMV called *synchronized IMV*, or *SIMV*, each of the machine-delivered breaths is

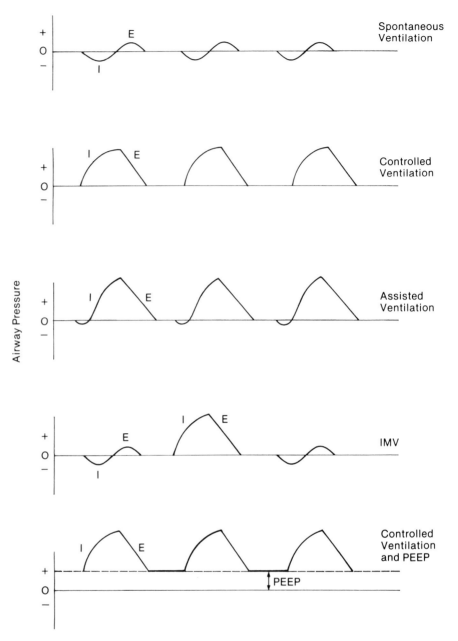

Figure 28–1. Airway pressure during spontaneous ventilation and during mechanical ventilation with several different ventilatory patterns. I = inspiration; E = expiration; IMV = intermittent mandatory ventilation; PEEP = positive end-expiratory pressure.

timed to coincide with and assist a patient–initiated breath. If the patient ventilated by IMV or SIMV changes his or her spontaneous respiratory rate significantly, the variation in minute ventilation is much less than in the assist-control mode of ventilation, since each breath has not been supplemented by a relatively large tidal volume delivered by the ventilator.

As we mentioned in our discussion of ARDS, an important option available for the intubated patient with hypoxemic respiratory failure is the use of *positive end-expiratory pressure (PEEP)*. When a patient is assisted by a mechanical ventilator without PEEP, airway (and alveolar) pressure falls during expiration from the positive level achieved at the height of inspiration down to zero. However, if we place the expiratory part of the tubing 10 cm under a column of water, then the expired gas bubbles through the column of water only until the airway pressure falls to 10 cm water. Alternatively, the expiratory portion of the tubing can be connected to a valve requiring a pressure of at least 10 cm H_2O to open it; once the pressure falls to this level, the valve closes and expiration ceases. Whatever the particular method used to obtain PEEP, the end-result is the same—airway pressure at the end of expiration does not fall to zero but remains at the level determined by the height of the column of water or the specifications of the expiratory valve. By changing the valve or adjusting the depth of the expiratory tubing in the column of water, the level of PEEP can be set as desired.

A variation of PEEP that works on the same principle is called *continuous positive airway pressure*, or *CPAP*. The term CPAP is used when the patient is breathing spontaneously (without a mechanical ventilator) and expiratory tubing is placed under a column of water or connected to a PEEP valve. To use CPAP, the patient can either be intubated or given a tightly fitting face mask. Though no positive pressure is provided by a mechanical ventilator during inspiration, inspired gas is delivered from a reservoir bag under tension or at a high enough flow rate to keep airway pressure positive during inspiration as well as expiration.

With PEEP or CPAP, the benefit comes from the positive pressure within airways and alveoli at the end of expiration. Functional residual capacity (FRC) is increased by the positive pressure, and closure of airways and alveoli at the end of expiration is diminished.

When the underlying problem precipitating the need for mechanical ventilation has improved, ventilatory support is discontinued, either rapidly or after a process of weaning. Indirect guidelines, which are essentially the converse of the indications for intubation, may be helpful in predicting the likelihood of successful weaning. A common method of weaning patients is to place them on an IMV mode of ventilation (if not already used) and gradually decrease the number of breaths and hence the proportion of total minute ventilation provided by the ventilator. Before patients are finally extubated, they are often allowed to breathe entirely on their own through the endotracheal tube. This procedure insures that they can maintain adequate gas exchange without any ventilatory assistance.

Complications of Mechanical Ventilation

Unfortunately, intubation and mechanical ventilation of patients in respiratory failure are not entirely without risks or complications (Table 28–1). The procedure of intubation can be complicated acutely by such problems as arrhythmias, laryngospasm, and malposition of the endotracheal tube (either in the esophagus or in a mainstem bronchus). When a tube remains in the trachea for days to weeks, complications affecting the larynx and trachea can be seen. Vocal cord ulcerations and laryngeal stenosis and granulomas may develop, while the trachea is subject to ulcerations, stenosis, and tracheomalacia (degeneration of supporting tissues in the tracheal wall) resulting from

Table 28–1. COMPLICATIONS OF INTUBATION AND MECHANICAL VENTILATION

Associated with intubation
    Malposition of tube
        Tube in esophagus
        Tube in mainstem bronchus (usually right)
    Arrhythmias
    Hypoxemia
    Laryngospasm
Associated with endotracheal or tracheostomy tubes
    Vocal cord ulcers
    Laryngeal stenosis/granulomas
    Tracheal stenosis
    Nasal necrosis
    Sinusitis/otitis media (with nasotracheal tubes)
    Occlusion or kinking of tube
    Infection
Associated with mechanical ventilation
    Decreased cardiac output/hypotension
    Barotrauma
        Pneumothorax
        Pneumomediastinum
        Subcutaneous emphysema
    Alveolar hypo- or hyperventilation

pressure applied by the inflated balloon at the end of the tube. As a precaution to decrease tracheal complications, tubes are now made with cuffs that minimize the pressure exerted on the tracheal wall and the resulting pressure necrosis. For prolonged ventilatory support (weeks to months), a tracheostomy tube, placed directly into the trachea through an incision in the neck, has some advantages over prolonged orotracheal or nasotracheal intubation, not the least of which is prevention of further vocal cord injury.

The administration of positive pressure by a mechanical ventilator has its own attendant problems. Patients receiving positive pressure ventilation are subject to *barotrauma*, i.e., traumatic changes such as pneumothorax or pneumomediastinum occurring as a result of high alveolar pressures. The development of a pneumothorax in these patients can have catastrophic consequences if not detected and treated quickly. The ventilator continues to deliver gas to the patient, and the pneumothorax can quickly be put under tension, thus severely diminishing venous return and cardiac output and causing rapid cardiovascular collapse. In such situations, a tube, catheter, or needle must be immediately inserted to decompress the pleural space, allow venous return to resume, and enable re-expansion of the lung.

Besides barotrauma, the other major adverse effect of positive pressure ventilation is a decrease in venous return to the heart. Whereas the normally negative intrathoracic pressure during inspiration promotes venous return from the periphery, positive inspiratory pressure from a ventilator impedes venous return. The hemodynamic consequences, low cardiac output and blood pressure, are even more likely when the patient is also on PEEP. In many cases, judicious administration of fluids can restore the effective intravascular volume and reverse the adverse hemodynamic consequences of positive pressure ventilation.

In patients receiving positive pressure ventilation, particularly those with hypoxemic respiratory failure who require PEEP, management becomes extremely tricky. In these patients, many factors interact in a complex way—specifically oxygenation, cardiac output, and fluid status. Optimal care of the patient requires both sophisticated monitoring of the patient and substantial expertise from the team responsible for patient care. Such care is necessary not only for proper support of vital functions but also to keep complications of therapy at the minimum possible level.

REFERENCES

Bone, R. C., and Strober, G.: Mechanical ventilation in respiratory failure. Med. Clin. North Am. 67:599–619, 1983.

Pick, R. A., Handler, J. B., Murata, G. H., and Friedman, A. S.: The cardiovascular effects of positive end-expiratory pressure. Chest 82:345–350, 1982.

Pontoppidan, H., Wilson, R. S., Rie, M. A., and Schneider, R. C.: Respiratory intensive care. Anesthesiology 47:96–116, 1977.

Popovich, J., Jr.: The physiology of mechanical ventilation and the mechanical zoo: IPPB, PEEP, CPAP. Med. Clin. North Am. 67:621–631, 1983.

Rizk, N. W., and Murray, J. F.: PEEP and pulmonary edema. Am. J. Med. 72:381–383, 1982.

Sahn, S. A., Lakshminarayan, S., and Petty, T. L.: Weaning from mechanical ventilation. JAMA 235:2208–2212, 1976.

Weisman, I. M., Rinaldo, J. E., and Rogers, R. M.: Positive end-expiratory pressure in adult respiratory failure. N. Engl. J. Med. 307:1381–1384, 1982.

Zwillich, C. W., Pierson, D. J., Creagh, C. E., Sutton, F. D., Schatz, E., and Petty, T. L.: Complications of assisted ventilation: a prospective study of 354 consecutive episodes. Am. J. Med. 57:161–170, 1974.

Index

Note: Page numbers in *italics* refer to illustrations; page numbers followed by (t) refer to tables.

Flexible fiberoptic bronchoscope, 46, *47*
Flow, in airways. See *Airflow* and *Flow-volume loops.*
Flow-volume loops, 57, *58*
  in obstructive disease, 57, *58*, *59*
Fluid, in alveoli, and outlining of air-filled bronchi, 38, 41, *41*
  in pleural space, 180–185, 181(t), *184*
    due to pneumonia, 182, *269*, 271
    sampling of, 50, 185
    with pneumothorax, 189, *189*
Forced expiration, *69*, 69–71
  measures of airflow during, 53, *54*. See also *Flow-volume loops.*
  in obstructive disease, 55
Friction rub, 34
Functional residual capacity, 52, *52*
  elastic recoil of chest wall and lung at, 5–6
Fungal infection, and pulmonary infiltrates, in immunosuppressed patients, 257, 257(t)
  identification of pathogens in, 50
  of lung, 281–286
Fungus ball, in lung, *285*, 285–286

Gas(es), dilution of, in determination of lung volumes, 53
  exchange of. See *Gas exchange.*
  in arterial blood. See specific entries under *Arterial blood.*
  partial pressure of, 10, 11. See also under *Carbon dioxide* and *Oxygen.*
  toxic, inhalation of, and adult respiratory distress syndrome, 302
Gas dilution tests, in determination of lung volumes, 53
Gas exchange, 1
  abnormal, 18–21
    in adult respiratory distress syndrome, 306
    in asthma, 81
    in COPD, 96–97
    in interstitial lung disease, 128–129
    in respiratory failure, 290, 291, 293. See also *Respiratory failure.*
    correction of, 311–319
    pathophysiology of, 293–295, *295*
    presentation of patients with, 293
  at alveolar surface, 2–3
  diffusion and, 9–10
  support of, in management of respiratory failure, 311–319
  tidal volume and, 7
  ventilation-perfusion ratios and, 15
Gel layer, of airway mucus, 250
Genetic susceptibility, to emphysema, 80–90, *90*
  to lung cancer, 229
Germ cell tumor(s), in anterior mediastinum, 194, *196*
Glands, mucous, bronchial, 65, 66
Goblet cells, of airway, 65, 66
Gold therapy, and interstitial lung disease, 141
Goodpasture's syndrome, lung involvement in, 152
Granuloma(s), eosinophilic, of lung, 152
  noncaseating, in sarcoidosis, *124*, 149

Granuloma(s) (*Continued*)
  of lung, 124, 152
    in coccidioidomycosis, 283
    in histoplasmosis, 281
    in sarcoidosis, *124*, 149
    in tuberculosis, 274
Granulomatosis, Wegener's, lung involvement in, 153
Granulomatous vasculitis, 153
Guillain-Barré syndrome, 218

Haldane effect, 14
Hampton's hump, 165
Heart, decreased venous return to, due to mechanical ventilation, 318
  output of, effect of, on tissue oxygen delivery, 312
Heart failure, congestive, Cheyne-Stokes breathing in, 212
  cough in, 28
Hemoglobin, oxygen saturation of, 11
  Po_2 and, 11, *12*, 311–312
  ventilatory response to, 205, *205*
Hemoptysis, 28–29
  causes of, 28–29, 29(t)
  conditions mimicking, 28
  in bronchiectasis, 107, 108
Hemosiderosis, pulmonary, 153
Heparin, for pulmonary embolism, 166, 167
Hereditary susceptibility, to emphysema, 88–90, *90*
  to lung cancer, 229
Hering-Breuer reflex, 203
Hernia, diaphragmatic, posterior, 195
Histamine, and asthma, 77
Histiocytosis X, 152
Histoplasmosis, 281–282
Hodgkin's disease, mediastinal mass in, 194
Honeycomb lung, 125, *125*
Hormones, ectopic production of, in lung cancer, 237
Humoral immunity, respiratory defense function of, 252, 253
  impairment of, 255
Hydropneumothorax, 189, *189*
Hypercapnia, 312
  causes of, 21
  correction of, mechanical ventilation in, 312
  in obesity, 224
  ventilatory response to, 203–204
  with hypoxemia, in respiratory failure, 292, 294–297
    response to oxygen administration in, 213
Hyperpnea, isocapneic, as challenge test, in diagnosis of asthma, 82
Hyperreactivity, of airways, and asthma, 73. See also *Asthma.*
Hypersensitivity pneumonitis, 138–140
Hypersomnolence, sleep apnea and, 214
Hypertension, pulmonary. See *Pulmonary hypertension.*
Hypertrophic pulmonary osteoarthropathy, 35
Hyperventilation, 23
  arterial Pco_2 in, 23
  central nervous system disease and, 210